Breast Imaging THE REQUISITES

SERIES EDITOR **James H. Thrall,** MD
Radiologist-in-Chief
Department of Radiology
Massachusetts General Hospital
Juan M. Taveras Professor of Radiology
Harvard Medical School
Boston, Massachusetts

OTHER VOLUMES IN THE REQUISITES™ SERIES

Gastrointestinal Radiology

Pediatric Radiology

Neuroradiology

Nuclear Medicine

Ultrasound

Musculoskeletal Imaging

Cardiac Imaging

Genitourinary Radiology

Thoracic Radiology

Vascular and Interventional Radiology

Breast Imaging

THE REQUISITES

Debra M. Ikeda, MD
Associate Professor
Department of Radiology
Stanford University School of Medicine
Stanford, California

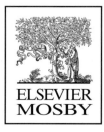

ELSEVIER
MOSBY

ELSEVIER
MOSBY

The Curtis Center
170 S Independence Mall W 300E
Philadelphia, Pennsylvania 19106

BREAST IMAGING: THE REQUISITES   ISBN: 0-323-01969-2
Copyright 2004, Elsevier Inc.

Notice

Radiology is an ever-changing field. Standard safety precautions must be followed, but as new
research and clinical experience broaden our knowledge, changes in treatment and drug therapy may
become necessary or appropriate. Readers are advised to check the most current product information
provided by the manufacturer of each drug to be administered to verify the recommended dose, the
method and duration of administration, and contraindications. It is the responsibility of the treating
physician, relying on experience and knowledge of the patient, to determine dosages and the best
treatment for each individual patient. Neither the Publisher nor the author assume any liability for
any injury and/or damage to persons or property arising from this publication.

The Publisher

Library of Congress Cataloging-in-Publication Data

Ikeda, Debra M.
    Breast Imaging: the requisites/Debra M. Ikdea.
        p. ; cm.
    ISBN 0-323-01969-2
    1. Breast–Radiography. 2. Breast–Imaging. 3. Breast–Diseases–Diagnosis. I. Title.
    [DNLM: 1. Mammography. WP 815 I26m 2004]
RG493.5.R33I346 2004
618.1′907572–dc22   2004050413

Acquisitions Editor: Hilarie Surrena
Developmental Editor: Christy Bracken
Design Manager: Ellen Zanolle
Project Manager: Linda Lewis Grigg

Printed in the United States of America

Last digit is the print number: 9   8   7   6   5   4   3   2   1

For my husband, Robert J. Pelzar;
my mom and dad, Dorothy and Otto;
and my brother, Clyde.

Contributors

Bruce L. Daniel, MD
Assistant Professor
Department of Radiology
Stanford University School of Medicine
Attending Radiologist
Stanford University Medical Center
Stanford, California

Frederick M. Dirbas, MD
Assistant Professor of Surgery
Stanford University School of Medicine
Attending Surgeon, Stanford Hospital
Stanford, California

R. Edward Hendrick, PhD
Research Professor, Department of Radiology
Northwestern University Feinberg School of Medicine
Director, Breast Imaging Research
Lynn Sage Comprehensive Breast Center
Northwestern Memorial Hospital
Chicago, Illinois

Debra M. Ikeda, MD
Associate Professor
Department of Radiology
Stanford University School of Medicine
Stanford, California

Yvonne Karanas, MD
Assistant Professor
Division of Plastic Surgery
Stanford University School of Medicine
Stanford University Medical Center
Stanford, California

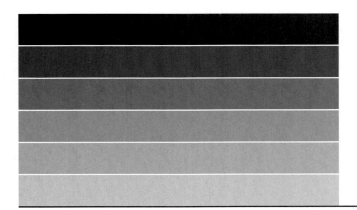

Foreword

Breast Imaging: The Requisites is the 11th book and the newest addition to the Requisites in Radiology series. Dr. Debra Ikeda has done a truly outstanding job in structuring the content and in writing her book. The topic of breast imaging is challenging because it encompasses screening, diagnostic, and interventional procedures that in turn are accomplished with a multiplicity of imaging methods. Dr. Ikeda's approach is logical, and readers will have no trouble in finding and going immediately to the chapter of interest.

The chapter organization and content of *Breast Imaging: The Requisites* clearly indicate the rapid development of technology for breast imaging. Breast imaging is no longer just or even predominantly x-ray mammography, but encompasses ultrasound and magnetic resonance imaging. In turn, these methods are playing important roles for guiding interventional procedures in the breast. Although ultrasound and MRI have been used to some extent for many years, their relative importance has increased significantly in contemporary practice, and this is well reflected in Dr. Ikeda's wonderful book.

Apart from any other aspect of radiology practice, breast imaging brings with it special challenges for both physician and patient. The critical stewardship of a patient's care in going from a screening study to a diagnostic study and then to an interventional procedure is simply unique in radiology practice. Dr. Ikeda and her invited co-authors capture this and provide not only the right information but the right outlook for the reader.

Dr. Ikeda has succeeded in producing a book that exemplifies the philosophy of the Requisites series. She has captured the important conceptual, factual, and practical aspects of breast imaging in a book that is at the same time concise and authoritative. She and her invited co-authors are to be congratulated on doing an outstanding job for the benefit of their readers and for the benefit of both physicians and patients engaged in providing and receiving breast imaging services.

The Requisites in Radiology series is now an old friend for a generation of radiologists. The original intent of the series was to provide the resident or fellow with a text that could be reasonably read within several days at the beginning of each rotation and perhaps reread several times during subsequent rotations or for board preparation. The books in the series are not intended to be exhaustive but to provide the material required for clinical practice. Each book is written by nationally recognized authorities, and each author is challenged to present material in the context of today's practice of radiology and practice of medicine.

Dr. Ikeda has done an outstanding job in sustaining the philosophy of the Requisites series. *Breast Imaging: The Requisites* is a truly outstanding and contemporary text for breast imaging. I believe it will serve residents in radiology as a concise and useful introduction to the subject. It will also serve as a very efficient source for reference or review by practicing radiologists and oncologists and surgeons involved in treating breast cancer.

James H. Thrall, MD

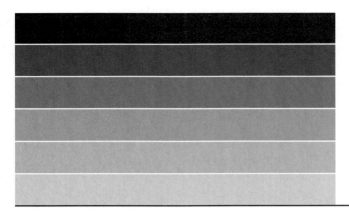

Preface

The specialty of breast imaging is a uniquely challenging and personal combination of imaging, biopsy procedures, clinical correlation, advances in technology, and, in part, psychology. A diagnosis of breast cancer is intensely personal and potentially devastating for the patient. The radiologist's job is to detect and diagnose the cancer and support the patient through the discovery period, the diagnosis, and the treatment. The role of the breast imager has changed in the past few decades from one of simply identifying the cancer to that of being deeply involved in both the biopsy and follow-up. Thus, instead of sitting alone in a dark room, the radiologist in breast imaging is truly part of a team, working with oncologic surgeons, pathologists, radiation oncologists, medical oncologists, and plastic surgeons.

This is a very simple book. It is meant to help the first-year resident understand why the mammogram, the ultrasound, and the MRI scan look the way they do in benign and malignant disease and to help residents in their final year pass their boards. I hope that with careful scrutiny of each chapter, residents will be able to know in which clinical scenarios cancers are more likely to occur; develop a systematic method of analyzing images; generate a differential diagnosis for masses, calcifications and enhancement; and be able to manage patients once certain imaging findings are detected.

The book is meant as an initial teaching guide. However, the pictures and tools within the book can be compared and adapted to patient findings in general clinical practice. Thus, when you come upon a tough case out in the "real world," look to the skills that you learned in this book as tools to use in a time of diagnostic adversity. Do all the tricks you learned on each tough case, because there will be tough cases. Adversity is inevitable. If you welcome adversity as your personal challenge and as an opportunity, and if you use *common sense,* you will most certainly succeed. Remember, the goal of your imaging endeavors is for the good of the patient—to diagnose and treat breast cancer so that the patient will live. Therefore, view the challenging case, the adversity of the difficult diagnosis, as your challenge and as an opportunity. As Bruce Daniel told me when I was flailing around in the most difficult of MRI-guided procedures, *within the realm of common sense* his motto is "Never give up!"

Debra M. Ikeda

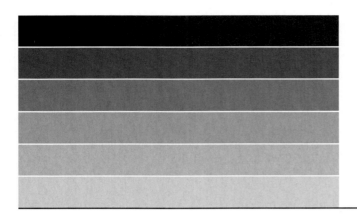

Acknowledgments

In both Ann Arbor and at Stanford, our residents and fellows kept me on my toes by asking "Why do you do it this way?" or "What is it about these findings that makes you say cancer?" You bet you have to have a pretty darned good reason for your answer, because they will always discover the hole in your answer. It was this continual questioning and constant requests for explanation from our trainees that made me write this book. So the first people I have to acknowledge are all the residents and fellows bugging me throughout the years, keeping my skills and my tiny brain sharp.

The first two people I'd like to acknowledge individually are Drs. William Martel and Ingvar Andersson. In the early 1980s, mammography was a specialty in radiology that was considered a "chest appendage." There were no fellowships. The American College of Radiology Boards breast case was a needle localization study shown during the chest section. In 1983, our chairman at the University of Michigan, Dr. William Martel, recruited a star mammographer of great fame from Sweden, Dr. Ingvar Andersson. Because of his vast experience in the Malmö Mammographic Screening Trial in Sweden and his patience, skill, and charm, Dr. Andersson trained and inspired many great mammographers who had their start during his 2-year tenure in Ann Arbor during my residency.

Two days before Christmas in my junior year as a resident, my mother's mammogram showed a 7-mm spiculated nonpalpable breast mass that was suspicious for breast cancer. It was probably detected because the University of Michigan had updated equipment, a QA program, and faculty trained by Dr. Andersson, who had by then returned to Sweden. My mother underwent a brand-new diagnostic technique brought from Sweden: fine-needle aspiration under x-ray guidance using a grid coordinate plate. The aspirate showed cancer. She had a second opinion for surgery on Christmas Eve and underwent mastectomy two days after Christmas. On New Year's Eve, we got the good news that she had a very small invasive tumor, her axillary lymph nodes were negative, and she had a good prognosis. After this experience, I wanted to learn about breast imaging. I knew first hand what happens within families with a new diagnosis of breast cancer. I knew that diagnosis and treatment of small breast cancers at an early stage can result in a long, healthy life for the woman. I knew that we as radiologists could train to find and diagnose early breast cancer and profoundly affect women and their families for the better.

I want to acknowlege my mentors. My fellowships in breast imaging were at the University of California, San Francisco, under Dr. Edward A. Sickles, where I was his first fellow in mammography, and in Sweden at Malmö General Hospital under Dr. Ingvar Andersson, where he ran his randomized, controlled population trial to screen for breast cancer by invitation to mammography. They were, and are, dedicated teachers with a vast knowledge base, patience, compassion, and integrity. They showed a curiosity to learn more about what makes breast cancers tick and taught me to never give up on tough cases.

For their help and inspiration, I also want to acknowledge my colleagues who were at the University of Michigan including Drs. Mark Helvie, Murray Rebner, David Pennes, Anne Smid, Naomi Kane, Kathy Chan, Dorit Adler, and others. At Stanford University, I want to acknowledge smart, visionary colleagues Drs. Robyn Birdwell, Robert J. Herfkens, Gary H. Glover, Bruce L. Daniel, Anne Sawyer-Glover, Judy Illes, Kim Butts, Daniel Spielman, Stefanie S. Jeffrey, Kent W. Nowels, Frederick Dirbas, Robert Carlson, Frank Stockdale, Don Goffinet, Anne Thrush, Sylvia Plevritis, and especially my chairman, Gary M. Glazer. I thank them for fighting the battles, making the diagnoses, and pushing the research envelope to answer questions for women who have no answers now.

I thank Mark Riesenberger for his unflagging support in helping get the best image for each illustration and Dr. Sunita Pal for helping to organize the illustrations. I also thank my co-authors Drs. Edward Hendrick, Yvonne Karanas, Bruce Daniel, and Frederick Dirbas for their contributions to the book chapters in their specialties. The Elsevier editors and corrections staff have also been quite helpful, and I thank Stephanie Donley, Hilarie Surrena, and Christy Bracken for keeping me on track.

I have to get back to my chairmen, Dr. William Martel and Dr. Gary Glazer. Who else but the chairmen had the vision so long ago, and also now, to realize how important breast imaging is to women's futures? Because of Dr. Martel's vision and foresight, a generation of great breast imagers were trained at the University of Michigan. And Dr. Gary Glazer brought together physicians, engineers, and physicists at Stanford 10 years ago to create a critical mass to continue to develop breast imaging technology, to help women and train a new generation of breast imagers at Stanford. Therefore, I have to acknowledge both my chairmen for their foresight and dedication to women's health, without which my career would have taken a much different tack.

Most important of all, I'd like to acknowledge and thank my husband, Robert J. Pelzar, who has asked "Isn't your book done yet?" "How long does it take to write a book?" "Now what do you have to do?" for a year and a half. He has supported and encouraged the completion of this project through my grumpy hours at the computer, my nights and weekends working on text, burning CDs, and looking for illustrations, hours on EndNote and PubMed, and his bike rides alone without me. He has been happy, cheerful, and unflaggingly supportive through the entire thing, and now he is just relieved. And so am I.

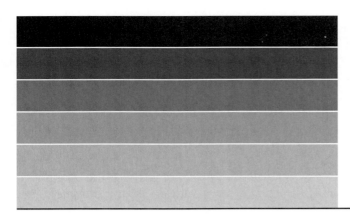

Contents

1 **Mammogram Acquisition: Screen-film and Digital Mammography, Computer-Aided Detection, and the Mammography Quality Standards Act**   1
Debra M. Ikeda and R. Edward Hendrick

2 **Mammogram Interpretation**   24
Debra M. Ikeda

3 **Mammographic Analysis of Breast Calcifications**   60
Debra M. Ikeda

4 **Mammographic and Ultrasound Analysis of Breast Masses**   90
Debra M. Ikeda

5 **Breast Ultrasound**   133
Debra M. Ikeda

6 **Image-Guided Breast Procedures**   163
Debra M. Ikeda

7 **Magnetic Resonance Imaging of Breast Cancer and MRI-Guided Breast Biopsy**   189
Bruce L. Daniel and Debra M. Ikeda

8 **The Postoperative Breast and Breast Cancer Treatment-Related Imaging**   225
Debra M. Ikeda and Frederick M. Dirbas

9 **Breast Implants**   252
Debra M. Ikeda and Yvonne Karanas

10 **Clinical Breast Problems and Unusual Breast Conditions**   279
Debra M. Ikeda

Index   321

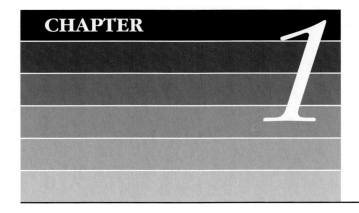

CHAPTER 1

Mammogram Acquisition: Screen-Film and Digital Mammography, Computer-Aided Detection, and the Mammography Quality Standards Act

DEBRA M. IKEDA

R. EDWARD HENDRICK

Introduction and the Mammography Quality Standards Act

Screen-Film Mammography

Technical Aspects of Image Acquisition

Quality Assurance

Digital Mammography

Technical Aspects of Image Acquisition

Quality Assurance

Computer-Aided Detection

Conclusion

Key Elements

INTRODUCTION AND THE MAMMOGRAPHY QUALITY STANDARDS ACT

Randomized controlled trials of women invited to mammography screening have shown that early detection and treatment of breast cancer lead to a 25% to 30% decrease in breast cancer mortality. These studies have demonstrated that image quality is a critical component of early detection of breast cancer. Currently, the American Cancer Society recommends that asymptomatic women 40 years and older have an annual mammogram and receive a clinical breast examination as part of a periodic health examination, preferably annually (Box 1-1).

To standardize and improve the quality of mammography, Congress passed the 1992 Mammography Quality Standards Act (MQSA) and the MQSA Reauthorization Act of 1998 (H.R. 4382) amending the Public Health Service Act to revise and extend the MQSA program. These laws mandate minimal requirements for facilities performing mammography. MQSA regulates all aspects of mammography, including accreditation of facilities; training and education of all technologists, physicians, and physicists involved in mammography; and mandated reporting of outcome data (Box 1-2). Enforced by the Food and Drug Administration (FDA), MQSA stipulates that all institutions performing mammography must be certified by the FDA. A prerequisite to FDA certification is to be accredited to perform mammography by an FDA-recognized accrediting body such as the American College of Radiology (ACR) or a state accrediting body. Currently, the states of Arkansas, California, Iowa, and Texas are approved to accredit mammography facilities in their own states. MQSA regulations are listed in a federal publication called *The Federal Register.* To keep facilities

---

Box 1-1 American Cancer Society Guidelines for Mammographic Screening of Asymptomatic Women

1. Annual mammography beginning at age 40
2. For women in their 20s and 30s, clinical breast physical examination at least every 3 years
3. For women 40 and older, clinical breast examination as part of a periodic health examination, preferably annually

---

Box 1-2 Mammography Quality Standards Act of 1992

Congressional act to regulate mammography

Regulations enforced by the FDA require yearly inspections of all U.S. mammography facilities

All mammography centers must comply; non-compliance results in corrective action or closure

Falsifying information submitted to the FDA can result in fines and jail terms

Regulations regarding equipment, personnel credentialing and continuing education, quality control, quality assurance, and day-to-day operations

posted on the latest regulation changes and updates, the FDA maintains a website on MQSA (http://www.fda.gov/cdrh/mammography/) and a website to guide users who have questions on compliance (http://www.fda.gov/cdrh/mammography/guidance-rev.html).

To perform mammography in the United States, facilities must document compliance with MQSA regulations. To do so, the facility must be accredited by an FDA-approved accrediting body and meet MQSA requirements regarding mammography equipment and processors, quality control, personnel, and outcome data. Certification involves an initial application and approval, continuous documentation of compliance, and yearly facility inspections by the FDA or another accrediting body. Non-compliance with regulations may result in FDA warnings, with time limits on correction of deficiencies. Serious non-compliance or deficiencies may lead to closure of the facility. Falsification of data submitted to the FDA can result in monetary fines and jail terms.

This chapter will outline the basics of image acquisition by screen-film and digital mammography, the essentials of computer-aided detection (CAD) in mammography, and review the quality assurance procedures and requirements for mammography stipulated by the MQSA.

SCREEN-FILM MAMMOGRAPHY

Technical Aspects of Image Acquisition

Mammograms are obtained on specially designed, dedicated x-ray machines using either x-ray film or digital detectors to capture the image. All screen-film mammography (SFM) units consist of a rotating anode of molybdenum or rhodium with matched molybdenum or rhodium filters for soft tissue imaging, a breast compression paddle, a moving grid, an x-ray film cassette holder, and an automatic exposure control (AEC) device that can be placed under the densest portion of the breast, all mounted on a rotating C-arm (Fig. 1-1). A technologist compresses the patient's breast between the image receptor and compression plate for a few seconds during each x-ray exposure. Breast compression is important because it separates normal glandular tissue away from cancers so that they can be seen better and it decreases breast thickness, thereby reducing exposure time (and the potential for image blurring as a result of patient motion) and limiting the radiation dose to the breast.

Women are worried about breast pain from breast compression and about the radiation dose from mammography. Patient pain during compression varies among individuals and can be decreased by obtaining the mammogram 1 week after the onset of menses when breasts are least painful or by taking oral analgesics such as acetaminophen before the mammogram.

Current mammography delivers a low dose of radiation to the breast. The best measure of breast dose is the mean glandular dose, or the average dose of ionizing radiation to glandular tissue, by far the most radiosensitive tissue in the breast. The mean glandular dose received by the average woman is approximately 2 mGy (0.2 rad) per exposure or 4 mGy (0.4 rad) for a typical two-view examination. Doses to thinner compressed breasts are substantially lower than those to thick breasts.

The main radiation risk from mammography is the possible induction of breast cancer years after exposure. The estimated risk of inducing breast cancer is linearly proportional to the radiation dose and inversely related to age at exposure. The lifetime risk for the development of fatal breast cancer as a result of two-view mammography in women 45 years of age at exposure is estimated to be about 1 in 100,000. For a woman 65 years of age at exposure, the risk is less than 1 in 5,000,000. The benefit of screening mammography is earlier detection of clinically occult breast cancer. The likelihood of such detection in a woman undergoing screening at age 45 is about 1 in 3500, for a benefit-to-risk ratio of about 25:1. For a woman aged 65 at screening, the likelihood of a mortality benefit from mammography is about 1 in 1000, for a benefit-to-risk ratio of about 5000:1. Of course, screening is only effective when combined with regular periodic examination.

The generator for a mammography system provides power to the x-ray tube. The peak kilovoltage (kVp) of mammography systems is lower than that of conventional x-ray systems because it is desirable to use softer x-ray beams to improve soft tissue contrast and increase absorption of x-rays in the cassette phosphor. Typical

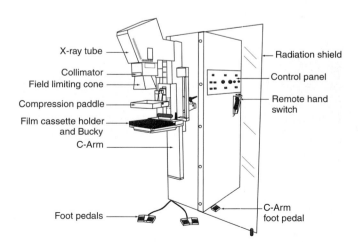

FIGURE 1-1 Components of an x-ray mammography unit.

kVp values for mammography are in the 24- to 32-kVp range for molybdenum targets and 26 to 35 kVp for rhodium or tungsten targets. A key feature of mammography generators is the electron beam current (mA) rating of the system. The higher the mA rating, the shorter the exposure time for total tube output (mAs). A compressed breast of average thickness (5 cm) would require about 150 mAs. If the tube rating is 100 mA (typical of the larger focal spots used for non-magnification mammography), the exposure time would be 1.5 seconds. A higher-output, 150-mA system would cut the exposure time to 1.0 second for the same compressed breast. Because of the wide range of breast thicknesses, exposure requires mA values ranging from 10 to several hundred mAs. Specifications for generators are listed in Box 1-3.

The most commonly used anode-filter combination is a molybdenum (Mo) anode (or target) and an Mo filter (25 to 30 μm thick), especially for thinner compressed breasts (<5 cm thick). Most current manufacturers also offer a rhodium (Rh) filter, to be used with the Mo target to produce a slightly more penetrating (harder) x-ray beam for use with thicker breasts. Some manufacturers offer other target materials, such as rhodium (Rh) paired with a rhodium filter, or tungsten (W) paired with an Rh or aluminum (Al) filter. These anode-filter combinations are designed for thicker (>5 cm) or denser breasts. Typically, higher kVp settings are also used with these target-filter combinations to produce a harder x-ray beam for thicker breasts because fewer x-rays are attenuated with a harder x-ray beam (Box 1-4). One of the best parameters to measure the hardness or penetrating capability of an x-ray beam is the half-value layer (HVL), which represents the thickness of aluminum that reduces the exposure by half. The harder the x-ray beam, the higher the HVL. The typical HVL for mammography is 0.3 to 0.4 mm of Al. An FDA requirement is that the HVL for mammography cannot be less than kVp/100 (in millimeters of Al) so that the x-ray beam is not too soft. For example, for 28 kVp, the HVL cannot be less than 0.28 mm of Al.

Box 1-4	**Anode-Filter Combinations for Mammography**
Mo/Mo	
Mo/Rh	
Rh/Rh	
W/Rh or W/Al	

Al, aluminum; Mo, molybdenum; Rh, rhodium; W, tungsten.

The size of the larger mammography focal spot used for standard, contact mammography is typically 0.3 mm. Magnification mammography requires a smaller focal spot, about 0.1 mm, to reduce penumbra (geometric blurring produced by placing the breast farther from the image receptor to produce magnification). The resolution of the focal spot is tested by a line pair pattern placed at a specific distance (4.5 cm) from the breast support surface. The larger mammography focal spot used for standard contact mammography should produce an image that resolves at least 11 line pairs/millimeter (lp/mm) with resolution pattern bars perpendicular to the anode-cathode axis and at least 13 lp/mm with bars parallel to the anode-cathode axis.

The x-ray tube and image receptor are mounted on opposite ends of a rotating C-arm to obtain mammograms in almost any projection. The source-to-image receptor distance (SID) for mammography units must be at least 55 cm for contact mammography. Most systems have SIDs of 65 to 70 cm.

Geometric magnification is achieved by moving the breast farther from the image receptor (closer to the x-ray tube) and switching to a small focal spot. Placing the breast halfway between the focal spot and image receptor would magnify the breast by a factor of 2.0. The MQSA requires that mammography units with magnification capabilities provide at least one fixed magnification factor of between 1.4 and 2.0 (Table 1-1). Geometric magnification makes small, high-contrast structures such as microcalcifications more visible by making them larger relative to the noise pattern in the image (increasing their signal-to-noise ratio). Optically magnifying a contact

---

Box 1-3	**Mammography Generators**

Provide 24-32 kVp, 5-300 mAs
Half-value layer between kVp/100 + 0.03 and kVp/100 + 0.12 (in mm of aluminum) for Mo-Mo anode-filter material
Average breast exposure is 26-28 kVp (lower kVp for thinner or fattier breasts, higher kVp for thicker or denser breasts)
Screen-film systems deliver an average absorbed dose to the glandular tissue of the breast that is 2 mGy (0.2 rad) per exposure

---

Table 1-1   Mammography Focal Spot Sizes and Source-to-Image Distances

Mammography Type	Nominal Focal Spot Size	Source-to-Image Distance
Contact film-screen	0.3 mm	≥55 cm
Magnification	0.1 mm	≥55 cm

The Mammography Quality Standards Act requires magnification factors between 1.4 and 2.0 for systems designed to perform magnification mammography.

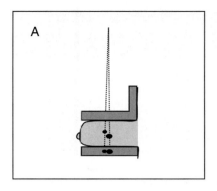

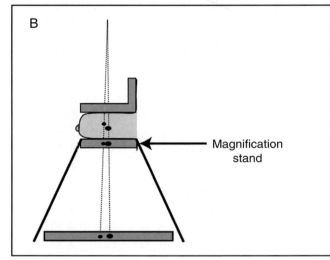

FIGURE 1-2 Magnification mammography improves resolution. **A,** With contact mammography, two small objects are shown as one structure on the image. **B,** With micro–focal spot magnification mammography, moving the breast further away from the image receptor results in geometric magnification and increased spatial resolution.

image, as would be done with a magnifier on a standard mammogram, does not increase the signal-to-noise ratio of the object relative to the background (Fig. 1-2). To avoid excess blurring of the image with geometric magnification, it is important to use a sufficiently small focal spot (usually 0.1 mm nominal size) and not too large a magnification factor (1.8 or less). A compromise inherent in using a small focal spot is decreased output (25 to 40 mA versus 80 to 150 mA for a large focal spot), which can extend imaging times for magnification mammography even though a grid is not used with magnification.

Collimators control the size and shape of the x-ray beam to limit patient exposure to tissues in the compressed breast. In mammography, the x-ray beam is collimated to match the image receptor (18 × 24 or 24 × 30 cm) rather than the breast contour. At the chest wall, the x-ray field can extend beyond the chest wall of the image receptor to accommodate posterior breast tissue,

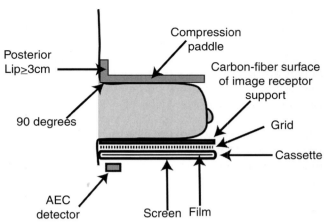

FIGURE 1-3 Schematic of a compression plate and image receptor showing the components of the cassette holder, the compression plate, and the breast. The film emulsion faces the screen. (Adapted from Farria DM, Kimme-Smith C, Bassett LW: Equipment, Processing, and Image Receptor. In Bassett LW (ed): Diagnosis of Diseases of the Breast. Philadelphia, WB Saunders, 1997, pp 32 and 34.

but not by more than 2% of the SID. Thus, for a 60-cm SID unit, the x-ray beam can extend beyond the chest wall edge of the image receptor by up to 1.2 cm.

The compression plate and image receptor hold the breast motionless during the exposure, decrease the thickness of the breast, and provide tight compression to separate the fibroglandular elements (Fig. 1-3). The compression plate has a posterior lip that is more than 3 cm high and oriented at 90 degrees to the plane of the compression plate at the chest wall. This lip keeps the chest wall structures from being superimposed on posterior breast tissue in the image. The compression paddle must be able to compress the breast for up to 1 minute with a compression force of 25 to 45 lb. The paddle can be advanced by a foot-controlled motorized device and adjusted manually (Box 1-5).

The image receptor holds the screen-film cassette in a carbon-fiber support, has a moving antiscatter grid, and has an automatic exposure control (AEC) detector placed under it. Screen-film image receptors are required

---

Box 1-5   Compression Plate and Imaging Receptor

Both 18 × 24- and 24 × 30-cm sizes are required
A moving grid is required for each image receptor size
The compression plate has a posterior lip >3 cm and oriented 90 degrees to the plane of the plate
Compression force of 25-45 lb
Paddle advanced by a foot motor with hand compression adjustments
Collimation to the image receptor, not the breast contour

to be 18×24 and 24×30 cm in size to optimally accommodate various-sized breasts. Each size of image receptor must have a moving antiscatter grid composed of lead strips with a grid ratio (defined as the ratio of the height of the lead strip to the distance between strips) between 3.5:1 and 5:1. The grid moves back and forth in the direction perpendicular to the grid lines during radiographic exposure to eliminate grid lines in the image by blurring them out. Use of a grid improves image contrast by decreasing the fraction of scattered radiation reaching the image receptor. Grids increase the exposure required to image the breast by approximately a factor of 2 (the Bucky factor) because of attenuation of primary as well as scattered radiation. Grids are not used with magnification mammography. Scatter is reduced in magnification mammography by collimation and by rejection of scatter via the significant air gap between the breast and the image receptor.

The AEC system, also known as the phototimer, is calibrated to produce a consistent film optical density (OD) by sampling the x-ray beam after it has passed through the breast support, grid, and cassette. The AEC detector is usually a D-shaped sensor that lies along the midline of the breast support and can be positioned away from or near the chest wall. If the breast is extremely thick or inappropriate technique factors are selected, the AEC will terminate at a specific backup time (usually 4 to 6 seconds) or mAs (300 to 750 mAs) to prevent tube overload or melting of the x-ray track on the anode.

The screen-film cassettes used in mammography have a spatial resolution of 20 lp/mm or greater. Such resolution is achieved by using a single-emulsion film placed emulsion side down against a single intensifying screen that faces upward toward the breast in the film cassette. The single-emulsion film with a single intensifying screen is used to prevent the parallax unsharpness and crossover exposure produced with double-screen systems. Most screen-film processing combinations have relative speeds of 100 to 270, with speed defined as the reciprocal of the exposure required to produce an OD of 1.0 above base plus fog (which is 0.15 to 0.20 OD).

Film processing involves development of the latent image on the exposed film emulsion. The film is placed in an automatic processor that takes the exposed film and rolls it through liquid developer to amplify the latent image on the film by reducing the silver ions in the x-ray film emulsion to metallic silver, thereby resulting in darkening of the film in exposed areas. The temperature of the developer ranges from 92°F to 96°F. The film is then run through a fixer, usually sodium thiosulfate (or hypo), to remove any unused silver and preserve the film. The film is then rinsed with water to remove residual fixer chemicals, which can cause the film to turn brown over time. The film is then dried with heated air.

Table 1-2 Variables Affecting Image Quality of Screen-Film Mammograms	
Film too dark	Developer temperature too high
	Wrong mammographic technique (excessive kVp or mAs)
	Excessive plus-density control
Film too light	Inadequate chemistry or replenishment
	Developer temperature too low
	Wrong mammographic technique
Lost contrast	Inadequate chemistry or replenishment
	Water to processor turned off
	Changed film
Film turns brown	Inadequate rinsing of fixer
Motion artifact	Movement by patient
	Inadequate compression applied
	Inappropriate mammographic technique (long exposures)

Film processing is affected by many variables, the most important of which are developer chemistry (weak or oxidized chemistry makes films lighter and lower in contrast), developer temperature (too hot may make films too dark), replenishment of developer (too little results in lighter, lower-contrast films), inadequate agitation of developer, and uneven application of developer to films (causing a mottled film background) (Table 1-2).

For positioning, the technologist tailors the mammogram to the individual woman's body habitus to get the best image. The breast is relatively fixed in its medial borders near the sternum and the upper part of the breast, whereas the lower and outer portions of the breast are more mobile. The technologist takes advantage of the mobile lower outer portion of the breast to obtain as much breast tissue on the mammogram as possible. The two mammograms usually obtained for screening mammography are the craniocaudal (CC) and mediolateral oblique (MLO) projections. The names for the mammographic views and abbreviations are based on the ACR Breast Imaging Reporting and Data System (ACR BI-RADS), a lexicon system developed by experts for standard mammographic terminology. The first word in the mammographic view indicates the location of the x-ray tube, and the second word indicates the location of the image receptor. Thus, a CC view would be taken with the x-ray tube pointing at the breast from the head (cranial) down through the breast to the image receptor in a more caudal position.

To pass accreditation, the MLO mammogram must show most of the breast tissue in one projection, with portions of the upper inner and lower inner quadrants

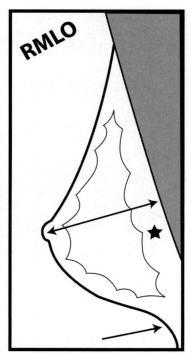

FIGURE 1-4   Positioning for a Normal Mediolateral Oblique (MLO) Mammogram. By convention, the view type and side (R, L) labels are placed near the axilla. On a properly positioned MLO view, the inferior aspect of the pectoralis muscle should extend down to the posterior nipple line, an imaginary line drawn from the nipple back to and perpendicular to the pectoral muscle *(double arrow)*. The anterior margin of the pectoralis muscle should be convex in a properly positioned MLO view. Ideally, the image shows fat posterior to the glandular tissue *(star)*. The open inframammary fold *(arrow)* and abdomen are displayed with the breast pulled up and away from the chest.

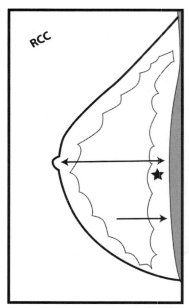

FIGURE 1-5   Normal Craniocaudal (CC) Mammogram. The posterior nipple line (PNL) on the CC view is the distance between the nipple and the posterior aspect of the image. The PNL on the CC view *(double arrow)* should be within 1 cm of the PNL on the mediolateral oblique (MLO) view. The goal is to include posterior medial tissue (excluded on the MLO view) *(arrow)* and as much retroglandular fat *(star)* as possible.

partially excluded (Fig. 1-4). Clinical evaluation of the MLO view should show fat posterior to the glandular tissue and a large portion of the pectoralis muscle, which should be concave and extend inferior to the posterior nipple line (PNL). The PNL is an imaginary line drawn from the nipple to the pectoralis muscle or film edge and perpendicular to the pectoralis muscle. The PNL should intersect the pectoralis muscle in more than 80% of women. Skin folds are to be avoided when possible, but they may be seen occasionally on the film and do not usually cause problems for the radiologist reading the film. The MLO view is also evaluated for adequate compression, exposure, contrast, and an open inframammary fold, and both the lower portion of the breast and a portion of the upper abdominal wall should be seen.

To pass accreditation, the CC view should include the medial posterior portions of the breast without sacrificing the outer portions (Figs. 1-5 and 1-6). With proper positioning technique, the technologist should be able to include the medial portion of the breast without rotating

the patient medially by lifting the lower medial breast tissue onto the image receptor. The pectoralis muscle should be seen when possible on the CC view. The PNL line on the CC view extends from the nipple to the pectoralis muscle or the edge of the film, whichever comes first, and is perpendicular to the pectoralis muscle or film edge. The length of the PNL line on the CC view should be within 1 cm of its length on the MLO view.

• Evaluation of clinical images takes into account positioning, compression, contrast, proper exposure, noise (radiographic mottle, usually quantum mottle produced by fewer x-rays used to make an image), sharpness, and artifacts. A phantom image is helpful in evaluating most of these factors, except for positioning and compression (Fig. 1-7). Adequate exposure (to achieve adequate film OD) and adequate contrast (OD difference) are important to ensure detection of subtle abnormalities (Fig. 1-8). Artifacts seen on clinical images include processing artifacts (roller marks, wet pressure marks, guide shoe marks), dust artifacts from dirt between the fluorescent screen and film emulsion, grid lines from incomplete grid motion, motion artifacts from patient movement (made more likely by longer exposure times), skin folds from positioning, tree static caused by static electricity from low humidity in the dark room, or film-handling artifacts (fingerprints, crimp marks, or pressure marks) (Figs. 1-9 through 1-12).

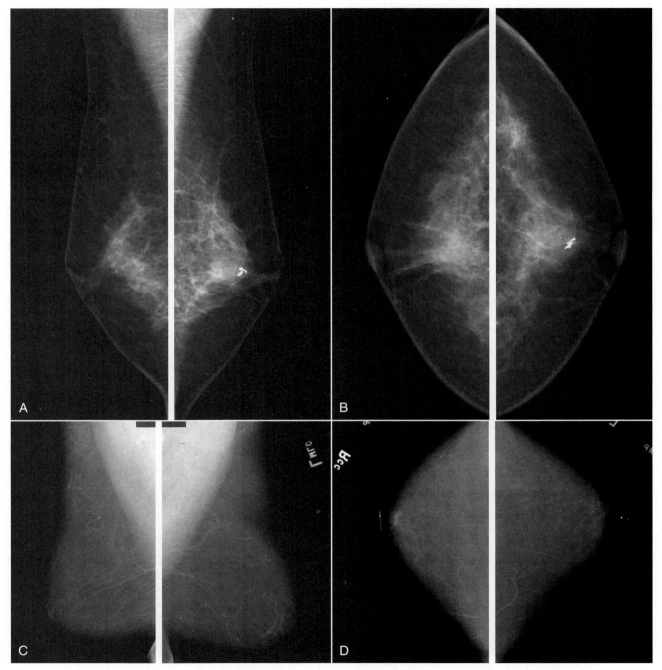

FIGURE 1-6   Improper Positioning. Inadequate pectoralis muscle and sagging breast tissue on this full-field digital mediolateral oblique view show that the posterior nipple line (PNL) requirements are not met (**A**), and the craniocaudal (CC) view is rotated laterally (**B**). Note the calcifying fibroadenoma on the *left*. In a second patient with a fatty breast, the pectoralis muscle is concave but just barely meets PNL requirements (**C**). The CC views are adequate (**D**).

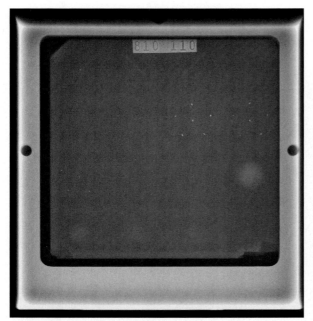

FIGURE 1-7   Phantom Image. Fibers, speck groups, and masses in graduated sizes embedded in a 4.5-cm-thick phantom are used to evaluate the mammography system; phantom images are obtained at least weekly and after calibration or servicing of equipment. Minimum score: four fibers, three speck groups, and three masses.

Film labeling is important because patients' original mammograms may be reviewed at other facilities (Box 1-6). Proper labeling ensures accurate identification of the facility, mammography unit, patient, laterality, and projection. Guidelines from the ACR Mammography Accreditation Program for labeling of mammograms include an identification label on the mammogram in which the date, view, and laterality are specified; numbers indicating the mammography unit and cassette used; and the technologist's initials. The patient's first and last name and unique identification number and the facility's name and address should be labeled clearly. The laterality and projection marker should be placed near the axilla on all screen-film views.

According to the MQSA, film viewing conditions should include hot lights or other illumination devices that can produce light levels brighter than the view box, as well as the ability to mask all unexposed areas of the film. Such masking minimizes the light that reaches the radiologist's eye without passing through the film of interest ("dazzle" glare), which could otherwise interfere with interpretation.

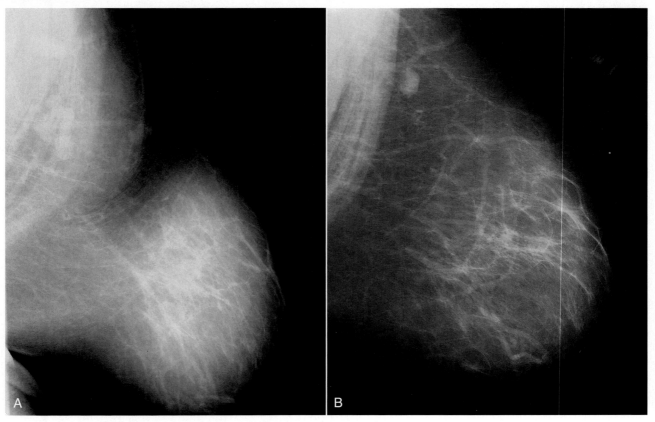

FIGURE 1-8   Underpenetration and an inadequately exposed and compressed breast produce a light film and poor separation of breast tissue; even though the pectoralis muscle is adequately included, skin folds are apparent in the lower portion of the image (**A**). A mammogram of a properly exposed and compressed breast shows normal glandular tissue (**B**).

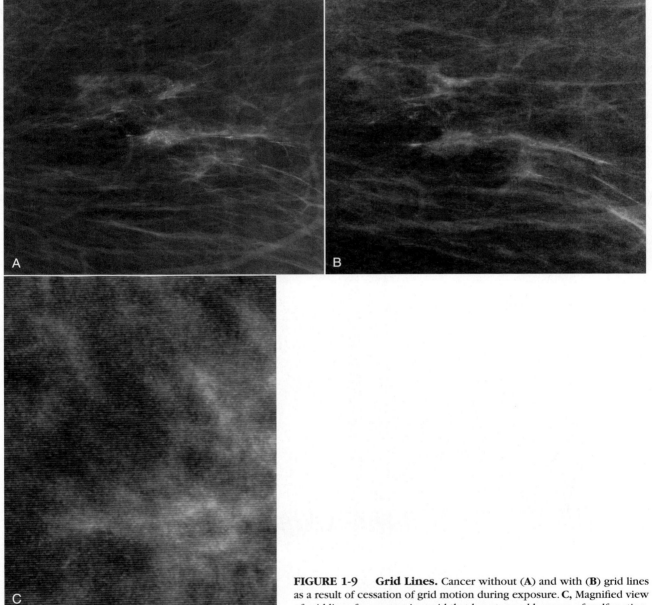

FIGURE 1-9   Grid Lines. Cancer without (**A**) and with (**B**) grid lines as a result of cessation of grid motion during exposure. **C,** Magnified view of grid lines from a moving grid that has stopped because of malfunction.

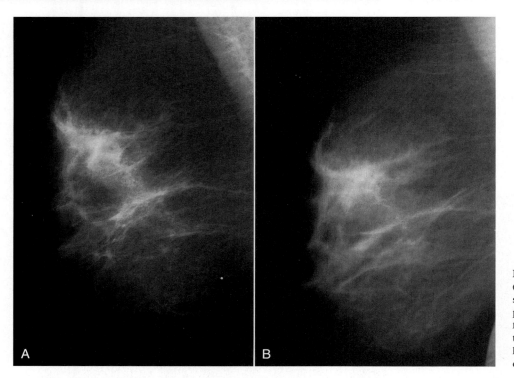

FIGURE 1-10   Dust. Blurring (**A**) is caused by a large dust particle shown as a white dot in the upper part of the breast and is due to poor film-screen contact as the dust lifts the film off the screen. After the large dust particle is removed, the dust artifact and blur are gone (**B**).

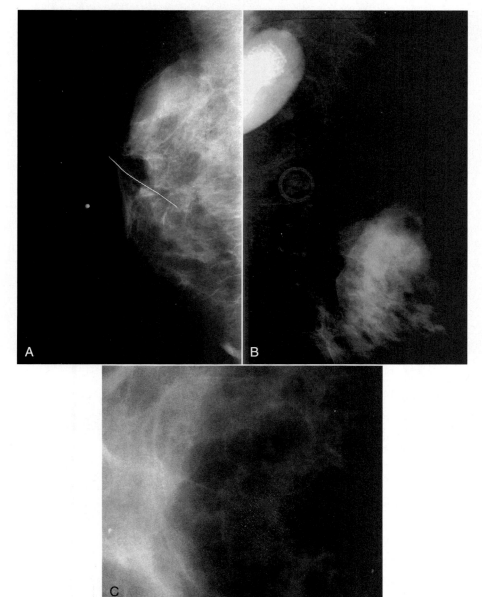

FIGURE 1-11   Artifacts. A, A medio-lateral oblique view after biopsy and radiation therapy shows tiny bright white specks over the biopsy scar compatible with dust on the film. Dust can interfere with a search for microcalcifications. Note the nipple marker and linear scar marker showing the previous biopsy site. **B,** Patient's fingertip is visible in the film. **C,** Magnified view of a minus-density (white) fingerprint artifact, usually caused by contact with the film before exposure.

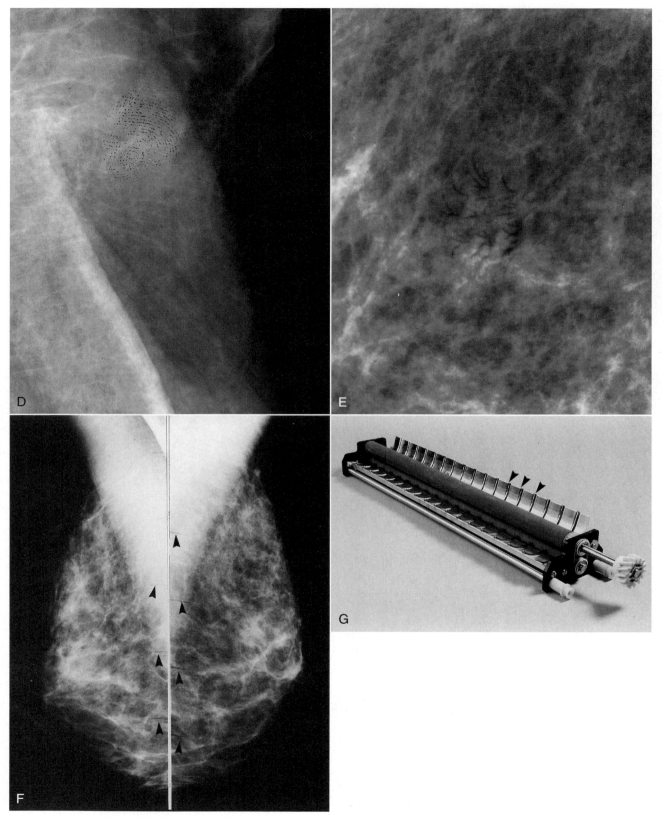

FIGURE 1-11 cont'd   **D,** Magnified view of a plus-density (dark) fingerprint artifact, usually caused by contact with the film after exposure but before processing. **E,** Subtle plus-density tree static artifacts caused by static discharge in a limited region of the film. The light emitted from the static discharge causes localized film exposure before processing. **F,** Guide shoe marks. Dark lines *(arrowheads)* at the edge of the film in the direction of film travel that are evenly spaced are caused by excessive pressure on the film emulsion from guide shoes as the film travels through the processor. Guide shoe marks can sometimes result in minus-density linear artifacts in the direction of film travel as well. **G,** A film guide that turns the film as it passes through the processor. Such guides (arrowheads) are located at the top and bottom of each tank. Improperly adjusted film guides can lead to excessive pressure on the film emulsion and result in guide shoe artifacts.

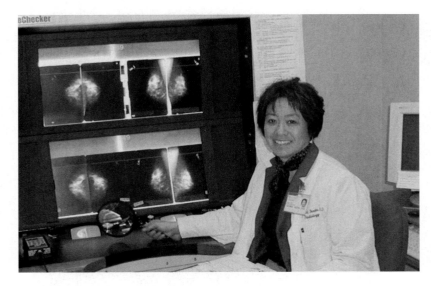

FIGURE 1-12   Viewing conditions.

Box 1-6   Film Labeling

Patient's first and last name
Unique patient identification number
Name and address of the facility
Mammography unit
Date
View and laterality placed near the axilla
Arabic number indicating the cassette
Technologist's initials

From 1999 ACR Mammography Quality Control Manual. American College of Radiology, Reston, VA, p27.

Quality Assurance

On October 1, 1994, regulations stipulated by the 1992 MQSA went into effect. National regulations for mammography facilities were established, and yearly inspections overseen by the U.S. FDA were required. All facilities performing mammography must be certified by the FDA. A prerequisite to being FDA certified is being accredited by an FDA-approved accreditation body. Currently, the ACR and several states (Arkansas, California, Iowa, and Texas) are designated by the FDA as accrediting bodies. Specific qualifications for radiologists, technologists, and medical physicists are outlined in Boxes 1-7 through 1-9. MQSA equipment requirements are summarized in Box 1-10. In addition, one radiologist is designated as the "supervising physician" to oversee the facility's quality assurance program (Boxes 1-11 and 1-12).

The supervising physician oversees assessment of mammography outcomes to evaluate the accuracy of interpretation. The facility must have a method for making

---

Box 1-7   MQSA Qualifications for Interpreting Physicians

Be licensed to practice medicine in the state
Be certified by a body approved by the FDA to certify interpreting physicians *or* have 3 months full-time training in mammography interpretation, radiation physics, radiation effects, and radiation protection *and*
Have 60 hours of documented mammography continuing medical education (CME) (time in residency will be accepted if documented in writing) and 8 hours of training in each modality (such as screen-film or digital mammography) *and*
Have read at least 240 examinations in the preceding 6 months under supervision *or* have read mammograms under the supervision of a fully qualified interpreting physician (see *The Federal Register* for exact requirements) *and*
Have read 960 mammograms over a period of 24 months
Have at least 15 category 1 CME credits in mammography over a 36-month period, with 6 credits in each modality used
To re-establish qualifications, either interpret or double-read 240 mammograms under direct supervision or bring the total to 960 over a period of 24 months and accomplish these tasks within the 6 months immediately before resuming independent interpretation. Regarding CME, if the requirement of 15 hours per 36 months is not met, the total number of CME hours must be brought up to 15 per 36 months before resuming independent interpretation
Note: to perform a new imaging modality, the interpreting physician must have 8 CME credits specific to that modality before starting the modality

Modified from *The Federal Register.* http://www.fda.gov/cdrh/mammography/.

Box 1-8 MQSA Qualifications for Radiologic Technologists

Have a license to perform radiographic procedures in their state *or*

Be certified by one of the bodies (such as the American Registry of Radiologic Technicians) approved by the FDA

Have undergone 40 hours of documented mammography training, with 8 hours of instruction in each modality used, and have completed at least 25 examinations *or*

Be exempted by being qualified under interim regulations

Complete 200 examinations in the previous 24 months and teach or complete at least 15 continuing education units (CEUs) in the past 36 months, including 6 in each modality used

To re-establish qualifications, must complete 25 examinations under direct supervision and complete 15 CEUs per 36 months

Modified from *The Federal Register.* http://www.fda.gov/cdrh/mammography/.

Box 1-9 MQSA Qualifications for Medical Physicists

Have a license or approval by a state to conduct evaluations of mammography equipment under the Public Health Services Act *or* have certification in an accepted area by one of the accrediting bodies approved by the FDA

Have a masters or higher degree in physics, radiologic physics, applied physics, biophysics, health physics, medical physics, engineering, radiation science, or public health with a bachelor's degree in the physical sciences *and*

Have 1 year in training in medical physics specific to diagnostic radiologic physics *and*

Have 2 years' experience in conducting performance evaluation of mammography equipment *and*

Teach or complete 15 hours of continuing medical education in mammography physics every 36 months

Modified from *The Federal Register.* http://www.fda.gov/cdrh/mammography/.

Box 1-10 MQSA Equipment Requirements for Mammography

Be specifically designed for mammography

Have a breast compression device and have additional hand-operated compression to augment motor-driven compression

Have provision for operation with a removable grid for either 18×24- or 24×30-cm image receptors

The mean glandular dose to a 4.5-cm-thick breast is less than 3 mGy (0.3 rad) when the site's clinical technique is used

Can angulate 180 degrees from CC orientation in at least one direction

Other minimum standards for beam limitation and light field, magnification capability, display of focal spot selection, technique factor selection and display, automatic exposure control, x-ray film, intensifying screens, film processing solutions, lighting and hot lights, film masking devices

Modified from *The Federal Register.* http://www.fda.gov/cdrh/mammography/.

Box 1-11 Quality Assurance Program for Equipment

All programs must establish and maintain a quality assurance (QA) program with periodic monitoring of the dose delivered by the examinations

For screen-film systems, the QA program is the same as described in the 1999 *Mammography Quality Control Manual Radiologist's Manual, Radiological Technologist's Manual,* and *Medical Physicist's Manual* prepared by the American College of Radiology Committee on Quality Assurance in Mammography at 1891 Preston White Drive, Reston, VA 22091-5431

Maintenance of log books documenting compliance and corrective actions for each unit

Establish and maintain radiographic images of phantoms to assess performance of the mammography system for each unit

Major changes from the interim regulations include weekly phantom image quality testing and mammography unit performance tests after each relocation of the mobile unit

Modified from *The Federal Register.* http://www.fda.gov/cdrh/mammography/.

a reasonable effort to record outcomes on interpretation of all abnormal mammographic findings and to tally these interpretations for each individual physician and for the group as a whole and provide feedback to each radiologist on a yearly basis (Box 1-13). A portion of the medical audit includes review of the pathology in cases recommended for biopsy.

One radiologic technologist designated the "QC technologist" oversees the quality control (QC) tasks outlined in Table 1-3, which specifies the minimum frequency of each QC test and action limits for test performance. One important test performed by the QC technologist and reviewed by the interpreting physician is evaluation of the mammography phantom image; this test is performed at least weekly and evaluates the entire imaging system. The phantom consists of fibers, speck clusters, and masses of various size embedded in a uniform phantom material. The technologist uses the site's clinical technique to take a mammogram of a 4.5-cm-thick compressed breast, the radiograph is processed on the site's film processor, and the image is evaluated for the number of objects seen in each category. To pass accreditation and meet MQSA requirements, the phantom should show a minimum of four fibers, three speck groups, and three masses. The phantom image should also be free of significant artifacts. The phantom image test evaluates the entire imaging chain (Box 1-14).

The medical physicist surveys the equipment after installation, after important major equipment repairs or upgrades, and annually, performing the QC tests outlined in Box 1-15. This report is an important component of the quality assurance program and is reviewed by the supervising physician to ensure high-quality mammography.

Each year, the mammography facility is inspected by state or federal officials for compliance with MQSA regulations. Non-compliance with guidelines may result in warnings requiring corrective action or, in extreme cases, closure of the facility.

Box 1-12   Quality Assurance for Clinical Images

Monitoring of repeat rate for repeated clinical images and their causes

Record keeping, analysis of results, and remedial actions taken on the basis of this monitoring

Modified from *The Federal Register.* http://www.fda.gov/cdrh/mammography/.

Box 1-13   Quality Assurance for Interpretation of Clinical Images

Establishment of systems for reviewing outcome data from mammograms, including
   Disposition of all positive mammograms
   Correlation of surgical biopsy results with mammogram reports
   Designation of a specific physician to ensure data collection and analysis and show that the analysis is shared with the facility and individual physicians

Modified from *The Federal Register.* http://www.fda.gov/cdrh/mammography/.

Box 1-14   Phantom Image

Evaluates the mammography imaging setup
Performed at least weekly
Must see 4 fibers, 3 speck groups, 3 masses
Must be free of significant artifacts

From 1999 ACR Mammography Quality Control Manual. American College of Radiology, Reston, VA, p 119.

Table 1-3   Technologist Quality Control Tests for Screen-Film Mammography

Periodicity	Quality Control Test	Desired Result
Daily	Darkroom cleanliness	No dust artifacts
Daily	Processor QC	Density difference and mid-density changes not to exceed control limits of ±0.15
Weekly	Screen cleanliness	No dust artifacts on films
Weekly	View box cleanliness	No marks on panels, uniform lighting
Weekly	Phantom image evaluation	Film density >1.4 with control limits of ±0.20. Densities do not vary over time or between units. Minimum test objects seen: 4 largest fibers, 3 largest speck groups, 3 largest masses
Monthly	Visual checklist	Each item on checklist present and functioning properly
Quarterly	Repeat analysis	Overall repeat rate of <5% Percent repeats similar for each category
Quarterly	Analysis of fixer retention	Residual sodium thiosulfate (hypo) ≤0.05 µg/cm^3
Semiannually	Darkroom fog	Fog ≤0.05 for 2-minute exposure in darkroom
	Screen-film contact	Large areas (>1 cm) of poor contact unacceptable
	Compression	Power mode: 25-45 lb Manual mode: >25 lb

From 1999 Mammography Quality Control Manual. American College of Radiology, Reston, VA, p. 119.

DIGITAL MAMMOGRAPHY

Technical Aspects of Image Acquisition

Digital x-ray image acquisition has several potential advantages in terms of image availability, image processing,

Box 1-15	Medical Physicist's Screen-Film Mammography Quality Control Tests (Annually and after Major Equipment Changes)

1. Unit assembly evaluation
2. Assessment of collimation
3. Evaluation of system resolution
4. Automatic exposure control (AEC) assessment of performance
5. Uniformity of screen speed
6. Artifact evaluation
7. Evaluation of image quality
8. kVp accuracy and reproducibility
9. Assessment of beam quality (half-value layer measurement)
10. Breast entrance exposure, AEC reproducibility, average glandular dose, and radiation output rate
11. View box luminance and room luminance

and CAD. Instead of using a screen-film cassette to capture the mammogram, a full-field digital mammography (FFDM) unit uses a fixed or removable digital detector (Fig. 1-13). The mammogram is obtained with the use of a compression paddle and an x-ray tube, just as for SFM, but the image receptor is a digital detector (Figs. 1-14 and 1-15).

FFDM detectors can be indirect or direct digital detectors. Indirect digital detectors use fluorescent screens such as cesium iodide (CsI) to convert each absorbed x-ray to hundreds of visible light photons. Behind the CsI screen are placed light-sensitive detector arrays made of materials such as amorphous silicon diodes or charge-coupled devices. These arrays measure the light produced pixel by pixel. The weak electronic signal from each pixel is amplified and sent through an analog-to-digital converter to enable computer storage of the measured detector signal. Direct digital detectors use detector elements that capture and count x-rays directly, although amplification and analog-to-digital conversion are still applied. Another method to produce digital mammograms involves amorphous selenium. An amorphous selenium plate is an excellent absorber of x-rays and an excellent capacitor that stores the charge created by ionization at sites where x-rays are absorbed. Unlike its use in xeromammography, in which a blue toner system produces the image on paper, an electronic readout must be used to record the charge distribution

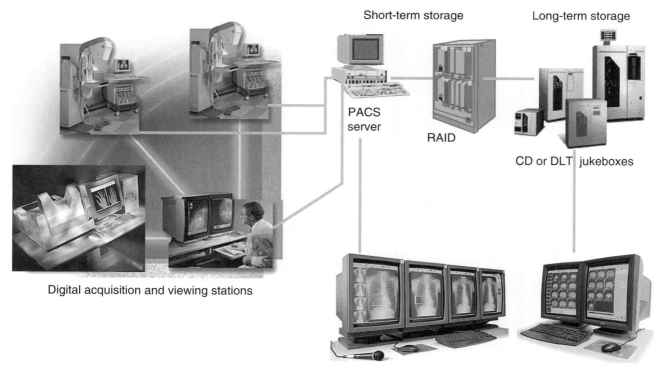

Short-term storage   Long-term storage

PACS server

RAID

CD or DLT jukeboxes

Digital acquisition and viewing stations

Hi-resolution multimodality workstations

FIGURE 1-13   Schematic of a full-field digital mammography unit and its components. (Adapted from figures provided by GE Medical Services, Waukasha, WI.)

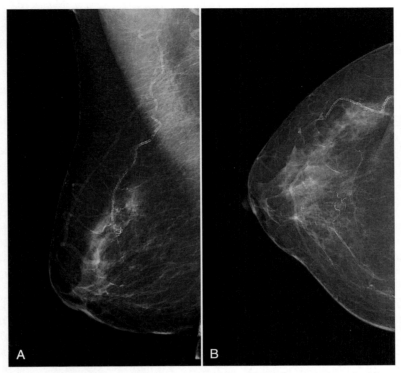

FIGURE 1-14   Full-Field Digital Mammography (FFDM). Mediolateral oblique (**A**) and craniocaudal (**B**) FFDM in a breast with scattered fibroglandular densities.

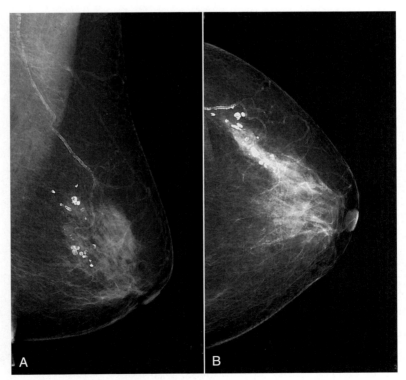

FIGURE 1-15   Calcifications seen on mediolateral oblique (**A**) and craniocaudal (**B**) full-field digital mammograms represent fat necrosis from previous trauma that was noted on a screening mammogram.

on the selenium plate for digital imaging. This can be done by scanning the selenium plate with a laser beam or by placing a silicon diode array in contact with one side of the plate to read out the stored charge. Each of these methods allows the production of high-resolution digital images.

Another approach to FFDM is the computed radiography approach, which uses a photo-stimulable phosphor (BaFlBr:Eu). The plate is used to absorb x-rays just as a screen-film cassette. However, rather than emitting light immediately after exposure through fluorescence, x-ray absorption causes electrons within the phosphor material to be promoted to higher energy levels within the crystal. A laser scans the phosphor plate, electrons are released, and higher-energy (blue) light is emitted in proportion to the x-ray exposure. Problems with this system include inefficient light collection and scatter of laser light in the phosphor material.

No matter which digital detector is used, its job is to detect x-rays passing through the breast, compression plate, and breast holder into a signal that is amplified and converted to a digital signal. The digital detector design determines how the summed attenuation signals will be distributed into the picture elements (pixels) that make up the reconstructed breast image.

The analog-to-digital converter determines how many bits of memory will be used to store the signal for each pixel. The more bits per pixel, the higher the dynamic range for the image, but at higher storage cost. Specifically, if 12 bits per pixel are used, 2^{12} or 4096 signal values can be stored. If 14 bits per pixel are used, 2^{14} or 16,384 signal values can be stored. Usually, 12 to 14 bits per pixel are used, or 2 bytes per pixel. The GE Senographe 2000D digital detector has $1920 \times 2304 = 4.4$ million pixels, which requires 8.8 million bytes (Mbytes) of storage per image. Other FFDM systems require up to 52 Mbytes of storage per image. These large amounts of data can be acquired, displayed, archived, and retrieved easily with current hardware and software.

Screen-film systems used for mammography have a line-pair resolution of about 20 lp/mm. To produce images equaling the spatial resolution of SFM, the digital system would require pixels spaced 25 µm apart, which produces a signal-to-noise, storage, and display issue for the large data sets required to produce such images. In 2003, FFDM systems had spatial resolution ranging from 5 to 10 lp/mm.

However, it has been argued that the lower spatial resolution of FFDM systems may in part be compensated by their increased contrast resolution. Unlike SFM, where the image cannot be manipulated after capture other than through film processing, FFDM images may be optimized after image capture by soft copy display and adjustment of window width and window level to change the contrast and brightness of the images, respectively. Second, screen-film images have a linear relationship between log (exposure) and film OD only in the central portion of the characteristic curve. In FFDM, signal value is linearly proportional to exposure over the entire dynamic range of the detector. Thus, digital images do not suffer contrast loss in underexposed or overexposed areas (as long as detector saturation does not occur) and instead show similar contrast over the full dynamic range of signals. FFDM also eliminates the variability and noise added as a result of film processing. Interestingly, when averaged over all breast types and sizes, FFDM is associated with a lower radiation dose than SFM is for specific equipment, especially those using slot-scanning techniques in which a narrow slot of detector elements is scanned under the breast in synchronization with a fan beam of x-rays swept across the breast. This design, though technically more difficult to implement, has the advantage of eliminating the need for a grid to reduce scattered radiation. Scatter is eliminated by the narrow slot itself, thereby reducing the amount of radiation delivered to the breast to obtain the same signal-to-noise ratio at the detector. Full area detectors with AEC systems have also been shown to use lower breast doses than those needed with SFM, especially for thicker breasts.

Once captured, the image data are transferred to a reading station and interpreted on high-resolution ($2K \times 2.5K$ or 5 Mpixel) monitors or printed on films by laser imagers (with 40-µm spot sizes) to be interpreted on film view boxes. The digital data are stored on optical disks, on a picture archiving and communication system (PACS), or on CD-ROMs for later retrieval.

The MQSA states that FFDM images must be made available to patients and that hard copy films must be available as needed, which means the facility must have an FDA-approved laser printer for mammography that has the ability to reproduce the gray scale and resolution of FFDM films.

A study evaluating FFDM versus SFM for screening asymptomatic women for breast cancer screened 6736 asymptomatic women with both FFDM and SFM. The results showed that FFDM was associated with a significantly lower recall rate (11.8% versus 14.9%, $P > .001$) and significantly lower biopsy rate (14 versus 21 per 1000 examinations, $P < .001$) than SFM. No statistically significant difference was found in sensitivity ($P > .1$) or receiver operating characteristic (ROC) curve areas (0.74 for FFDM versus 0.80 for SFM, $P = .18$). A larger paired study with similar design, the American College of Radiology Imaging Network Digital Mammographic Imaging Screening Trial (ACRIN-DMIST), has recently recruited 49,500 asymptomatic women for screening with both FFDM and SFM, but final results are not yet available.

Quality Assurance in Digital Mammography

To comply with MQSA requirements, all personnel must have 8 hours of training specific to digital mammography documented in writing before clinical use in that facility (Box 1-16). Specifically, the radiologist must receive 8 hours of training in interpretation of digital mammography, with a strong recommendation from the FDA that training include instruction from a radiologist experienced in interpretation of digital mammography on the specific system used. Technologists and medical physicists must also have documented training by appropriately qualified individuals, for example, by the manufacturer's application specialists for technologists and by medical physicists qualified in digital mammography and be able to conduct hands-on training for medical physicists. After initial certification, all personnel must have 6 hours of Category 1 continuing medical education or continuing educational units every 3 years, which can be part of the required 15 hours of continuing education required in mammography.

The ACR and the state of Iowa began accrediting FFDM systems in 2003, and all new FFDM systems must be accredited before use. Such accreditation involves submitting a medical physicist's equipment evaluation, a laser-printed phantom image, registration of the digital equipment, documentation of personnel qualifications, and a fee. Sites already accredited to perform mammography may begin using new digital units, just as they would a new SFM unit, after submission of the aforementioned items. *New facilities* seeking certification should apply to their accreditation body and submit the items just mentioned, but they must wait to perform mammography on patients until they receive a 6-month provisional certificate from the FDA. This usually takes about a week after submission of all data to the accreditation body. During the provisional 6-month period, the facility must submit clinical images and phantom images to the accreditation body to receive accreditation and become fully certified by the FDA.

Quality assurance testing for FFDM is stipulated by the image receptor manufacturer and includes tests that if found to be out of compliance, must be corrected immediately before that component of the FFDM system can be used. Test failures that must be corrected immediately include phantom image quality, contrast-to-noise ratio, radiation dose, and calibration of the review workstation. Correction of other test failures such as repeat analysis, assessment of collimation, and other physics tests is permitted within 30 days after identification of the problem. These tests are listed in Box 1-17.

COMPUTER-AIDED DETECTION

Radiologists are trained to detect early, subtle signs of breast cancer such as pleomorphic calcifications and spiculated masses on mammograms. CAD systems use algorithms to review mammograms for bright clustered specks or converging lines, which represent possible early signs of breast cancer such as pleomorphic calcifications or spiculated masses, respectively. The reason that these programs were developed was to help radiologists search for signs of cancer against the complex background of dense breast tissue and fat.

Some facilities use CAD as a "second reader." "Double reading" in screening mammography involves two observers reviewing the same mammograms to increase detection of cancer, decrease the false-negative rate, or in some facilities, decrease the false-positive recall rate by

---

Box 1-16 Educational Requirements for New Personnel Using Digital Mammography

8 hours of training specific to digital mammography before its use

6 hours of Category 1 continuing medical education or continuing education unit credits every 3 years

The 6 hours can be part of the required 15 hours of continuing education in mammography required by the MQSA

Modified from *The Federal Register*. http://www.Fda.gov/cdrh/mammography/.

Box 1-17 Medical Physicist's Digital Quality Control Tests (Annually and after Major Equipment Changes)

1. Full-field digital mammography (FFDM) unit assembly evaluation
2. Flat-field uniformity test*
3. Artifact evaluation
4. Automatic exposure control (AEC) mode and signal-to-noise ratio (SNR) check*
5. Phantom image quality test*
6. Contrast-to-noise ratio (CNR) test*
7. Modulation transfer function (MTF) measurement*
8. Assessment of collimation
9. Evaluation of focal spot size
10. kVp accuracy and reproducibility
11. Assessment of beam quality (half-value layer measurement)
12. Breast entrance exposure, mean glandular dose,* and radiation output rate
13. Image quality of the display monitor

*Indicates immediate correction required before use of the FFDM unit.

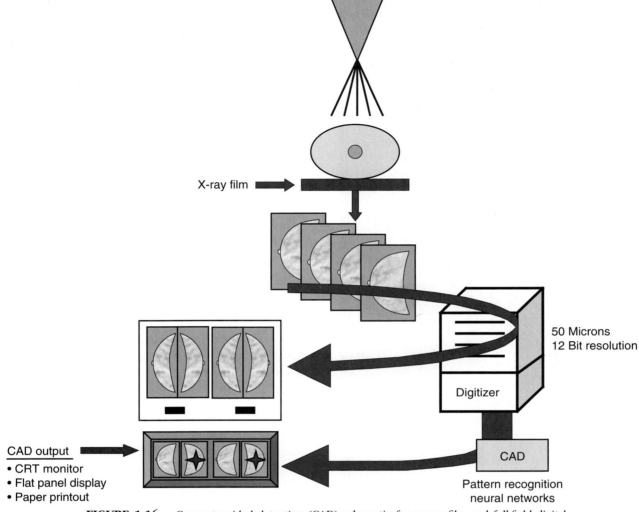

X-ray film

50 Microns
12 Bit resolution

Digitizer

CAD output
- CRT monitor
- Flat panel display
- Paper printout

CAD

Pattern recognition
neural networks

FIGURE 1-16   Computer-aided detection (CAD) schematic for screen-film and full-field digital mammograms. (Courtesy of R. Castellino, R2 Technology, San Jose, CA).

using a consensus. Studies have shown that double reading, depending on its implementation, increases the rate of detection of cancer by 5% to 15%. However, the expense and logistic problems of implementing a second interpreting radiologist limit the practice of double-reading mammography in clinical practice.

Mammographic data used for CAD algorithms are obtained digitally from FFDM units or are digitized from screen-film mammograms. The digitized mammograms undergo analysis by computer schemes, which mark potential abnormal findings on paper or on a low-resolution monitor image (Fig. 1-16). The radiologist interprets and analyzes the findings identified, and the patient is recalled for further work-up or the findings are dismissed as insignificant (Fig. 1-17).

CAD algorithms detect microcalcifications, masses, and parenchymal distortions on mammograms by using computer schemes derived from large numbers of mammograms in which the biopsy results are known. The computer scheme's ability to mark true cancers is optimized by reviewing the "true-positive" and "false-positive" marks on the training set of mammograms. These optimized algorithms are later tested on both known subtle and obvious cancers. With the use of optimized schemes, commercial CAD systems mark abnormalities that represent cancer ("true-positive" marks, a measure of CAD sensitivity) and findings that do *not* represent cancer or in which no known cancer has occurred ("false-positive" marks, a measure of CAD specificity) (Fig. 1-18). Because detection of masses or calcifications by the CAD

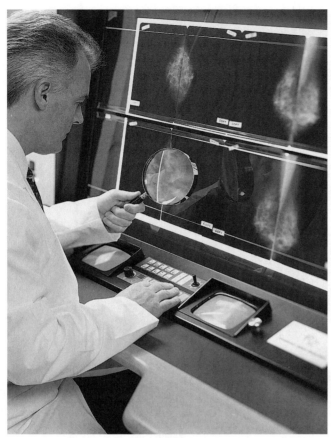

FIGURE 1-17   Mammograms and computer-aided detection output. For screen-film mammography, the technologist digitizes the mammograms and then mounts the images on an alternator for the radiologist to interpret. A computer marks potential findings on the mammogram and displays the findings on low-resolution images on the monitor below the films. (Courtesy of R. Castellino, R2 Technology, San Jose, CA.)

scheme is directly affected by the quality of the image, good-quality mammograms are required to obtain good CAD output. Mammograms of suboptimal quality will result in poor CAD output. CAD output also can be affected by the type and reproducibility of the digitizer if image data have been derived from digitized screen-film mammograms. Thus, it is essential to have high-quality mammograms because CAD cannot "make up" for poor image quality.

The FDA has approved CAD systems for detection of breast cancer in both screening and diagnostic mammography.

A retrospective study of breast cancers found on mammography by Dr. Linda Warren Burhenne et al. determined that a CAD program marked 77% (89/115) of screening-detected breast cancers. Dr. Robyn Birdwell et al. reviewed "negative" mammograms obtained the year before the diagnosis of 115 screen-detected cancers in 110 patients. They reported that a CAD program marked findings in 77% (88/115) of false-negative mammograms; specifically, the program marked calcifications in 86% (30/35) and marked masses in 73% (58/80).

Freer and Ulissey reported that in a prospective community breast center study of 12,860 women undergoing screening mammography, CAD increased their cancer detection rate by 19.5%. Radiologists detected 41 of 49 cancers and missed 8 cancers found by a CAD system (7 of 8 were calcifications). CAD detected 40 of the 49 cancers, but it did not mark 9 radiologist-detected masses that were proven cancers.

It is important to note that CAD systems do not diagnose all cancers, nor should they be used as the only evaluator of screening mammograms. In Freer and Ulissey's study, radiologists initially made a decision about the mammogram and *then* used CAD and re-reviewed the marked mammogram. The radiologist's decision to recall a potential abnormality could not be changed by failure of the CAD system to identify the potential finding. Findings marked by CAD could be recalled even if the finding was not initially detected by the radiologist but was judged to be abnormal in retrospect. This means that radiologists should read the mammogram first so that they are not influenced by the CAD marks initially because not all cancers are identified by CAD.

CAD marks have low specificity inasmuch as approximately 97.6% of the CAD marks were dismissed by the interpreting radiologists in the paper of Freer and Ulissey. The radiologist had identified almost all of the 2.4% of CAD-marked findings that were selected for recall, which means that high-sensitivity CAD systems will mark significant potential findings as well as numerous nonsignificant findings, thus identifying tumors but marking a number of normal findings that must be dismissed. Accordingly, it is expected that many insignificant findings will be marked by the CAD system, most of which can be dismissed readily, and yet the radiologists' attention will still be drawn to overlooked suspicious areas.

CAD programs have the potential to increase detection of cancer. In the end, however, it is the radiologist's knowledge and interpretive skill that have an impact on detection of cancer.

CONCLUSION

Mammogram acquisition is affected by multiple complex interactions of the x-ray equipment, processing, technologist, patient, and interpreting radiologist. It is important to understand equipment requirements and the effect of imaging parameters on image quality. It is

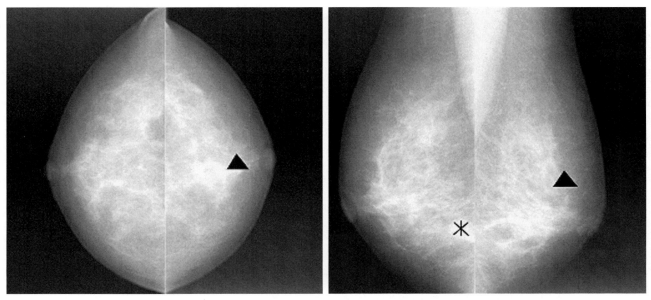

FIGURE 1-18   Magnified view of low-resolution images with computer scheme marks for detecting microcalcifications *(triangle)* or masses *(star)* by computer-aided detection on digitized mammograms or on directly acquired digital mammograms. (Courtesy of R. Castellino, R2 Technology, San Jose, CA.)

also important to understand the technology of breast imaging and be able to solve problems that occur in the everyday clinical practice of breast imaging. MQSA regulations were put into effect to mandate many of the factors that are known to affect image quality and to improve the quality of mammography. Every radiologist who performs breast imaging must understand the MQSA requirements and be able to supervise a high-quality mammography practice.

KEY ELEMENTS

American Cancer Society Guidelines for breast cancer screening of asymptomatic women includes annual mammography starting at age 40.

The Mammography Quality Standard Act of 1992 is a congressional act enforced by the FDA under which mammography facilities in the United States are regulated.

The usual exposure for a mammogram is 24 to 32 kVp at 25 to 200 mAs.

Screen-film systems deliver an average absorbed dose of 2 mGy per exposure to the glandular tissue of the breast.

Anode-filter combinations for mammography are Mo/Mo, Mo/Rh, Rh/Rh, and W/Rh.

Screen-film image receptors are 18 × 24 cm and 24 × 30 cm in size.

Focal spot sizes for contact mammography and magnification mammography are nominally 0.3 and 0.1 mm, respectively.

Magnification mammography should produce 1.4× to 2.0× magnification.

Moving grids with grid ratios between 3.5:1 and 5:1 are used for contact mammography; no grid is used for magnification mammography.

The phantom image evaluates the entire mammography imaging chain, is performed weekly, and at a minimum should detect four fibers, three speck groups, and three masses.

Film labeling includes the patient's first and last name and unique identification number, the name and address of the facility, the date, the view and laterality positioned near the axilla, numbers indicating the cassette and the mammography unit, and the technologist's initials.

The mediolateral oblique view should show good compression, contrast, exposure, sharpness, little noise, a posterior nipple line that intersects a concave pectoralis muscle, and an open inframammary fold.

The craniocaudal view should show good compression, contrast, exposure, sharpness, little noise, and a posterior nipple line (PNL) that has a distance within 1 cm of the mediolateral oblique PNL length, and it should include medial breast tissue without sacrificing lateral breast tissue.

The MQSA requires specific training, experience, and continuing education for technologists, radiologists, and medical physicists.

To use a new modality, personnel are required to have an initial 8 hours of training in that modality plus 6 hours of Category 1 continuing medical education or continuing education unit credits every 3 years.

Digital mammography detectors are composed of amorphous silicon diodes, arrayed charge-coupled devices, or a charged selenium plate read by silicon diodes.

Digital mammograms may be interpreted on printed films or on high-resolution 2K × 2.5K (5 Mpixel) monitors.

CAD programs can detect subtle but suspicious mammographic findings in dense or complex breast tissue.

CAD programs do not detect every breast cancer.

When CAD is used for interpretation of mammograms, the decision to recall a finding on a mammogram rests solely on the radiologist's experience and judgment in interpretation of films.

SUGGESTED READINGS

Baker JA, Rosen EL, Lo JY, et al: Computer-aided detection (CAD) in screening mammography: Sensitivity of commercial CAD systems for detecting architectural distortion. AJR Am J Roentgenol 181:1083-1088, 2003.

Bassett LW, Feig SA, Hendrick RE, et al: Breast Disease (Third Series) Test and Syllabus. Reston, VA, American College of Radiology, 2000.

Berns EA, Hendrick RE, Cutter GR: Performance comparison of full-field digital mammography to screen-film mammography in clinical practice. Med Phys 29:830-834, 2002.

Birdwell RL, Ikeda DM, O'Shaughnessy KF, Sickles EA: Mammographic characteristics of 115 missed cancers later detected with screening mammography and the potential utility of computer-aided detection. Radiology 219:192-202, 2001.

Ciatto S, Del Turco MR, Risso G, et al: Comparison of standard reading and computer aided detection (CAD) on a national proficiency test of screening mammography. Eur J Radiol 45:135-138, 2003.

Compliance Guidance: The Mammography Quality Standards Act Final Regulations Document #1; availability. Food and Drug Administration, HHS. Notice. Fed Reg 64(53):13590-13591, 1999.

Curry TS, Dowdy JE, Murray RC: Christensen's Physics of Diagnostic Radiology, 4th ed. Malvern, PA, Lea & Febiger, 1990.

Freer TW, Ulissey MJ: Screening mammography with computer-aided detection: Prospective study of 12,860 patients in a community breast center. Radiology 220:781-786, 2001.

Galen B, Staab E, Sullivan DC, Pisano ED: Congressional update: Report from the Biomedical Imaging Program of the National Cancer Institute. American College of Radiology Imaging Network: The digital mammographic imaging screening trial—an update. Acad Radiol 9:374-375, 2002.

Hemminger BM, Dillon AW, Johnston RE, et al: Effect of display luminance on the feature detection rates of masses in mammograms. Med Phys 26:2266-2272, 1999.

Hendrick RE, Bassett LW, Botsco MA, et al: Mammography Quality Control Manual. Reston, VA, American College of Radiology, 1999.

Hendrick RE, Berns EA. Digital Mammography Quality Control Manual. Chicago, Phantom Image Press, 2001, revised edition 2003.

Lewin JM, D'Orsi CJ, Hendrick RE, et al: Clinical comparison of full-field digital mammography and screen-film mammography for detection of breast cancer. AJR Am J Roentgenol 179:671-677, 2002.

Lewin JM, Hendrick RE, D'Orsi CJ, et al: Comparison of full-field digital mammography with screen-film mammography for cancer detection: Results of 4,945 paired examinations. Radiology 218:873-880, 2001.

Linver MN, Osuch JR, Brenner RJ, Smith RA: The mammography audit: A primer for the Mammography Quality Standards Act (MQSA). AJR Am J Roentgenol 165:19-25, 1995.

Markey MK, Lo JY, Floyd CE Jr: Differences between computer-aided diagnosis of breast masses and that of calcifications. Radiology 223:489-493, 2002.

Monsees BS: The Mammography Quality Standards Act. An overview of the regulations and guidance. Radiol Clin North Am 38:759-772, 2000.

1998 MQSA (Mammography Quality Standards Act) final rule released. American College of Radiology. Radiol Manage 20:51-55, 1998.

Nass SJ, Henderson IC, Lashof LJ (eds): Mammography and Beyond: Developing Technologies for the Early Detection of Breast Cancer. Washington, DC, National Academy Press, 2001.

Pisano ED, Cole EB, Kistner EO, et al: Interpretation of digital mammograms: Comparison of speed and accuracy of soft-copy versus printed-film display. Radiology 223:483-488, 2002.

Pisano ED, Cole EB, Major S, et al: Radiologists' preferences for digital mammographic display. The International Digital Mammography Development Group. Radiology 216:820-830, 2000.

Pisano ED, Yaffe MJ, Hemminger BM, et al: Current status of full-field digital mammography. Acad Radiol 7:266-280, 2000.

Quek ST, Thng CH, Khoo JB, Koh WL: Radiologists' detection of mammographic abnormalities with and without a computer-aided detection system. Australas Radiol 47:257-260, 2003.

Rong XJ, Shaw CC, Johnston DA, et al: Microcalcification detectability for four mammographic detectors: Flat-panel, CCD, CR, and screen/film. Med Phys 29:2052-2061, 2002.

Smith RA, Saslow D, Sawyer KA, et al: American Cancer Society guidelines for breast cancer screening: Update 2003. CA Cancer J Clin 53:141-169, 2003.

State certification of mammography facilities. Final rule. Fed Reg 67(25):5446-5469, 2002.

Vedantham S, Karellas A, Suryanarayanan S, et al: Breast imaging using an amorphous silicon–based full-field digital mammographic system: Stability of a clinical prototype. J Digit Imaging 13:191-199, 2000.

Vedantham S, Karellas A, Suryanarayanan S, et al: Full breast digital mammography with an amorphous silicon–based flat panel detector: Physical characteristics of a clinical prototype. Med Phys 27:558-567, 2000.

Venta LA, Hendrick RE, Adler YT, et al: Rates and causes of disagreement in interpretation of full-field digital mammography and film-screen mammography in a diagnostic setting. AJR Am J Roentgenol 176:1241-1248, 2001.

Warren Burhenne IJ, Wood SA, D'Orsi CJ, et al: Potential contribution of computer-aided detection to the sensitivity of screening mammography. Radiology 215:554-562, 2000.

Zheng B, Shah R, Wallace L, et al: Computer-aided detection in mammography: An assessment of performance on current and prior images. Acad Radiol 9:1245-1250, 2002.

Zhou XQ, Huang HK, Lou SL: Authenticity and integrity of digital mammography images. IEEE Trans Med Imaging 20:784-791, 2001.

CHAPTER 2

Mammogram Interpretation

Introduction
Breast Cancer Risk Factors
Signs and Symptoms of Breast Cancer
The Normal Mammogram
Mammographic Findings of Breast Cancer
An Approach to the Mammogram
Diagnostic versus Screening Mammography
Additional Views to Confirm or Exclude the Presence of a
True Lesion
Triangulation
Visualizing Findings in Specific Expected Locations
Additional Views to Characterize True Findings
Summary
Key Elements

INTRODUCTION

To detect breast cancer on mammograms, the reader detects and differentiates signs of cancer from the normal complex background of heterogeneous dense and fatty breast tissue. The incidence of breast cancer in women in the United States has continued to rise, although the rate of increase has slowed recently, with the exception of in situ breast cancer, which has continued to increase. Breast cancer death rates have decreased since the early 1990s, with decreases of 2.5% per year among white women. The American Cancer Society recommends annual screening mammography for women 40 years or older, and the U.S. Preventive Services Task Force recommends screening mammography every 1 to 2 years for the same age group. These guidelines have been promulgated only recently after much debate about the benefit of breast cancer screening with mammography to decrease breast cancer mortality. Decreased breast cancer deaths have been attributed in part to breast cancer screening, adjuvant chemotherapy, and adoption of a healthy standard of living that excludes obesity, a sedentary lifestyle, and the use of alcohol and hormone replacement therapy. Randomized controlled screening trials for breast cancer in women invited to screening mammography have shown about a 30% reduction in breast cancer deaths in the invited group. This chapter will review risk factors and signs and symptoms of breast cancer, the normal mammogram, mammographic findings of breast cancer, basic interpretation of screening mammograms, and work-up of findings detected at screening with additional mammographic views.

BREAST CANCER RISK FACTORS

Risk factors for breast cancer are an important consideration in patient evaluation, and compiling this information on the breast history sheet helps in the evaluation. Breast cancer risk factors are listed in Box 2-1. The most important risk factors are older age and gender.

Box 2-1   Breast Cancer Risk Factors

Female
Age
Personal history of breast cancer
First-degree relative with breast cancer
Early menarche
Late menopause
Nulliparous
First birth after age 30
Atypical ductal hyperplasia
BRCA1, BRCA2
Radiation exposure
Lobular carcinoma in situ

Female gender is the most important risk factor for breast cancer, and U.S. statistics indicate that breast cancer will develop in one in eight women during a 90-year life span. One percent of all breast cancers occur in men.

The risk for breast cancer increases with age and drops off at 80 years of age. Women with a personal history of breast cancer have a higher risk for breast cancer in the ipsilateral or contralateral breast than does the general population. In women undergoing breast conservation, the conservatively treated breast has a 1% per year risk of breast cancer developing.

A family history of breast or ovarian cancer is particularly important, with the age, number, and cancer type in relatives being of special significance. Women with a first-degree relative with breast cancer (mother, daughter, or sister) are at higher risk than is the general population, particularly if cancer developed in the relative before menopause or if the cancer was bilateral. If many relatives had breast or ovarian cancer, the woman may be a carrier of *BRCA1* or *BRCA2* (autosomal dominant breast cancer susceptibility gene). Although genetic testing for these genes is possible, it is most appropriate after proper counseling and evaluation in a genetic screening center. Carriers of the breast cancer susceptibility gene *BRCA1* on chromosome 17 have a breast cancer risk of 85% and ovarian cancer risk of 63% by 70 years of age. Women with *BRCA2* on chromosome 15 have a high risk of breast cancer and low risk of ovarian cancer. These genes account for 5% of all breast cancers in the United States, but for 25% in women younger than 30 years with breast cancer. Women of Ashkenazi (Eastern European) Jewish heritage have a slightly higher risk of breast cancer than does the general population (Box 2-2), but additional work is being done to determine whether this population has a higher rate of breast and ovarian cancer with *BRCA1* and *BRCA2* mutations. Other genetic risk factors include the Li-Fraumeni, Cowden, and ataxia-telangiectasia syndromes.

Early menarche, late menopause, nulliparity, and first live birth after the age of 30 bestow a higher risk for the development of breast cancer, perhaps because of long unopposed estrogen exposure. Data from a 2003 study of the Women's Health Initiative, a randomized controlled trial of the effects of estrogen plus progestin (combination hormone replacement therapy [CHRT]) versus placebo, showed a 24% greater incidence of breast cancer in women receiving CHRT versus the control group. Whereas previous data showed an adjusted relative risk of 1.46 for the development of breast cancer in women receiving CHRT for more than 5 years, the 2003 analysis showed the risk for breast cancer rising within 5 years of starting CHRT, more difficulty in detecting cancers by mammography, and breast cancers that were detected at a more advanced stage. Thus far, no evidence has indicated that the frequency of breast cancer is increased by estrogen replacement therapy alone, but more definitive results and the effects of estrogen replacement alone on heart disease await further study.

A biopsy specimen showing atypical ductal hyperplasia increases the risk for breast cancer to four to five times that of the general population, and lobular carcinoma in situ (LCIS) increases the risk for breast cancer 10-fold. LCIS is a misnomer because it is a high-risk marker and not a real breast cancer. The finding of LCIS indicates that the risk for the development of invasive ductal or lobular cancer in the ipsilateral or contralateral breast is 27% to 30% over a 10-year period. Detection of LCIS results in management consisting of either "watchful waiting" with increased surveillance by imaging and physical examination or bilateral mastectomy.

Women with early exposure to radiation, such as radiation therapy for Hodgkin's disease, multiple fluoroscopic examinations for tuberculosis, or ablation of the thymus or treatment of acne with radiation, have an increased risk for breast cancer.

Quantitative statistical models can be used to evaluate the short-term or lifetime risk for breast cancer, the more common models being the Claus model and the Gail statistical model, which evaluate individual risk factors and combine them into an estimate of the lifetime risk for breast cancer.

Despite all these risk factors, 70% of all women with breast cancer have none of these risk factors other than older age and gender.

Box 2-2   Family History Suggesting an Increased Risk of Breast Cancer

>2 relatives with breast or ovarian cancer
Breast cancer in relative <50 years old
Relatives with breast and ovarian cancer
Relatives with 2 independent breast cancers or breast plus ovarian cancer
Male relative with breast cancer
Family history of breast or ovarian cancer and Ashkenazi Jewish heritage
Li-Fraumeni syndrome
Cowden's syndrome
Ataxia-telangiectasia

SIGNS AND SYMPTOMS OF BREAST CANCER

Breast cancer is often manifested as a palpable hard breast lump, most often found by the woman herself or her partner, and it is a common symptom for which women seek advice (Box 2-3). Of particular concern are new, growing, or hard masses. Masses that are stuck to the skin or chest wall are particularly worrisome.

Nipple discharge is another breast cancer symptom. However, many types of nipple discharge are benign, particularly discharge occurring after nursing or whitish, green, or yellow nipple discharge produced from several ducts when the discharge is expressed. On the other hand, spontaneous discharge is of particular concern. Nipple discharge is also worrisome if it is new and bloody, serosanguineous, or a spontaneous, copious serous discharge.

Although inverted nipples can occur at birth and are not uncommon, new nipple inversion is of concern for a retroareolar tumor producing nipple retraction. Similarly, skin retraction or dimpling is another sign of breast cancer and is due to tethering of the skin by cancer. Skin retraction or tethering may be seen with the patient's arms at her sides, but occasionally, tethering may be observed only when the patient's arms are raised or on her hips so that the pectoralis muscle or tumor is pulled in and the skin is retracted.

Peau d'orange is a physical finding indicating breast edema; it is caused by skin edema rising around the bases of tethered hair follicles and results in apparent skin pitting or "orange peel" skin. Breast edema is a nonspecific finding and may indicate inflammatory cancer, mastitis, or lymph node obstruction.

In some women, breast cancer has no physical findings or symptoms at all and is detected on screening mammography.

Breast pain is a common cause of morbidity and, if cyclic, is usually endocrine in nature. Although breast pain is not generally caused by cancer, both breast pain and breast cancer are common. The physician's goals are to reassure a patient with breast pain, search for treatable causes of breast pain such as cysts, and exclude coexistent malignancy.

THE NORMAL MAMMOGRAM

A normal breast is composed of a honeycomb fibrous structure of Cooper's ligaments that supports fatty tissue, which in turn supports the glandular elements of the breast tissue (Fig. 2-1A). The glandular elements are composed of lactiferous ducts leading from the nipple and branching into excretory ducts, interlobular ducts, and terminal ducts leading to the acini that produce milk. The ducts are lined throughout their course by epithelium composed of an outer myoepithelial layer of cells and an inner secretory cell layer. The ducts and glandular tissue extend posteriorly in a fan-like distribution consisting of 15 to 20 lobes draining each of the lactiferous ducts, with most of the dense tissue found in the upper outer quadrant. Posterior to the glandular tissue is retroglandular fat, described by Dr. Laslo Tabar as "no man's land" in which no glandular tissue should be seen. The pectoralis muscle lies behind the fat on top of the chest wall.

On the craniocaudal projection the pectoralis muscle is seen as a half-moon–shaped density near the chest wall (Fig. 2-1B). Fat lies anterior to the muscle. In older women, most of the glandular tissue in the medial part of the breast undergoes fatty involution, and therefore most of the dense glandular tissue remaining is located in the outer portion of the breast. On occasion, the sternalis muscle may be seen on the craniocaudal view as a muscular density near the medial aspect of the chest wall and should not be mistaken for a mass (Fig. 2-1C and D). If there is a question about a mass versus the sternalis muscle, a cleavage view mammogram or ultrasound may show the muscle as a normal structure.

On the mediolateral oblique mammogram the pectoralis muscle is a concave structure posterior to the retroglandular fat near the chest wall. Normal lymph nodes are often seen in the axilla and overlying the pectoralis muscle on the mediolateral oblique view (Fig. 2-1E). A normal lymph node is an oval or lobulated dense mass with a radiolucent fatty hilum that is most often found in the upper outer quadrant along blood vessels. Lymph nodes also occur normally within the breast and are known as normal "intramammary" lymph nodes. If the lymph node has the typical kidney bean shape and a fatty hilum, it should be left alone. If one is uncertain about whether a mass represents an intramammary lymph node, mammographic magnification views may help display the fatty hilum, or ultrasound may show the typical hypoechoic appearance of the lymph node and the echogenic fatty hilum.

The ratio of glandular to fatty tissue varies considerably in normal breasts. A mammogram of a normal breast displays relative amounts of age-related dense glandular tissue and fat that reflect the natural history of normal

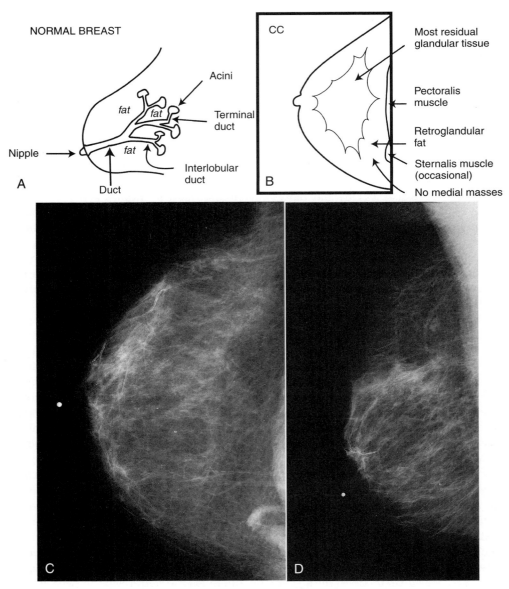

FIGURE 2-1   Normal Breast Anatomy and Correlative Mammograms. A, Schematic of a normal breast showing the nipple, ducts, and acini containing glands producing breast milk. **B,** Schematic of a normal craniocaudal (CC) mammogram. Note the normal fat in the medial and retroglandular regions, the location of the pectoralis muscles. Most of the residual glandular and sternalis tissue remains in the upper outer quadrants. **C** and **D,** Sternalis muscle. The breast is composed of scattered fibroglandular density. A muscle-like density seen in the right breast medial to the half-moon shape of the pectoralis muscle near the chest wall on the CC view (**C**) but not seen on the mediolateral oblique (MLO) view (**D**) represents the sternalis muscle.

breast tissue. The American College of Radiology Breast Imaging and Reporting and Database System (BI-RADS) categories of breast density are fatty, scattered fibroglandular densities, heterogeneously dense, and dense (Box 2-4). In young women, breast tissue is highly glandular, dense, and white on a normal mammogram (Fig. 2-1F). As women age, the glandular tissue involutes to fat, with relatively greater amounts of dense glandular tissue remaining in the upper outer portion of the breast and darker fatty areas in the medial and lower part of the breast; in some women, mostly fatty tissue is left (Fig. 2-1G). Knowledge of the relative decrease in breast tissue and breast density over time is important. Increases in breast density in normal women are seen only in those who are pregnant, lactating, or starting exogenous hormone replacement therapy. Unexplained increases in breast density or new focal density should prompt investigation because a developing density or focal densities may indicate cancer.

Breast tissue is usually symmetrical or mirror image from left to right, but 3% of women have normal asymmetrical glandular tissue. Normal asymmetrical glandular tissue is characterized by a larger volume of normal fibroglandular tissue in one breast than in the other but not necessarily one breast being larger than the other. One method of evaluating for symmetry is to view the left and right mediolateral oblique mammograms back to back and the craniocaudal mammograms back to back (Fig. 2-1H). The glandular tissue pattern is usually fairly symmetrical from side to side, and asymmetries are easily identified with this technique (Fig. 2-2A-C).

A normal mammogram does not usually change from year to year after taking into account the normal involution of glandular tissue over time. It is important to compare old studies with current examinations to evaluate for new or developing changes (Fig. 2-2D-H). For this reason, older films of good quality are placed adjacent to the new films to look for subtle change. Because subtle changes may take over a year to become evident, films older than 2 years may be beneficial for comparison, as well as the most recent studies.

If the mammograms are screen-film studies, the images are viewed on a high-intensity view box with the light parts of the films masked to optimize viewing conditions. For full-field digital mammograms (FFDMs) viewed on soft copy, the images are displayed on high-resolution bright monitors in a dark room with no ambient light.

MAMMOGRAPHIC FINDINGS OF BREAST CANCER

Mammographic detection of breast cancer depends on the sensitivity of the test, the experience of the radiologist, the morphologic appearance of the tumor, and the background on which it is displayed.

Breast cancers are most often identified on screening mammography by detection of pleomorphic calcifications or spiculations produced by the tumor. Other mammographic signs of breast cancer are architectural distortion, asymmetric density, a developing density, a round mass, breast edema, lymphadenopathy, or a single dilated duct. The mammographic signs of breast cancer are listed in Table 2-1 and are discussed in further detail in Chapter 3 on breast calcification, Chapter 4 on breast masses, and Chapter 10 on clinical problems.

Ten percent to 15% of breast cancers are mammographically occult, which means that breast cancer is present but the mammogram is normal. Accordingly, if suspicious clinical symptoms or physical findings are present and the mammogram is negative, the decision for biopsy should be based on clinical grounds alone.

The ability of mammography to depict breast cancer is optimized by good mammographic technique and positioning, which produces the best chance to display suspicious findings against the normal breast background. Mammographic signs of breast cancer are not seen as well against a dense or fibroglandular background because masses or subtle developing densities may be hidden or tiny pleomorphic calcification clusters may be overlooked. Similarly, suspicious masses may be lost in a "busy" background of round benign cysts, which may hide a tumor or draw the radiologist's attention away from the finding. Therefore, a systematic approach to examining the mammogram that involves a consistent, reproducible search pattern for signs of cancer and re-review of "danger zones" in which cancers are commonly missed increases the likelihood of detecting cancers on the mammogram.

AN APPROACH TO THE MAMMOGRAM

A systematic approach to evaluating the mammogram includes a review of the breast history and physical findings and a consistent, reproducible systematic review

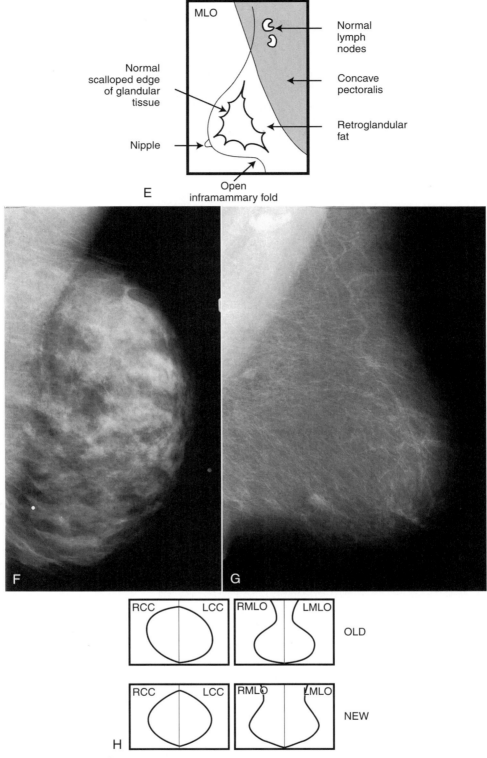

FIGURE 2-1 cont'd   **E,** Schematic of a normal MLO mammogram. Note the normal scalloped edge of glandular tissue, retromammary fat, concave pectoralis muscle, and normal lymph nodes. **F** and **G,** Mammograms of normal breast density. Dense glandular tissue of greater than 75% breast tissue by volume in a young woman categorized in BI-RADS terms as "dense" (**F**), a woman with "heterogeneously dense" breast tissue with 50% to 75% glandular tissue (see Fig 2-4B and C), a woman with "scattered fibroglandular densities" with 25% to 50% glandular tissue (see Fig 2-1C and D), and an older woman with a "fatty" breast composed of less than 25% glandular tissue (**G**). **H,** Schematic of viewing normal mammograms to judge the symmetry and change over time. The CC and MLO mammograms are viewed with the right and left sides placed back to back. Older mammograms are placed above to check for change from year to year.

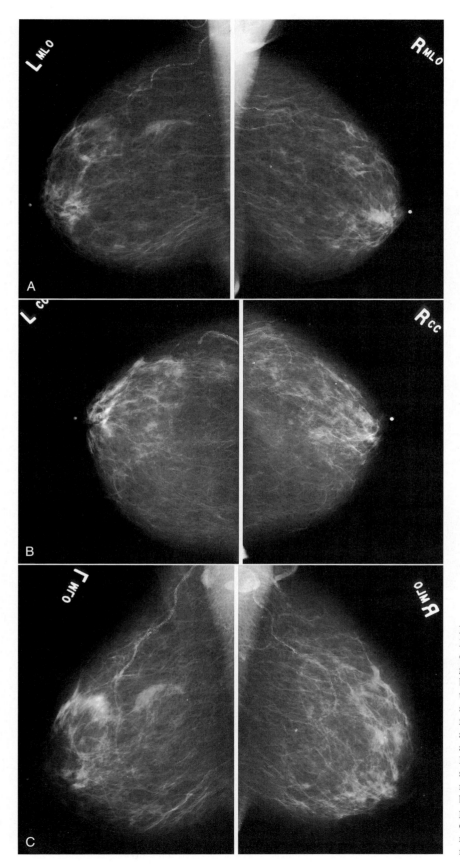

FIGURE 2-2   Normal Focal Asymmetry.
Mediolateral oblique (MLO) (**A**) and craniocaudal (CC) (**B**) views show more white glandular tissue in the upper part of the left breast on the MLO view than on the right. On the CC view no definite mass is seen, with the same shape and density at the same distance from the nipple. The different appearance of the asymmetric tissue on the two views suggests an asymmetry of normal fibroglandular tissue. Repeat MLO views (**C**) show that the density has started to separate into the components of normal tissue and that the density was produced by a summation shadow that looked like a possible mass. Ultrasound was negative, the diagnosis of asymmetric glandular tissue was made, and this finding was unchanged for the next 3 years.

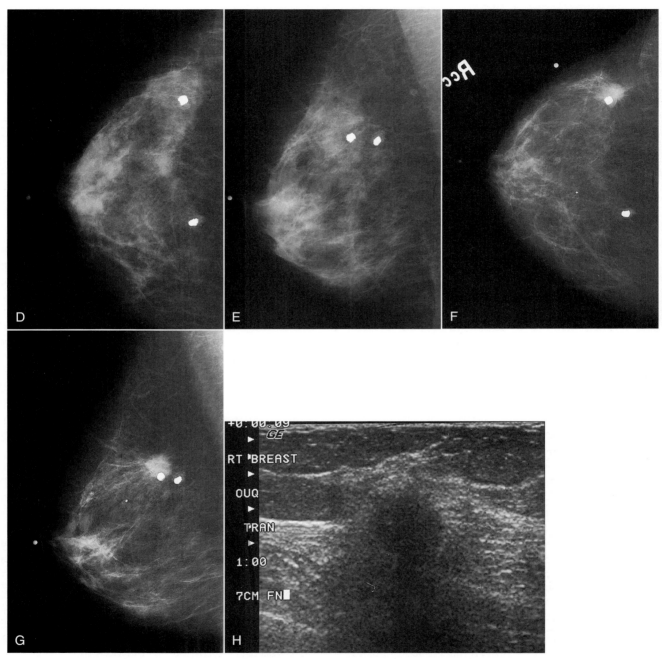

FIGURE 2-2 cont'd   D-H, Developing density. CC (**D**) and MLO views (**E**) show two degenerating calcified fibroadenomas. A developing density formed near the outer calcifying "fibroadenoma" on the CC (**F**) and MLO views (**G**) and was later seen on ultrasound as an irregular mass (**H**). Invasive ductal cancer was diagnosed.

Table 2-1 Mammographic Findings of Breast Cancer

Finding	Differential Diagnosis
1. Pleomorphic calcifications	Cancer (most common), benign disease, fat necrosis
2. Spiculated mass	Cancer, post-surgical scar, radial scar, fat necrosis
3. Round mass	Cyst, fibroadenoma, cancer, papilloma, metastasis
4. Architectural distortion	Post-surgical scarring, cancer
5. Developing density	Cancer, hormone effect, focal fibrosis
6. Asymmetry: focal or global	Normal asymmetric tissue (3%), cancer (suspicious: new, palpable, a mass, contains suspicious calcifications or spiculation)
7. Breast edema	Unilateral—mastitis, post-radiation therapy, inflammatory cancer Bilateral—systemic disease: liver disease, renal failure, congestive heart failure
8. Lymphadenopathy	Unilateral—mastitis, cancer Bilateral—systemic disease: collagen vascular disease, lymphoma, leukemia, infection, adenocarcinoma of unknown primary
9. Nothing	10% of all cancers are false negative on mammography

Table 2-2 Tools Used for Interpretation of Mammograms

Tool	Use
Breast history, risk factors	Evaluate patient's complaint and risks
Technologist's marks	Show skin lesions, scars, problem areas
Put images back to back	Detection of asymmetry Look for whitest part of study
Bright light (screen film)	View skin, dark parts of film
Window/level (FFDM)	Contrast for masses, calcifications
Magnifying lens or magnifier	Magnify for visualization of mass borders, calcifications
Old films	Compare for changes
CAD (if available)	Look for CAD marks *after* initial interpretation

CAD, computer-aided detection; FFDM, full-field digital mammogram.

of the mammograms (Table 2-2). The breast history sheet alerts the radiologist to the patient's risk factors for cancer and the patient's pre-test probability of cancer (Fig. 2-3A). The patient's clinical history of breast biopsies and their location and results aid in mammographic interpretation and patient management once findings are discovered.

The location of any palpable finding is marked on the breast history sheet, and its position in the breast is noted. The position may be described in quadrants, with the upper outer quadrant denoting breast tissue nearest the axilla. Another way to describe a breast location is by using the clock face method, in which the location of breast findings is described as though a clock were superimposed on each breast as the woman faces the examiner (Fig. 2-3B). Hence, the upper outer quadrant in the *right* breast would be between the 9- and 12-o'clock positions, but the upper outer quadrant in the *left* breast would be between the 12- and 3-o'clock positions.

The radiologist then reviews the breast history sheet and accompanying technologist marks indicating skin moles, scars, or implants. Markers placed for the examination draw the radiologist's attention, and an explanation of their meaning on the breast history sheet guides the subsequent work-up.

When viewing the mammogram, the radiologist first does an overall search of the mammographic technique for good positioning, contrast, and compression. Next, the radiologist reviews the dense breast tissue for fibroglandular symmetry between the left and right breasts. The radiologist then looks at the whitest, or densest, part of the mammogram to see whether a mass or distortion is apparent in the white part.

A targeted systematic review of each film involves inspection of all edges of the glandular tissue for tethering (the "tent sign") or masses, the skin/nipple/areolar complex for thickening or retraction, the retroareolar region, the axilla, retroglandular fat, breast tissue at the film edge, and the skin. The next step is to use a magnifying lens on screen-film mammograms or an optical magnifier for digital mammograms reviewed on monitors to search for calcifications. The radiologist then compares the new films with older films of the same quality to evaluate for changes. If computer-aided detection devices are used, they are used after the radiologist's interpretation of the mammogram, and computer-provided marks are evaluated as a "second look."

The following section describes the individual components of a systematic approach to the mammogram (Table 2-3). The first step is to look at the mammographic technique to ensure that the films are of good quality and then inspect for symmetry between the breasts. An asymmetric density may consist of a normal asymmetric volume of breast tissue, which is present in 3% of women and characterized by more fibroglandular tissue in one breast than the other. Asymmetry can also be caused by removal of fibroglandular tissue from one breast by biopsy. Breasts with normal asymmetry should be without suspicious calcifications, spiculations, or palpable masses; be stable when compared with older

STANFORD HOSPITAL AND CLINICS
DEPARTMENT OF RADIOLOGY
MAMMOGRAM HISTORY

Tech: _____

KVP: _____ Density: _____

DAY TELEPHONE#: (   ) _____

PLEASE CHECK

YES	NO	Do you have any current breast complaints or problems?

Indicate below any scars, lumps, moles, and/or areas of concern:

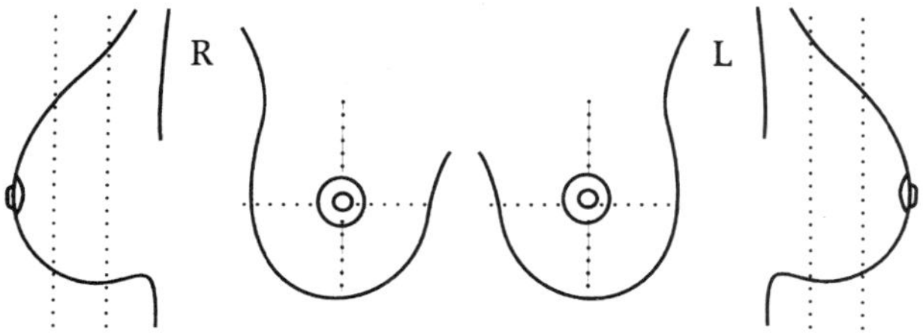

Right   Left

☐ Scars _____ _____
☐ Lump or Mass _____ _____
☐ Moles _____ _____
☐ Tissue Thickening _____ _____
☐ Skin Thickening or Retraction _____ _____
☐ Nipple Discharge _____ _____
☐ Nipple Inversion or Retraction _____ _____
☐ Pain _____ _____
☐ Other _____ _____ _____
☐ Comments _____ _____ _____

YES	NO	Have you had a mammogram before? Location: _____ Date: _____ If your last mammogram was NOT at Stanford, please complete a FILM RELEASE FORM
YES	NO	Have you had a breast *physical* examination by a health care professional? If yes when? _____ If you have *not* had a breast *physical* exam, *you should have one within a month* of this mammogram by your own health care professional to complete the evaluation of your breasts.
YES	NO	Do you have children? *Your* age at the birth of your first child _____
		Date of the beginning of your last period, or _____ Date of menopause, or _____ Date of your hysterectomy _____

DO YOU HAVE BREAST IMPLANTS?

YES _____   NO _____

YES	NO	Are you taking birth control or fertility drugs? If yes, began in 19 _____
YES	NO	Are you taking hormones (estrogen/Premarin)? If yes, began in 19 _____ IF YES, WHY? ☐ menopause ☐ heart condition ☐ osteoporosis ☐ prior hysterectomy ☐ other
YES	NO	Do you have rheumatoid arthritis?
YES	NO	Have you or anyone in your family ever had breast cancer? ☐ Don't know ☐ MYSELF at age _____ ☐ MOTHER at age _____ ☐ GRANDMOTHER at age _____ ☐ SISTER at age _____ ☐ AUNT at age _____ ☐ DAUGHTER at age _____
YES	NO	Have you had cancer? If yes, please describe what type: _____ Type of treatment: ☐ Radiation ☐ Chemotherapy ☐ Surgery
YES	NO	Have you ever had breast surgery? IF YES, SEE BELOW.

If you answered yes to the question above, please indicate date, reason for surgery, and type of surgery below:

	Right	Date and reason, benign or malignant	Left	Date and reason, benign or malignant
Surgical biopsy	Right	_____	Left	_____
Needle biopsy	Right	_____	Left	_____
Cyst aspiration	Right	_____	Left	_____
Lumpectomy	Right	_____	Left	_____
Mastectomy	Right	_____	Left	_____
Breast Implants	Right	_____	Left	_____
Breast Reduction	Right	_____	Left	_____

FIGURE 2-3   A, A breast history sheet includes a diagrammatic breast template and places to record the patient's history and current problems or complaints.

Continued

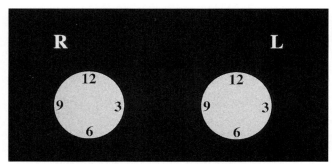

FIGURE 2-3 cont'd   B, Clock face description of breast lesion locations. The clock face location of breast findings is described by imaging a clock on both the left and the right breast as the woman faces the examiner. Note that the outer portion of the breast on the *right* is at the 9-o'clock position and the outer portion on the *left* is at the 3-o'clock position.

studies; and be composed of fibroglandular tissue rather than a three-dimensional mass. If the asymmetry is palpable, has suspicious calcification or spiculation, is new, or is a mass, the asymmetry may represent cancer and should prompt a work-up.

The next step is to look in the glandular tissue for masses, which are often whiter than the surrounding tissue or are detected because of a round or spiculated mass edge seen against fat. If a possible mass is seen on one projection, the radiologist looks for the finding on the orthogonal view by measuring the distance from the nipple to the finding and searching the orthogonal view for the finding at this distance (Fig. 2-4). If the finding is seen on two views, it is considered a mass. If it is seen on only one view, it is called a "density" and represents either a summation shadow (Fig. 2-4B and C) or a mass (Fig. 2-4D and E) that is obscured on the second view. The decision to recall this type of finding and prompt a work-up is based on the radiologist's experience and the degree of suspicion of the one-view finding.

The radiologist next looks at all normal glandular tissue edges where they interface with fat. These edges should be gently curving, scalloped, and without tethering. Masses at the glandular edge or in breast tissue may produce a "pulling in" or "tent sign" caused by productive fibrosis from cancer retracting the surrounding Cooper ligaments and ducts. In other cases, tumor spiculation produces straight lines extending into the glandular tissue that draw attention to a mass at the center of the radius (Fig. 2-4F and G). Detection of subtle equal-density cancers can be difficult, but looking for secondary signs of cancer such as straight lines in glandular tissue or tethering of the glandular edge guides the radiologist to the cancer. Similarly, the glandular tissue should not produce a concave border suggesting the edge of a mass.

Table 2-3   Systematic Approach to Interpretation of Mammograms

Search Pattern	Normal Findings
Overall Search	
Evaluation of technique	Good technique
Fibroglandular symmetry	Breast tissue usually symmetrical
	Asymmetric tissue in 3%—be alert for new, palpable, three-dimensional masses or suspicious calcifications
White areas in glandular tissue	No mass or distortion; white areas look like normal tissues not seen on the orthogonal view
Targeted Search	
Edge of glandular tissue	No "pulling in" or "tent" sign, no concave masses
Nipple/areolar complex	Nipple everted, no skin thickening
Retroareolar region	Normal ducts, vessels, nipple in profile on at least one view
Skin	2-3 mm in thickness, no edema
Axilla	Normal lymph nodes, normal variant axillary breast tissue
Retroglandular fat	All fat, no masses between glandular tissue and chest wall
Medial breast	Mostly fat, normal variant medial sternalis muscle
Film edge	No mass or spiculation from findings outside the field of view
Use magnifying lens or magnifier	No pleomorphic calcifications, subtle distortion, or masses
Use bright light (screen film)	Evaluate dark areas as needed; for FFDM, the window/level should have been adjusted in step 1
Compare with old films	No change; be alert for a developing density, new or changing calcifications or masses
CAD	Do a second look of the marked areas; CAD comes last because it does not pick up all cancers

CAD, computer-aided detection; FFDM, full-field digital mammogram.

The nipple is usually everted, and it should be seen in profile on at least one mammographic view. Such images allow for evaluation of both the nipple and the complex structures of ducts and vessels in the normal retroareolar region. If the nipple is not in profile on at least one view, the nipple may overlie the retroareolar region and prevent evaluation or detection of a mass. The nipple can be inverted at birth as a normal variant, as noted on the breast history sheet. New nipple inversion is of concern for a retroareolar tumor being the source of the inversion.

Normal breast skin is about 2 to 3 mm thick, and normal subcutaneous fat is dark. Skin thickening greater than 2 to 3 mm that is asymmetric with respect to the contralateral side is abnormal and should be investigated.

The axilla normally contains lymph nodes consisting of smooth oval or kidney bean–shaped masses containing

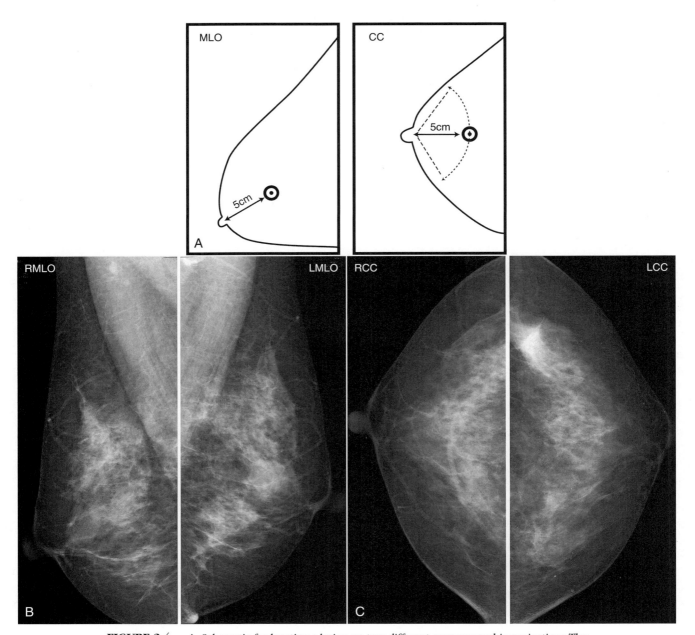

FIGURE 2-4   A, Schematic for locating a lesion on two different mammographic projections. The radiologist measures the distance from the finding to the nipple *(left image)* and then inspects the second view at the same distance from the nipple *(right image)* for the finding. **B** and **C,** Abnormal screening mammograms with a summation shadow on one view. Mediolateral (MLO) (**B**) and craniocaudal (CC) (**C**) screening mammograms show an asymmetric density in the outer left CC view. Review of the MLO view shows no mass of the same shape or density at the same distance from the nipple, thus suggesting a confluence of shadows because the asymmetry has no spiculations or calcifications, was not associated with a palpable finding, and did not appear to be a mass. Work-up showed that the density represented a summation shadow.

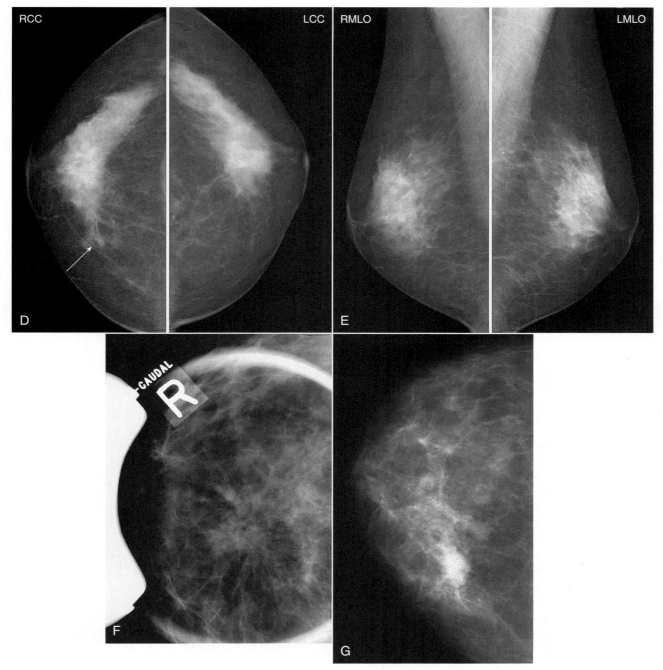

FIGURE 2-4 cont'd   **D** and **E,** Abnormal screening mammograms with cancer seen as an asymmetrical density on the CC view only. CC (**D**) and MLO views (**E**) show more breast tissue in the medial aspect of the right breast on the CC view *(arrow)* than in the medial aspect of the right breast *(arrow)*. Closer examination shows the density to have a slightly round shape and possible spiculations, unlike the asymmetric density in **A** and **B.** It is not seen on the MLO view. Follow-up examination confirmed the density to be a true mass and invasive ductal cancer. **F** and **G,** Use of the surrounding architecture to detect masses. A CC spot magnification view shows an equal-density spiculated mass (radial scar at biopsy) producing subtle distortion of the tissue with straightening of Cooper's ligaments (**F**). In another patient, a dense mass in the medial part of the breast has spiculated borders that are distorting the surrounding glandular tissue (**G**). Note that most of the glandular tissue remains in the outer portion of the breast and that medial breast densities are in a "danger zone."

fatty hila (Fig. 2-4H). Lymph nodes that grow larger, more dense, or round and lose their fatty hila represent lymphadenopathy (Fig. 2-4I).

Axillary breast tissue is a normal variant and consists of breast tissue in the axilla along the normal developmental nipple line that extends in animals from the axilla along the chest to the abdomen; it is rarely attached to an extra nipple. Noncompressed axillary breast tissue can simulate a mass, but it can be separated into its normal fibroglandular components by spot compression (Fig. 2-4J and K). Spiculated masses can also hide in the axilla behind the pectoralis muscle and mimic normal lymph nodes or axillary breast tissue, so the axilla should be scrutinized carefully in a systematic fashion (Fig. 2-4L-N).

A layer of fat typically surrounds the cone of normal fibroglandular tissue and should contain no masses. As part of the systematic review, the radiologist checks the fat all around the glandular tissue to make sure that no masses are present. A few locations in the breast usually contain fat and deserve both special mention and a second look. The medial portion of the breast becomes more fatty over time, and most of the residual glandular tissue remains in the upper outer quadrant. Masses or densities in the medial part of the breast are in a "danger zone" and should be scrutinized carefully because asymmetric or isolated residual normal glandular tissue in the medial aspect of the breast is unusual. Retroglandular fat, or fat between the cone of normal fibroglandular tissue and the chest wall, is another "danger zone" because it should include only fatty tissue and no masses, except for the medial sternalis muscle on the craniocaudal view. A film edge in which fat extends to the boundary of the field of view is another "danger zone." Here, the hint of a mass edge or spiculations may indicate a tumor not imaged on the mammogram that requires special mammographic views to display the cancer.

After the mammogram has been evaluated in this systematic fashion, the radiologist looks for pleomorphic calcifications with a magnifying lens for screen-film studies or a magnifier for FFDMs. Radiologists look at screen-film mammograms with the magnifying lens until they detect dust, which ensures that the film has been scrutinized enough to detect the tiny calcifications that form in breast cancer. For screen-film mammography, a hot light can be used to illuminate dark portions of the film edge or the skin as needed at this point. For FFDMs, the images are viewed at a proper window and level for detection of calcification, and the radiologist views all portions of the images under magnification.

During interpretation the radiologist compares abnormalities on the mammogram with findings on the breast history sheet. The current mammogram is then compared with older films of the same quality for detection of developing densities or new or progressive changes.

Finally, the radiologist uses computer-aided detection if available and re-evaluates findings marked on the mammograms by the computer algorithm.

By law, all mammograms are given a summary BI-RADS code to indicate the final assessment of the study, and the words must be spelled out in the report. Assessments include "0—Assessment incomplete, needs additional imaging evaluation;" "1—Negative;" "2—Benign;" "3—Probably benign;" "4—Suspicious;" "5—Highly suggestive of malignancy;" and "6—Known cancer" (Box 2-5).

The first category "0" is used for screening recalls or when more studies are needed at the end of a case to make a final assessment. Categories 1 and 2 are used for normal mammograms or findings requiring no action. Category 3 is used for findings thought to have a less than a 2% chance of malignancy and for which a short-term 6-month follow-up may be implemented, with the expectation that the finding will be stable. Specifically, this category is often used for smooth noncalcified benign-appearing masses, benign-appearing clustered punctate calcifications, or benign-appearing focal densities in appropriate clinical settings. Category 4 encompasses a wide variety of findings for which biopsy is recommended. Category 4 can be further subcategorized into 4A, 4B, and 4C for lesions that require biopsy but with a low, intermediate, or moderate suspicion for cancer, respectively. Category 5 is reserved for mammographic findings highly suggestive of cancer, with a greater than 95% likelihood of cancer. Category 6 is intended for cancers for which a known diagnosis has been established before definite therapy such as surgery or chemotherapy. For example, women with large breast cancers diagnosed by percutaneous core biopsy who will be undergoing subsequent neoadjuvant chemotherapy are probable candidates for Category 6.

DIAGNOSTIC VERSUS SCREENING MAMMOGRAPHY

Diagnostic mammography is used for symptomatic women or women with findings detected on screening mammography (Table 2-4). Additional mammographic views are used in diagnostic studies to confirm or exclude the presence of a true lesion suspected on screening, to characterize real lesions, and to triangulate a finding's location in the breast. In contradistinction, screening mammography is performed on asymptomatic women. In the United States, screening includes two views of each breast—craniocaudal and mediolateral oblique projections. Ten percent to 15% of all cancers may not be detected by screening mammography, and some palpable

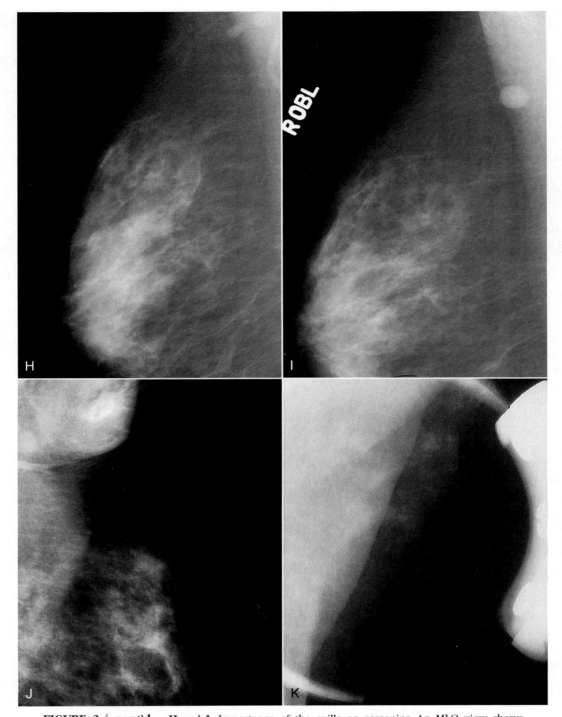

FIGURE 2-4 cont'd **H** and **I,** Importance of the axilla on screening. An MLO view shows heterogeneously dense tissue and normal axillary lymph nodes seen as two oval equal-density masses projected on the pectoralis muscle high in the axilla (**H**). The following year one of the lymph nodes was rounder and more dense and did not have any fatty hilum (**I**), findings characteristic of lymphadenopathy in lymphoma. If the axilla had not been reviewed, this finding would have been missed. **J** and **K,** Normal axillary breast tissue. A left screening MLO view shows a density high in the axilla over the pectoralis muscle, possibly representing a mass versus normal axillary breast tissue (**J**). A spot compression film shows that the density represents normal axillary breast tissue because the density does not persist in the same dense shape and pattern seen on the original screening study (**K**).

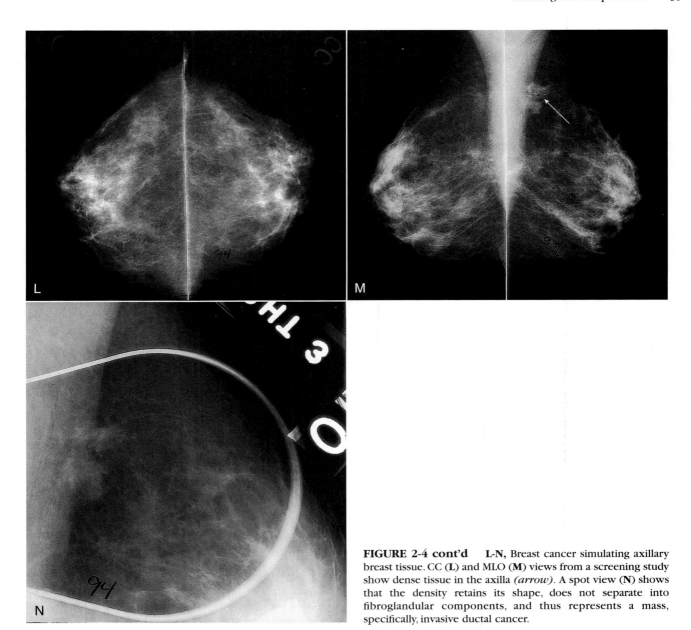

FIGURE 2-4 cont'd   L-N, Breast cancer simulating axillary breast tissue. CC (**L**) and MLO (**M**) views from a screening study show dense tissue in the axilla *(arrow)*. A spot view (**N**) shows that the density retains its shape, does not separate into fibroglandular components, and thus represents a mass, specifically, invasive ductal cancer.

Box 2-5   BI-RADS Code Assessment Categories

0—Assessment incomplete, need additional imaging evaluation and/or previous mammograms for comparison
1—Negative
2—Benign finding(s)
3—Probably benign, but initial short-interval follow-up suggested*
4—Suspicious
5—Highly suggestive of malignancy
6—Known cancer

*Noncalcified circumscribed mass, focal asymmetry, and clustered punctate calcifications in the appropriate clinical setting.
From American College of Radiology: ACR BI-RADS—Mammography, 4th ed. *In* ACR Breast Imaging Reporting and Data System, Breast Imaging Atlas. Reston, VA, American College of Radiology, 2003.

Table 2-4   Screening versus Diagnostic Studies

Screening	Asymptomatic women
	CC and MLO mammograms
Diagnostic	Symptomatic women or mammographic finding
	CC and MLO mammograms
	Additional mammograms tailored to the problem
	With or without breast ultrasound

CC, craniocaudal; MLO, mediolateral oblique.

cancers may be revealed by tangential views, spot views, or ultrasound. Therefore, in women with lumps or problems, diagnostic mammography targeted to their specific problems is performed rather than screening studies.

ADDITIONAL VIEWS TO CONFIRM OR EXCLUDE THE PRESENCE OF A TRUE LESION

Additional mammographic views are used in three common scenarios: to confirm or exclude a real lesion, to localize or triangulate a true lesion, or to characterize a true lesion (Box 2-6). A very common reason for obtaining a diagnostic mammogram is to evaluate a possible finding seen on only one view at screening mammography. Specifically, the radiologist may detect a finding on one view and not see the finding on the orthogonal view. Additional fine-detail mammograms tailored to this problem help determine whether the finding is real. The first step is to estimate the finding's location on the orthogonal view by measuring the distance from the nipple to the finding. The breast tissue is scrutinized along a radius of the same distance on the orthogonal view to identify the finding (see Fig. 2-4A). If it is seen on the second view, the finding is a true finding and additional views are used to characterize the lesion. If the finding is not seen on the second view, the finding may represent a true finding hidden on the second view, or it may represent a fortuitous summation of normal breast elements.

Box 2-6   Use of Additional Mammographic Views

Confirm or exclude the presence of a real lesion
Characterize a true lesion
Triangulate or localize a true lesion

Box 2-7   Views Used to Confirm or Exclude a Lesion (Commonly a One-View-Only Finding)

Lateral view
Spot compression
Spot compression magnification
Rolled views
Repeat the same view

Table 2-5   Mammographic Views Used to Visualize and Characterize Findings

Mammographic Problem	Mammographic View
True finding versus summation	Rolled views, spot view, step oblique views
Triangulation	Line up CC, MLO, and LM views and draw an imaginary line through the lesion. Use rolled views to determine whether the mass is upper or lower
Outer breast finding	XCCL, Cleopatra
Inner breast finding	XCCM, cleavage view, spot view
Upper breast finding	Compression from below (or caudal-cranial view), upper-breast-only view
Retroareolar finding	Spot compression with the nipple in profile
Lower inner finding	Superior-inferior oblique
Palpable finding	Spot compression over the mass or a tangential view
Characterization of a mass or calcification	Magnification, spot magnification views

CC, craniocaudal; LM, lateral-medial; MLO, mediolateral oblique; XCCL, laterally exaggerated craniocaudal; XCCM, medially exaggerated craniocaudal.

A variety of fine-detail mammographic views may be used to determine whether a one-view finding is a true lesion or a summation shadow (Box 2-7, Table 2-5).

Rolled views may separate normal fibroglandular elements into their individual components (Table 2-6). These views are performed by "rolling" the breast tissue and compressing the breast in the same projection in which the finding was first discovered. For example, to evaluate a finding on the craniocaudal view, the technologist would roll the top of the breast toward the axilla and the bottom of the breast toward the sternum and compress the breast the same as though it were for the craniocaudal view (Fig. 2-5A). On the rolled view a

Table 2-6 Mammographic Views and Abbreviations Used to Describe Them	
View	**Abbreviation**
Craniocaudal	CC
Mediolateral oblique	MLO
Medial-lateral	ML
Lateral-medial	LM
Laterally exaggerated craniocaudal	XCCL
Medially exaggerated craniocaudal	XCCM
Cleavage view	CV
Rolled view laterally	RL
Rolled view medially	RM
From below	FB

From 1999 ACR Mammography Quality Control Manual. American College of Radiology, Reston, VA.

summation shadow should be separated into its normal fibroglandular components (Fig. 2-5B-G). Unlike summation shadows, true masses will retain their shape and size and persist on the spot view or rolled view. Some facilities combine all three techniques into a spot compression–rolled view.

Spot compression involves the use of a small compression paddle directed over the finding to provide greater compression on the area of interest. A small spot paddle with or without magnification produces greater compression over the area of interest, and if applied to the view on which the finding was first detected, it may separate summation shadows into the normal fibroglandular components creating the shadow (Figs. 2-6 and 2-7). It is important to perform the spot view in the projection in which the finding is best seen or displayed against fat to increase the likelihood of showing that the finding is a true lesion (Fig. 2-8). On a spot view a true mass will retain its shape, size, and density, whereas a summation shadow will disperse into its fibroglandular components.

Another technique is the use of step oblique views, which produce slightly oblique studies (60, 50, 45 degrees, etc.) to confirm or exclude a lesion, similar to rolled views. True lesions should persist on multiple step oblique views and be distinguished from summation shadows, which separate into their fibroglandular components.

In all cases in which a mass is suspected, ultrasound may be helpful to confirm the presence of a mass when directed to areas suggested on the mammogram. Repeat mammograms with a marker over the ultrasound-detected mass may then display mammographic findings not previously suspected.

TRIANGULATION

Triangulation, or localizing a finding within the breast on two orthogonal views, is important to provide a clear three-dimensional position of a finding for subsequent imaging or biopsy. Triangulation is a common problem when a finding is seen on only two of the three standard mammographic views (craniocaudal, mediolateral, and lateral views). For example, a finding might be seen on a lateral view and a mediolateral oblique mammogram but not seen on a craniocaudal mammogram. Similarly, work-up for preoperative needle localization often involves a finding seen on screening craniocaudal and mediolateral oblique views but not on the lateral view. To predict a finding's location, place the craniocaudal and mediolateral oblique views so that the breast faces the same direction and the nipple is at the same level. If craniocaudal, mediolateral oblique, and mediolateral views are available, place the mediolateral oblique between the craniocaudal and mediolateral views, with the nipple at the same level on each view (Figs. 2-9 to 2-11). An imaginary line drawn through the lesion on the craniocaudal and mediolateral oblique views will predict the lesion's location on the mediolateral view.

Sometimes suspicious findings are thought to be true findings but are seen *only* on the craniocaudal view and not on the mediolateral or mediolateral oblique views. Rolled craniocaudal views can provide information regarding the location of true masses in either the upper or lower part of the breast by comparing the rolled view with the standard craniocaudal view. The "rolled laterally" view is performed by rolling the top of the breast toward the axilla and the bottom of the breast medially. If the mass moves toward the axilla on the "rolled laterally" view when compared with the standard craniocaudal mammogram, the mass must be in the upper portion of the breast. If the mass moves medially on the "rolled laterally" view when compared with the standard craniocaudal mammogram, the mass must be in the lower portion of the breast (Figs. 2-12 and 2-13).

VISUALIZING FINDINGS IN SPECIFIC EXPECTED LOCATIONS

The following section details standard mammographic projections modified to visualize findings in specific locations. It is not uncommon to identify a suspicious lesion on one view and not be able to see it on the orthogonal projection because of the patient's body configuration or the location of the finding. Some lesions have an expected location in the outer part of the breast as predicted by triangulation from the mediolateral oblique and mediolateral views but are not seen on

Text continued on p. 47

ROLLED VIEW SUMMATION SHADOW

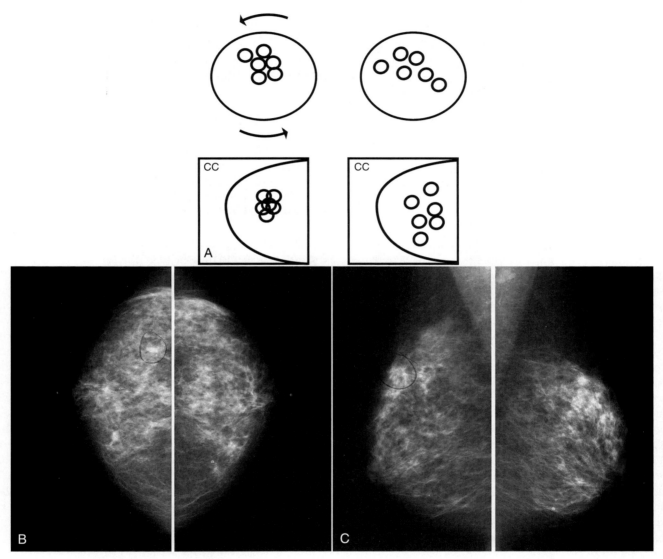

FIGURE 2-5 **A,** Schematic of a rolled view separating summation shadows into their fibroglandular components. The initial craniocaudal view on the *lower left* shows a "mass" composed of overlapping glandular tissue. The rolled view on the *lower right* shows the fibroglandular components separated into normal structures. In contradistinction, a mass should retain the same shape, form, and density as seen on the original mammogram. (Modified from Sickles EA: Practical solutions to common mammographic problems: Tailoring the examination. AJR Am J Roentgenol 151: 31-39, 1988.) **B-G,** Rolled views. Craniocaudal (**B**) and mediolateral oblique (**C**) screening mammograms show a possible mass in the outer portion of the right breast.

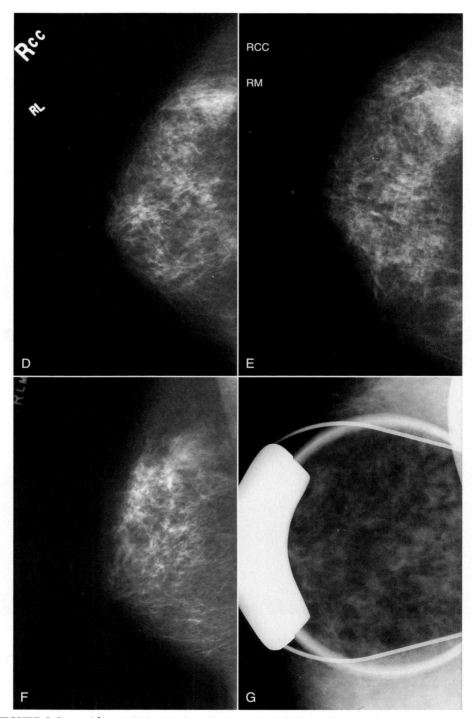

FIGURE 2-5 cont'd   Rolled views laterally (**D**) and medially (**E**) show no focal density. Because no mass is seen on the lateral view (**F**) or on the double spot compression view (**G**), this possible mass actually represents overlapping tissue.

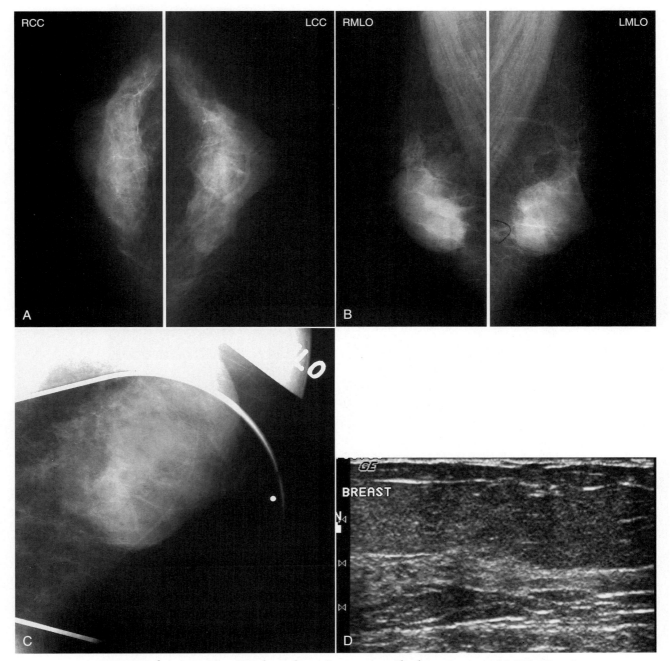

FIGURE 2-6   Spot View Work-up for a Summation Shadow. Craniocaudal (CC) **(A)** and mediolateral oblique (MLO) **(B)** screening mammograms show a possible mass in the lower part of the left breast on the MLO view near the chest wall that is not seen on the CC view *(circle)*. A spot compression film **(C)** shows no mass. Ultrasound in this region shows fatty and scant fibroglandular tissue **(D)**.

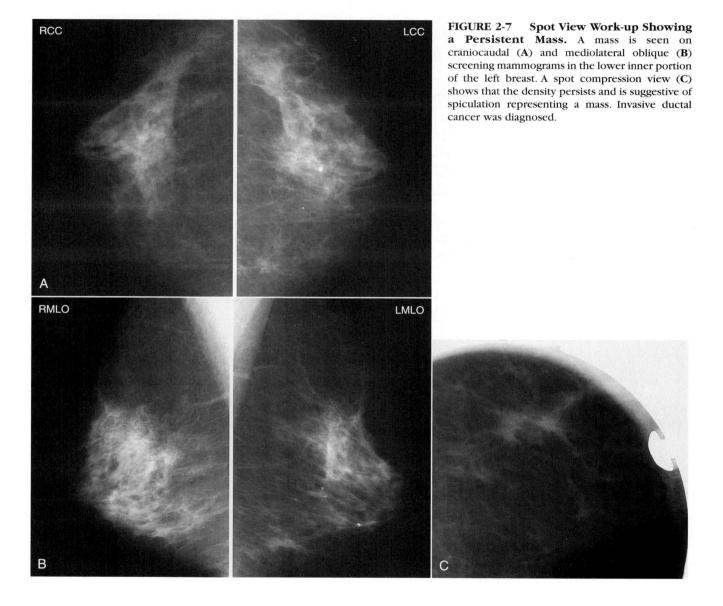

FIGURE 2-7   Spot View Work-up Showing a Persistent Mass. A mass is seen on craniocaudal (**A**) and mediolateral oblique (**B**) screening mammograms in the lower inner portion of the left breast. A spot compression view (**C**) shows that the density persists and is suggestive of spiculation representing a mass. Invasive ductal cancer was diagnosed.

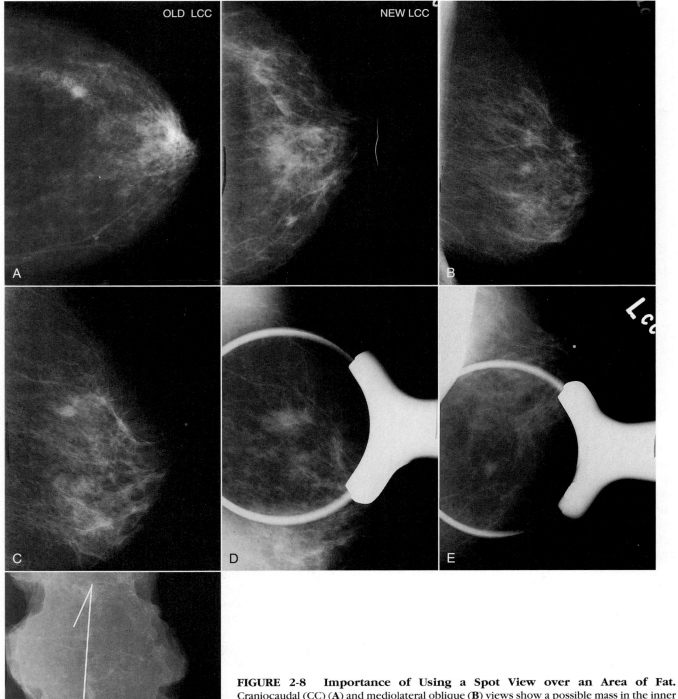

FIGURE 2-8 Importance of Using a Spot View over an Area of Fat.
Craniocaudal (CC) (**A**) and mediolateral oblique (**B**) views show a possible mass in the inner portion of the breast only on the CC view that was new from the previous year. It is seen in the upper part of the breast on the lateral view (**C**). A spot compression film in the lateral-medial view is taken over glandular tissue but (**D**) shows no mass. When the spot view is repeated over the fatty area on the CC view, it shows a spiculated mass against the dark fat that was hidden against the glandular tissue on the mediolateral spot view (**E**). The specimen shows the mass, which was invasive ductal cancer (**F**).

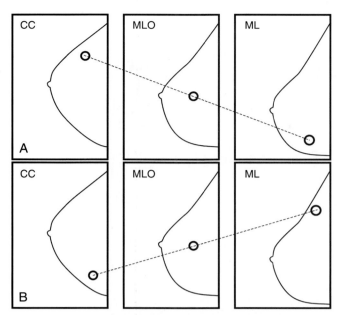

FIGURE 2-9   **A** and **B,** Schematic of how to triangulate findings on the craniocaudal (CC), mediolateral oblique (MLO), and lateral-medial (LM) views. Each view area is oriented with the nipples at the same level and the breasts pointing the same way. An *imaginary line* drawn through the lesions will predict its location on the third view. (Modified from Sickles EA: Practical solutions to common mammographic problems: Tailoring the examination. AJR Am J Roentgenol 151:31-39, 1988.)

the standard craniocaudal view. Craniocaudal views exaggerated laterally (abbreviated XCCL) are obtained by rotating the patient's body to display the outer breast tissue better than possible with a standard craniocaudal view. Specifically, the XCCL view is a modification of the craniocaudal projection that includes the outer tissue while excluding the medial portion of the breast (Fig. 2-14). This projection allows visualization of more of the outer breast tissue than seen on the standard craniocaudal view (Fig. 2-15). A modification of the XCCL view to include more outer breast tissue is the "Cleopatra" view, in which the patient rotates laterally as in the XCCL view, but also leans obliquely like Cleopatra reclining on a bed of pillows (Fig. 2-15E). The Cleopatra view also includes much of the outer part of the breast while excluding inner breast tissue, but it is slightly oblique, unlike the XCCL view, in which the patient stands upright and orthogonal to a lateral-medial projection.

For inner breast lesions, craniocaudal views exaggerated medially (abbreviated XCCM) image the medial portion of the breast while excluding the outer breast tissue (Fig. 2-16A and B). The inner portion of the breast may also be seen on cleavage views, which include the medial portions

of both breasts on the image receptor in a modified craniocaudal projection. Such views allow visualization of even more of the inner part of the breast than seen on standard craniocaudal views. When the XCCM or cleavage view fails to display an inner breast lesion, spot compression paddles can get closer to the chest wall to image extremely inner or deep lesions by compressing tissue near the chest wall that is excluded by standard compression paddles.

Some lesions in the upper part of the breast are difficult to visualize on the craniocaudal view because they are excluded from the field of view by the compression paddle (Fig. 2-17). This problem can be solved by using a view in which the image receptor is placed on the midportion of the breast with the lower portion excluded, as described by Sickles et al. This modified view incorporates more of the upper portion of the breast because the compression paddle effectively includes more upper breast tissue in the field of view. Another approach for imaging lesions high on the chest wall is to perform a caudal-cranial view. For this view, the image receptor is placed on the upper part of the breast. The breast is then compressed from below, called the "from-below view," to exclude the lower part of the breast but include tissue high on the chest wall.

Lesions behind the nipple can be hidden by adjacent blood vessels and ducts. Spot compression can help identify lesions in the retroareolar region by compressing normal ducts, blood vessels, and tissue away while pulling the nipple into profile (Fig. 2-18A and B). The nipple should be in profile on at least one view to see the retroareolar region; otherwise, the nipple may obscure this region.

Lesions in the lower inner part of the breast are especially problematic, but they can occasionally be seen with a superior-inferior oblique or "reverse oblique" view in which the imaging receptor is placed on the medial part of the breast, the compression plate is placed superior to the breast, and the patient leans medially (Fig. 2-19A and B). The compression paddle approaches the breast from the superior axillary side to allow more of the inner breast tissue to be visualized.

Palpable findings not seen on the mammogram constitute a special category of findings because 10% to 15% of breast cancers are mammographically occult. If the palpable mass is near the periphery of the breast, a spot compression view tangential to the palpable finding may push the mass against subcutaneous tissue and allow it to be seen. Alternatively, spot compression directly over the palpable mass, previously known as a "lumpogram," may show a mass by compressing the surrounding glandular tissue away from the suspicious finding (Fig. 2-20).

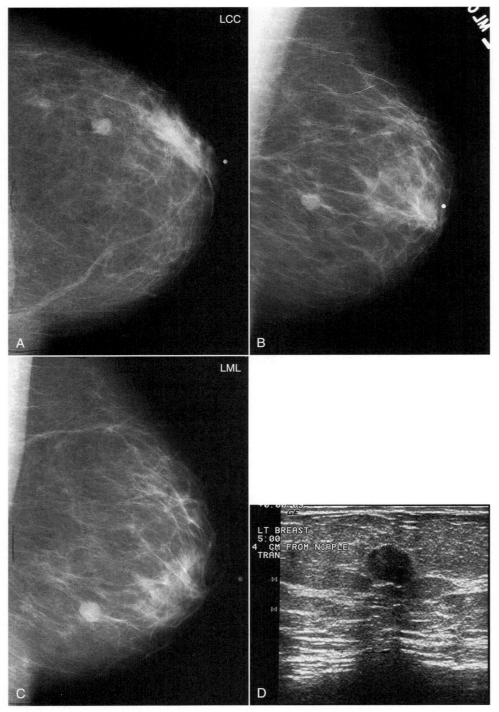

FIGURE 2-10   Triangulation of an Outer Breast Mass to Its Location on the Lateral View. A mass in the outer portion of the left breast on the craniocaudal view (**A**) is lower on the mediolateral oblique (MLO) view (**B**). Putting these two images together and drawing an imaginary line through the masses predicts an even lower position of the mass on the lateral view (**C**). Note that even though the mass is at nipple level on the MLO view, its actual location on the lateral view is at the 5-o'clock position, not the 3-o'clock position. Ultrasound shows a round microlobulated mass in the lower outer portion of the breast (**D**) that was diagnosed as invasive ductal cancer.

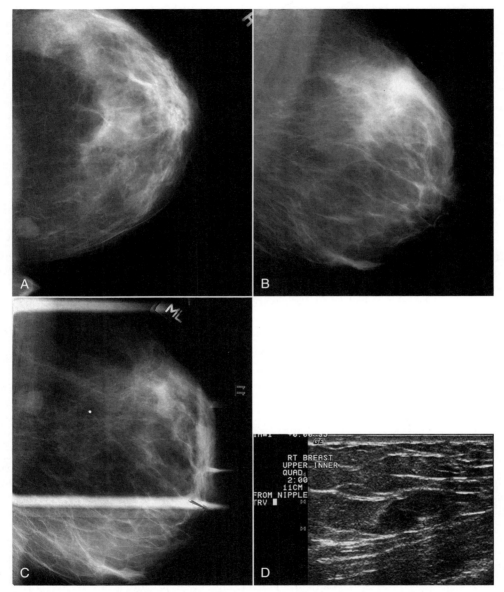

FIGURE 2-11   Triangulation of an Inner Breast Mass to Its Location on the Lateral View. A craniocaudal view (**A**) shows a mass in the inner portion of the breast that was not seen on the mediolateral oblique (**B**) or mediolateral views (not shown); therefore, the mass could be in the upper or lower part of the breast. Without a second view to guide additional views, more tissue close to the chest wall was visualized in the lateral-medial projection by using a smaller compression paddle that can compress closer to the pectoralis muscle and reveal the mass (**C**). Ultrasound could now be directed to the upper inner part of the left breast and showed a slightly hypoechoic, lobulated, oval smooth mass (**D**) that was diagnosed as fibroadenoma after biopsy.

ROLLED VIEW REAL LESION

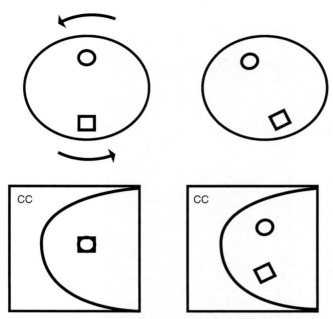

FIGURE 2-12 Schematic showing a rolled craniocaudal (CC) view predicting whether a lesion is in the upper or lower part of the breast. The initial CC view on the *left* superimposes two lesions on each other. When the top of the breast is rolled laterally, the superior lesion rolls with the top of the breast. The inferior lesion moves medially with the lower part of the breast. Comparing whether the lesion moves laterally on the rolled view with respect to the standard view will help predict whether the lesion is in the upper or lower part of the breast. (Modified from Sickles EA: Practical solutions to common mammographic problems: Tailoring the examination. AJR Am J Roentgenol 151:31-39, 1988.)

ADDITIONAL VIEWS TO CHARACTERIZE TRUE FINDINGS

Once a true mass or cluster of calcifications is determined to represent a true finding and has been triangulated within the breast, other views help characterize the finding (Box 2-8). Micro–focal spot magnification views of clustered calcifications may depict calcifications not detected on the initial screening study and the shapes and distribution of the calcifications. Magnification can also better evaluate the shape and borders of breast masses detected at screening by showing spiculated or irregular margins not discernible at lower resolution (Fig. 2-21). Spot compression magnification views provide not only greater visualization of the region of interest by pushing fibroglandular tissue away from the finding but also higher resolution of mass borders and margins or clustered calcifications.

SUMMARY

Evaluation of patients by mammography requires knowledge of breast cancer risk factors, the signs and symptoms of breast cancer, and a systematic approach to the mammogram to avoid diagnostic mistakes. The approach to the mammogram should include a standard review of normal mammographic structures and re-review of mammographic "danger zones" in which cancers are commonly missed. Once a finding is discovered, the radiologist has three duties: determine whether the finding is real, specify its location within the breast, and characterize its imaging findings to make a diagnosis. Additional modifications of standard views and fine-detail mammograms help the radiologist make these determinations.

KEY ELEMENTS

Breast cancer screening in women invited to undergo mammography decreases breast cancer mortality by about 30%.

Risk factors for breast cancer include age older than 50 years, personal history of or first-degree relative with breast cancer, nulliparous status, early menarche, late menopause, first birth after 30 years of age, radiation treatment, atypical ductal hyperplasia, lobular carcinoma in situ, and *BRCA1* or *BRCA2* breast cancer susceptibility genes.

Seventy percent of women who have breast cancer have no risk factors other than being female and older.

Signs and symptoms of breast cancer include a breast lump, bloody or new spontaneous nipple discharge, new nipple or skin retraction, *peau d'orange,* and symptoms from metastasis.

Signs of breast cancer on mammography include a spiculated mass, pleomorphic calcifications, a round mass, architectural distortion, a developing density, an asymmetric density, a single dilated duct, lymphadenopathy, breast edema, and no mammographic signs (occult cancer).

A normal mammogram is dense in young women and becomes replaced by fatty involution over time.

Increasing breast density is due to pregnancy or hormone replacement therapy; unexplained increasing breast density should prompt a work-up to determine its etiology and exclude breast edema or cancer.

Evaluation of a normal mammogram includes routine inspection for fibroglandular symmetry and examination of the periglandular edges, skin, retroareolar region and nipple, retroglandular fat, medial part of the breast, chest wall, and axilla.

Asymmetric glandular tissue occurs in 3% of women and is manifested as an asymmetry in normal glandular tissue without a palpable mass, suspicious calcifications or spiculations, a three-dimensional mass, or new findings.

Text continued on p. 58

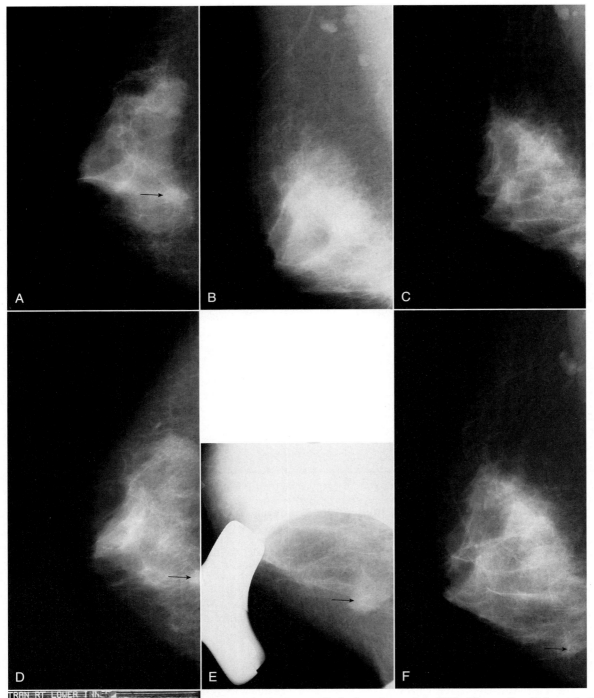

FIGURE 2-13   Rolled Craniocaudal (CC) Views for Triangulation. CC (**A**) and mediolateral oblique (MLO) (**B**) views show a density in the posterior medial aspect of the breast *(arrow)* that was not seen on the MLO view at the time of interpretation. In retrospect, spiculation is seen extending into the lower part of the breast from outside the field of view at the edge of the film. The lateral-medial (LM) view (**C**) does not show a definite mass at the time of interpretation. A CC view with the top of the breast rolled laterally (**D**) shows that the mass is medial in comparison to that seen on the original CC view *(arrow)*, thus indicating that it rolled medially with the lower part of the breast. Spot compression in the lower portion of the breast reveals a spiculated mass *(arrow)* (**E**), and a repeat LM view with more tissue (**F**) now shows the mass in the lower part of the breast as a rounded structure *(arrow)*. Ultrasound directed to the lower portion of the breast shows a hypoechoic irregular mass (**G**) that was diagnosed as invasive ductal cancer.

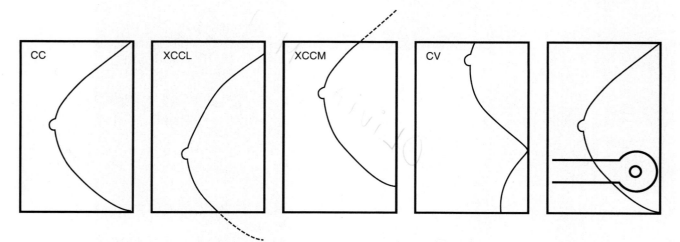

FIGURE 2-14   Schematic of Variations of the Craniocaudal (CC) View to Visualize Lesions in Specific Locations. The craniocaudal view exaggerated laterally (XCCL) includes outer breast tissue but excludes medial breast tissue. The XCCM view includes medial breast tissue while excluding outer breast tissue. The cleavage view (CV) includes the medial portions of both breasts on the mammogram. Spot compression may visualize findings close to the chest wall that are excluded by a larger compression paddle.

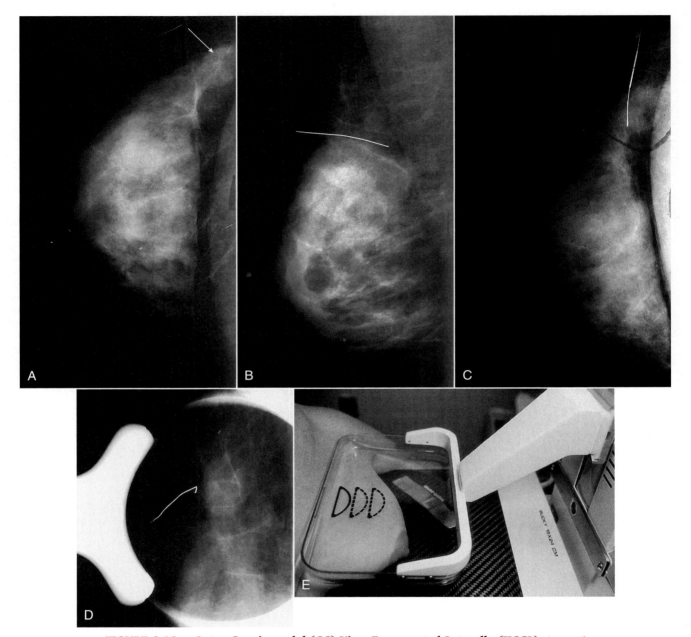

FIGURE 2-15   Outer Craniocaudal (CC) View Exaggerated Laterally (XCCL). A round density suggestive of a mass in the outer portion of the left breast is seen on the CC view under the scar marker *(arrow)* (**A**) but not seen on the mediolateral oblique view (**B**). An XCCL view shows the mass better (**C**), and it is also shown on a spot magnification view (**D**). **E,** Cleopatra view. For this view the patient leans outward and back, essentially performing an XCCL view with a degree of obliquity to image more outer tissue.

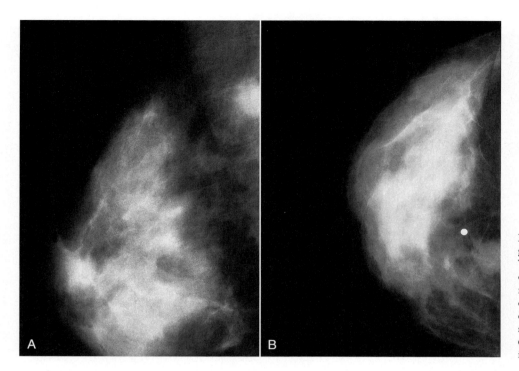

FIGURE 2-16   Medially Exaggerated Inner Craniocaudal View (XCCM). A mediolateral oblique view shows a round mass near the high chest wall that is excluded on the standard craniocaudal view (**A**). An XCCM view shows the round inner breast mass (**B**), which was diagnosed as invasive ductal cancer.

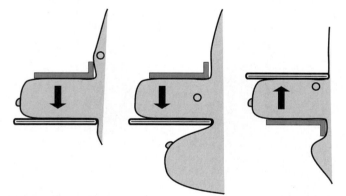

FIGURE 2-17   Methods to Visualize High Breast Lesions. The compression paddle may exclude high breast masses by compressing them out of the field of view *(left image)*. The *middle image* shows a view with the cassette holder above the nipple to allow compression of only the upper breast tissue. The *right image* shows a "from below" view where the image receptor is placed over the upper part of the breast and the compression paddle approaches the receptor from the lower part of the breast. (Modified from Sickles EA: Practical solutions to common mammographic problems: Tailoring the examination. AJR Am J Roentgenol 151:31-39, 1988.)

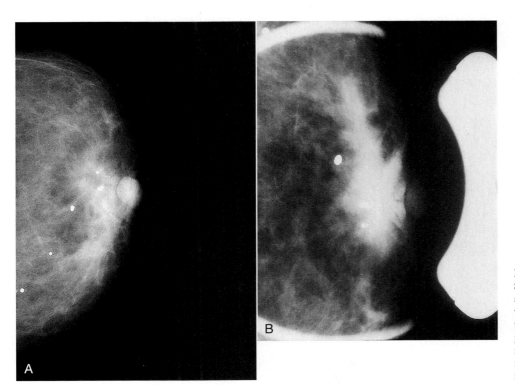

FIGURE 2-18 Spot View Showing a Mass in the Retroareolar Region. A craniocaudal view shows a vague density behind the nipple, but the nipple is not in profile (**A**). A spot view with the nipple in profile shows a spiculated mass (**B**) that was diagnosed as invasive lobular cancer.

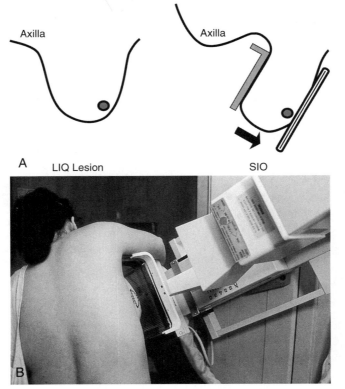

FIGURE 2-19 Superior-Inferior Oblique (SIO) View. A, A schematic shows a lower inner quadrant (LIQ) lesion in the *left image.* The SIO view is obtained with the image receptor next to the inner breast lesion and the compression plate compressing from the superior axillary side. **B,** Model demonstrating positioning for the SIO view.

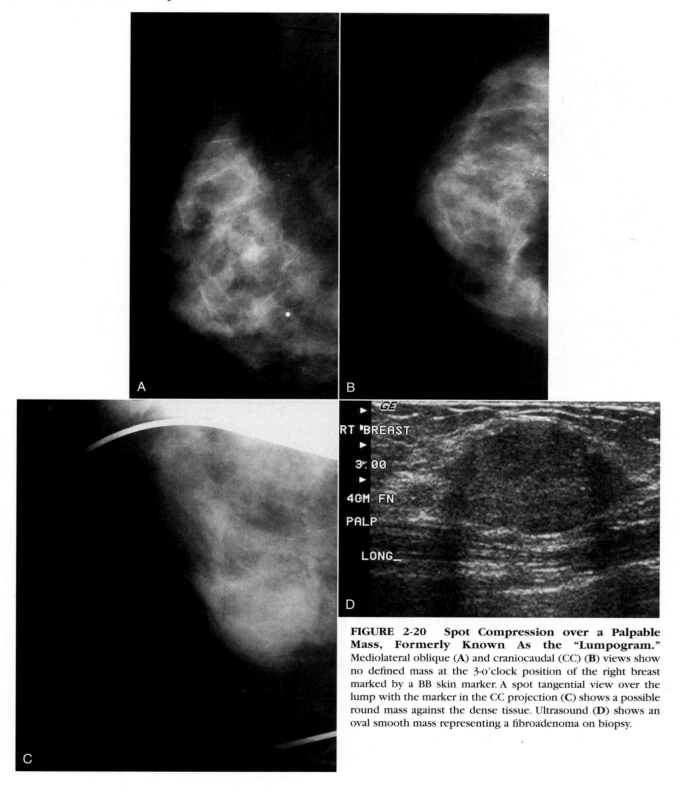

FIGURE 2-20   Spot Compression over a Palpable Mass, Formerly Known As the "Lumpogram." Mediolateral oblique (**A**) and craniocaudal (CC) (**B**) views show no defined mass at the 3-o'clock position of the right breast marked by a BB skin marker. A spot tangential view over the lump with the marker in the CC projection (**C**) shows a possible round mass against the dense tissue. Ultrasound (**D**) shows an oval smooth mass representing a fibroadenoma on biopsy.

Box 2-8   Views to Characterize a True Lesion
Magnification Spot compression magnification

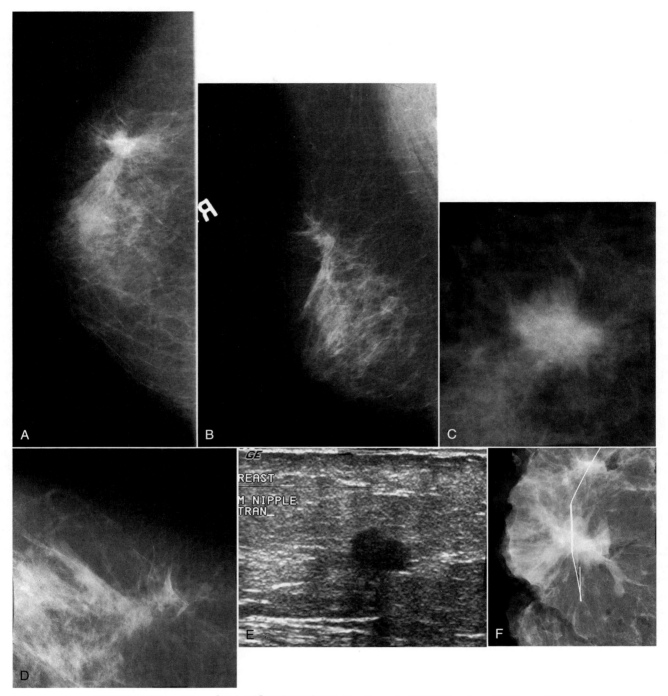

FIGURE 2-21   Use of Magnification Views. Craniocaudal (CC) (**A**) and mediolateral oblique (MLO) (**B**) mammograms show a spiculated mass seen better on the CC view than the MLO view. Distortion and the "tent" sign are evident in the upper part of the breast. Spot magnification views show the spiculated mass to better advantage on both the CC (**C**) and MLO (**D**) views. Ultrasound shows an oval, but very hypoechoic mass that has no acoustic spiculation or shadowing (**E**) corresponding to the mass on the mammogram. The mass was localized by ultrasound and was removed as shown by the specimen (**F**). Invasive ductal cancer was the diagnosis.

Be alert for findings in the medial part of the breast; the normal sternalis muscle variant is the one exception.

To detect developing densities, change, or asymmetries, view films back to back and compare them with old films.

Review both the breast history and the technologist's physical sheet before interpretation of the mammogram to identify previous biopsies, the meaning of skin markers, and patient complaints.

Ten percent to 15% of women with breast cancer have normal mammograms.

The skin should normally be 2 to 3 mm thick.

Diagnostic mammograms are used to confirm or exclude questionable findings seen on screening mammography, characterize true lesions, and triangulate the location of a lesion.

Rolled views, compression views, and step oblique views are used to distinguish true lesions from summation shadows.

Magnification spot compression views characterize mass, margins, and shape.

Magnification views are used to evaluate the shape and number of calcifications.

Laterally exaggerated craniocaudal and Cleopatra views are used to view the outer part of the breast.

Medially exaggerated craniocaudal and cleavage views are used to view the inner portion of the breast.

"From-below" and upper breast views are used to view the upper part of the breast.

Spot compression and nipple-in-profile images are used to view the nipple and retroareolar region.

The lower inner portion of the breast is best imaged by the superior-inferior oblique view (reverse oblique).

The breast location most often excluded by screening mammograms is the upper inner quadrant.

Lesions displayed at the nipple level on the mediolateral oblique view may be in the upper, lower, or midportion of the breast on the mediolateral view.

Triangulation with the craniocaudal and mediolateral oblique views can be used to predict the location of the lesion on the lateral view.

Magnification or spot magnification views can be used to further characterize breast calcifications or mass shapes and margins.

SUGGESTED READINGS

16-year mortality from breast cancer in the UK Trial of Early Detection of Breast Cancer. Lancet 353:1909-1914, 1999.

Alexander FE, Anderson TJ, Brown HK, et al: 14 years of follow-up from the Edinburgh randomised trial of breast-cancer screening. Lancet 353:1903-1908, 1999.

American College of Radiology: ACR BI-RADS—Mammography, 4th ed. *In* ACR Breast Imaging Reporting and Data System, Breast Imaging Atlas. Reston, VA, American College of Radiology, 2003.

Andersson I, Janzon L: Reduced breast cancer mortality in women under age 50: Updated results from the Malmö Mammographic Screening Program. J Natl Cancer Inst Monogr 22:63-67, 1997.

Beyer T, Moonka R: Normal mammography and ultrasonography in the setting of palpable breast cancer. Am J Surg 185:416-419, 2003.

Birdwell RL, Ikeda DM, O'Shaughnessy KF, Sickles EA: Mammographic characteristics of 115 missed cancers later detected with screening mammography and the potential utility of computer-aided detection. Radiology 219:192-202, 2001.

Bjurstam N, Bjorneld L, Duffy SW, et al: The Gothenburg breast screening trial: First results on mortality, incidence, and mode of detection for women ages 39-49 years at randomization. Cancer 80:2091-2099, 1997.

Bradley FM, Hoover HC Jr, Hulka CA, et al: The sternalis muscle: An unusual normal finding seen on mammography. AJR Am J Roentgenol 166:33-36, 1996.

Brenner RJ, Sickles EA: Acceptability of periodic follow-up as an alternative to biopsy for mammographically detected lesions interpreted as probably benign. Radiology 171:645-646, 1989.

Claus EB, Risch N, Thompson WD: Genetic analysis of breast cancer in the cancer and steroid hormone study. Am J Hum Genet 48:232-242, 1991.

Claus EB, Risch N, Thompson WD: Autosomal dominant inheritance of early-onset breast cancer. Implications for risk prediction. Cancer 73:643-651, 1994.

Colditz GA, Egan KM, Stampfer MJ: Hormone replacement therapy and risk of breast cancer: Results from epidemiologic studies. Am J Obstet Gynecol 168:1473-1480, 1993.

Colditz GA, Willett WC, Hunter DJ, et al: Family history, age, and risk of breast cancer. Prospective data from the Nurses' Health Study. JAMA 270:338-343, 1993.

Cook KL, Adler DD, Lichter AS, et al: Breast carcinoma in young women previously treated for Hodgkin disease. AJR Am J Roentgenol 155:39-42, 1990.

Faulk RM, Sickles EA: Efficacy of spot compression-magnification and tangential views in mammographic evaluation of palpable breast masses. Radiology 185:87-90, 1992.

Gail MH, Brinton LA, Byar DP, et al: Projecting individualized probabilities of developing breast cancer for white females who are being examined annually. J Natl Cancer Inst 81:1879-1886, 1989.

Goergen SK, Evans J, Cohen GP, MacMillan JH: Characteristics of breast carcinomas missed by screening radiologists. Radiology 204:131-135, 1997.

Gunhan-Bilgen I, Bozkaya H, Ustun EE, Memis A: Male breast disease: Clinical, mammographic, and ultrasonographic features. Eur J Radiol 43:246-255, 2002.

Hartge P, Struewing JP, Wacholder S, et al: The prevalence of common *BRCA1* and *BRCA2* mutations among Ashkenazi Jews. Am J Hum Genet 64:963-970, 1999.

Homer MJ: Proper placement of a metallic marker on an area of concern in the breast. AJR Am J Roentgenol 167:390-391, 1996.

Homer MJ, Smith TJ: Asymmetric breast tissue. Radiology 173:577-578, 1989.

Ikeda DM, Andersson I, Wattsgard C, et al: Interval carcinomas in the Malmö Mammographic Screening Trial: Radiographic appearance and prognostic considerations. AJR Am J Roentgenol 159:287-294, 1992.

Kopans DB: Negative mammographic and US findings do not help exclude breast cancer. Radiology 222:857-858, author reply 858-859, 2002.

Kopans DB, Swann CA, White G, et al: Asymmetric breast tissue. Radiology 171:639-643, 1989.

Larsson LG, Andersson I, Bjurstam N, et al: Updated overview of the Swedish Randomized Trials on Breast Cancer Screening with Mammography: Age group 40-49 at randomization. J Natl Cancer Inst Monogr 22:57-61, 1997.

Li CI, Malone KE, Porter PL, et al: Relationship between long durations and different regimens of hormone therapy and risk of breast cancer. JAMA 289:3254-3263, 2003.

Logan WW, Janus J: Use of special mammographic views to maximize radiographic information. Radiol Clin North Am 25:953-959, 1987.

Lynch HT, Watson P, Conway T, et al: Breast cancer family history as a risk factor for early onset breast cancer. Breast Cancer Res Treat 11:263-267, 1988.

Miki Y, Swensen J, Shattuck-Eidens D, et al: A strong candidate for the breast and ovarian cancer susceptibility gene BRCA1. Science 266:66-71, 1994.

Miller AB, To T, Baines CJ, Wall C: Canadian National Breast Screening Study-2: 13-year results of a randomized trial in women aged 50-59 years. J Natl Cancer Inst 92:1490-1499, 2000.

Miller AB, To T, Baines CJ, Wall C: The Canadian National Breast Screening Study-1: Breast cancer mortality after 11 to 16 years of follow-up. A randomized screening trial of mammography in women age 40 to 49 years. Ann Intern Med 137(Part 1):305-312, 2002.

Nystrom L, Andersson I, Bjurstam N, et al: Long-term effects of mammography screening: Updated overview of the Swedish randomised trials. Lancet 359:909-919, 2002.

Pearson KL, Sickles EA, Frankel SD, Leung JW: Efficacy of step-oblique mammography for confirmation and localization of densities seen on only one standard mammographic view. AJR Am J Roentgenol 174:745-752, 2000.

Roberts MM, Alexander FE, Anderson TJ, et al: The Edinburgh randomised trial of screening for breast cancer: Description of method. Br J Cancer 50:1-6, 1984.

Rosen EL, Sickles E, Keating D: Ability of mammography to reveal nonpalpable breast cancer in women with palpable breast masses. AJR Am J Roentgenol 172:309-312, 1999.

Schubert EL, Mefford HC, Dann JL, et al: BRCA1 and BRCA2 mutations in Ashkenazi Jewish families with breast and ovarian cancer. Genet Test 1:41-46, 1997.

Shapiro S, Venet W, Strax P, et al: Ten- to fourteen-year effect of screening on breast cancer mortality. J Natl Cancer Inst 69:349-355, 1982.

Sickles EA: Mammographic features of 300 consecutive nonpalpable breast cancers. AJR Am J Roentgenol 146:661-663, 1986.

Sickles EA: Practical solutions to common mammographic problems: Tailoring the examination. AJR Am J Roentgenol 151:31-39, 1988.

Sickles EA: Periodic mammographic follow-up of probably benign lesions: Results in 3,184 consecutive cases. Radiology 179:463-468, 1991.

Smith RA, Cokkinides V, Eyre HJ: American Cancer Society guidelines for the early detection of cancer, 2003. CA Cancer J Clin 53:27-43, 2003.

Smith RA, Saslow D, Sawyer KA, et al: American Cancer Society guidelines for breast cancer screening: Update 2003. CA Cancer J Clin 53:141-169, 2003.

Tabar L, Vitak B, Chen HH, et al: The Swedish Two-County Trial twenty years later. Updated mortality results and new insights from long-term follow-up. Radiol Clin North Am 38:625-651, 2000.

Tabar L, Yen MF, Vitak B, et al: Mammography service screening and mortality in breast cancer patients: 20-year follow-up before and after introduction of screening. Lancet 361:1405-1410, 2003.

Warren Burhenne LJ, Wood SA, D'Orsi CJ, et al: Potential contribution of computer-aided detection to the sensitivity of screening mammography. Radiology 215:554-562, 2000.

Wolverton DE, Sickles EA: Clinical outcome of doubtful mammographic findings. AJR Am J Roentgenol 167:1041-1045, 1996.

Wooster R, Neuhausen SL, Mangion J, et al: Localization of a breast cancer susceptibility gene, BRCA2, to chromosome 13q12-13. Science 265:2088-2090, 1994.

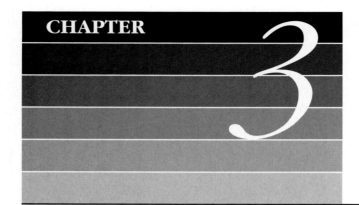

CHAPTER 3

Mammographic Analysis of Breast Calcifications

Introduction
Technique for Evaluating Calcifications
Anatomy
    Individual Calcification Forms
    Calcification Group Shape or Distribution
Benign Calcifications
    Artifacts Simulating Calcifications
    Round Calcifications (0.5 mm or Less Is Punctate)
    Calcifications with Radiolucent Centers
    Dermal Calcifications
    Milk of Calcium
    Plasma Cell Mastitis, Secretory Disease, Duct Ectasia (Large
        Rod-like Calcifications)
    Calcifying Fibroadenomas (Coarse or Popcorn-like)
    Dystrophic Calcifications
    Vascular Calcifications
    Calcifications from Foreign Bodies (Silicone Injections, Other)
Calcifications Developing in Malignancy
    Stability of Pleomorphic Calcifications
Indeterminate Calcifications and Management
    Ultrasound in Evaluation of Calcifications
Key Elements

INTRODUCTION

Calcifications without an associated mass are important because they may be the only sign of malignancy on mammography. At histologic examination, 50% to 80% of breast cancers contain calcifications, and a smaller percentage have calcifications detectable on mammography.

Calcifications form in breast cancers as a result of central necrosis or secretions by malignant cells. Most mammograms show calcifications, but the vast majority are the result of benign processes. Careful, systematic analysis will distinguish between characteristic benign calcifications, which can be dismissed immediately *with no further action necessary,* and suspicious pleomorphic calcifications, which require biopsy. Radiologists can recognize and dismiss characteristic benign calcifications by analyzing the individual calcification forms, the shape of the group or cluster, and their location and change over time, thereby leaving fewer indeterminate calcific groups requiring either follow-up or biopsy. The systematic approach to breast calcifications presented in this chapter will enable radiologists to classify breast calcifications into benign, malignant-appearing, or indeterminate categories.

TECHNIQUE FOR EVALUATING CALCIFICATIONS

High-quality images are essential for detecting and analyzing breast calcifications. For detection of calcifications, the images should have good contrast and be well penetrated. In film-screen mammography, radiologists use a hand-held magnifying lens or viewer to search for calcifications, with the assistance of a bright light for darker portions of the film. In digital mammography, image contrast and brightness are optimized for display of both masses and calcifications on high-resolution monitors or appropriately windowed printed films. On monitors, the viewing algorithm or scenario should include electronically magnified images of each projection with appropriate windows and levels to detect and analyze calcifications, as well as additional magnification or inversion as needed.

A hand-held or electronic magnifier enlarges calcifications on standard mammograms, but the magnifier does not improve image sharpness. Air-gap magnification with a 0.1-mm focal spot increases the resolving power of the imaging system by about 1.8 and thereby provides fine detail of each calcific particle and depicts smaller calcifications undetectable on nonmagnified views. Magnification separates closely grouped calcifications into their individual forms, displays faint calcifications not detected at screening, and improves visualization of the shape of calcifications for analysis. Magnification views may be obtained with standard compression paddles or spot compression paddles to provide increased focal compression over the area of interest.

The American College of Radiology (ACR) Breast Imaging Reporting and Database System (BI-RADS) lexicon has a good section on description and assessment of calcifications. In the mammography report, radiologists describe the shape or distribution and size of the calcification cluster or group, their location, the forms of the individual calcifications in the cluster or group, associated findings and whether any change has occurred since the previous study, and the final BI-RADS assessment and recommendation for patient management (Boxes 3-1 and 3-2).

The location of calcifications is important. Because breast cancer calcifications are almost always found in the parenchyma of the breast, calcifications localized to the skin, muscle, or nipple are almost invariably benign and can be dismissed. Skin calcifications are especially important to recognize because they can easily be mistaken for intraparenchymal calcifications and lead to unnecessary preoperative needle localization. Calcifications in the nipple are almost always benign unless associated with Paget's disease of the nipple.

In general, clustered calcifications are more suspicious than scattered calcifications. Superimposed scattered calcifications may simulate a cluster of calcifications. To prove that clustered calcifications are grouped, the radiologist looks for similar-appearing clustered calcifications over the same volume of tissue on orthogonal views. If the cluster is tightly packed on one view and scattered on the other view, it represents a superimposition of calcifications.

ANATOMY

Calcifications forming in breast ducts (Fig. 3-1), in lobules (Fig. 3-2), or within breast tumors can be benign or malignant. Calcifications forming in the interlobular stroma, in periductal locations, or in blood vessels, fat, or skin are usually benign, and some have a classic pathognomonic appearance as outlined in the section "Benign Calcifications." Because calcifications in *malignancy* develop within breast ducts or within an

---

Box 3-1 Calcification Report

Size of the cluster or calcific group
Location (right or left breast, quadrant or clock position, centimeters from the nipple)
Cluster or group shape
Overall characteristic of the worst-looking individual calcifications in the group
Associated findings
Change, if previous films are compared
BI-RADS code
Management recommendation

From American College of Radiology: ACR BI-RADS—Mammography, 4th ed. *In* ACR Breast Imaging Reporting and Data System, Breast Imaging Atlas. Reston, VA, American College of Radiology, 2003.

Box 3-2 Associated Findings with Calcifications

Mass
Architectural distortion
Axillary adenopathy
Skin retraction
Nipple retraction
Skin thickening
Trabecular thickening (breast edema)

From American College of Radiology: ACR BI-RADS—Mammography, 4th ed. *In* ACR Breast Imaging Reporting and Data System, Breast Imaging Atlas. Reston, VA, American College of Radiology, 2003.

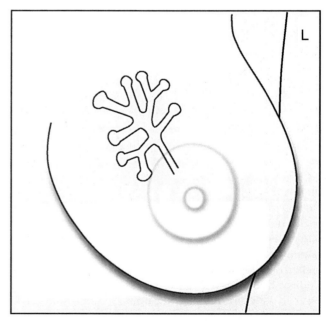

FIGURE 3-1 Schematic of a Normal Breast Duct. The breast has 9 to 22 ducts. Each duct branches into smaller ducts, with the ducts terminating in a terminal ductal lobular unit. Note that the branching duct extends over almost an entire breast quadrant.

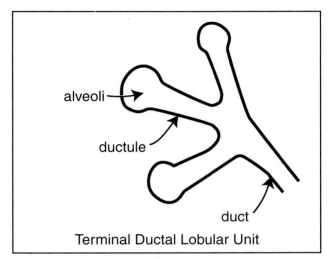

FIGURE 3-2   Schematic Magnification of a Terminal Ductal Lobular Unit (TDLU). The ducts branch into smaller ducts, similar to bronchioles and alveoli in the lung, and end in terminal ductal lobular units (TDLUs). Each duct and lobule are lined by breast epithelium, where breast cancer starts. Cancer grows in the ducts and, if confined to the duct as in ductal carcinoma in situ, produces linear and branching forms. Cancer can grow from the duct back into the lobule, a process called cancerization of lobules.

individual tumor, analysis of both the *individual* calcification *forms* and the *shape* of the calcification cluster or group is equally important.

Individual Calcification Forms

Knowledge of the underlying anatomic structure in which each calcific particle forms is important for understanding why some calcific shapes suggest benign or malignant disease. Some classic benign calcification morphologies are so characteristic that they require no further investigation. Calcifications forming in the round terminal breast acini or lobules in benign parenchymal breast disease take on the round shape of the acini (Fig. 3-3A-C) and can be dismissed. Most of these benign calcifications are round or punctate, regular in shape, densely calcified, and sharply marginated.

The BI-RADS terms "amorphous or indistinct" describe indeterminate calcifications that are tiny, roundish "flake-shaped" particles too small and vague to characterize further. Benign fibrocystic disease and sclerosing adenosis produce blunt duct extension and ductal dilatation that result in indeterminate amorphous or indistinct calcifications (Fig. 3-3D-F). However, some of the calcifications are so small that their shapes cannot be clearly identified as benign; for example, early granular-type calcifications forming in ductal carcinoma in situ (DCIS) mimic fibrocystic change and sclerosing adenosis (Fig. 3-3G and

H). This overlap between benign- and malignant-appearing calcifications partly explains the "false-positive" biopsy results found in up to 75% of procedures prompted by detection of calcifications.

Generally, calcifications forming in breast cancers are pleomorphic and vary in size, shape, and density (Box 3-3). On screening mammography, pleomorphic calcifications often herald the presence of DCIS, which is the diagnosis in 25% to 48% of all cancers found at screening. DCIS develops in breast duct epithelium, remains within the duct basement membrane, and grows within and along the duct, where it expands and assumes the configuration of the duct. Individual calcifications form in the middle of the DCIS tumor as a result of either secretions or cell death and necrosis; such calcifications are usually 0.5 mm or less in size. Suspicious calcifications in DCIS and invasive breast cancer are irregular in form, may be both faint and dense and very small (almost indiscernible), and vary in shape. The number of calcifications is also important. Sigfusson et al. reviewed thousands of calcification clusters on mammograms and showed that fewer than five calcifications in a cluster rarely represent cancer. Based on this observation, biopsy of fewer than five clustered calcifications is unlikely to yield cancer and should be undertaken only if the individual calcification forms are extremely suspicious or the calcifications are in an appropriate clinical scenario.

Linear, branching, or pleomorphic calcifications develop in DCIS growing in branching, tubular-like ducts or in invasive cancer (Fig. 3-4A and B). The ACR BI-RADS term for these calcifications is "fine linear or fine linear branching (casting) calcifications" because the calcifications form an irregular cast of the duct, often seen in the comedo form of DCIS. The calcifications may look like little broken needles with pointy ends or may have a "dot-dash" appearance with both round and linear shapes. X-, Y- or Z-shaped calcifications may be seen because of calcific casts of necrotic tumor in branching ducts. Radiologists describe these classic suspicious calcifications as "casting" or "pleomorphic" in the report to reflect a concern for cancer. They are much smaller, less dense, and less well defined than the linear calcifications in benign secretory disease, which can be mistaken for DCIS (Fig. 3-4C).

Another suspicious calcification form described by the ACR BI-RADS lexicon is "pleomorphic or heterogeneous calcifications (granular)"; this term reflects more rounded, but very tiny, irregularly shaped calcific particles that look like bizarre broken glass shards formed in small rounded pockets of necrotic tumors such as micropapillary or cribriform DCIS or in fibrocystic change or sclerosing adenosis (Fig. 3-5). The individual calcification forms are roughly round in shape but are irregular and can be faint, are smaller than 0.5 mm, and vary in size and density. A cluster containing granular

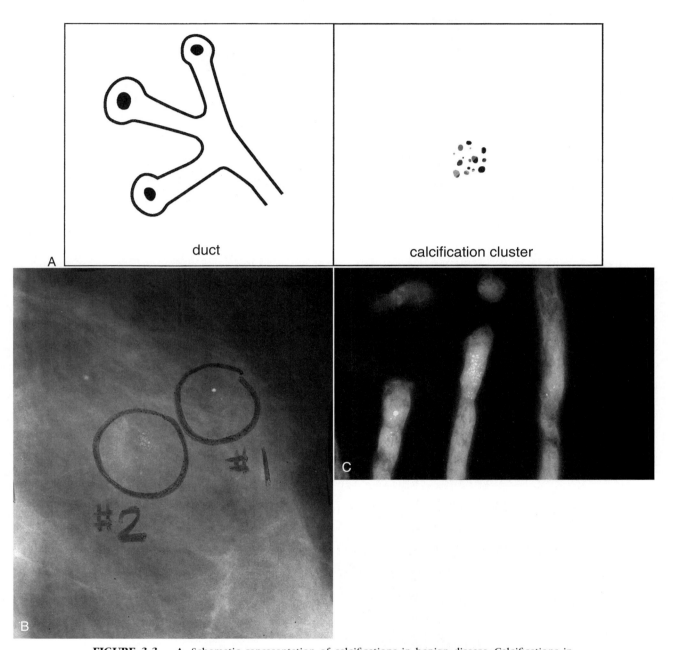

FIGURE 3-3   A, Schematic representation of calcifications in benign disease. Calcifications in benign disease form in the acini or lobuli of the duct, so they look round *(left box)*. On the mammogram, these calcifications will be sharply marginated, round, dense, and punctate because they form in round structures *(right box)*. These round, benign-appearing calcifications are the result of benign fibrocystic change. **B** and **C,** Mammogram and core biopsy specimen of two groups of round calcifications in proliferative fibrocystic change; biopsy was performed because of change in their appearance since the previous screening mammogram.

Continued

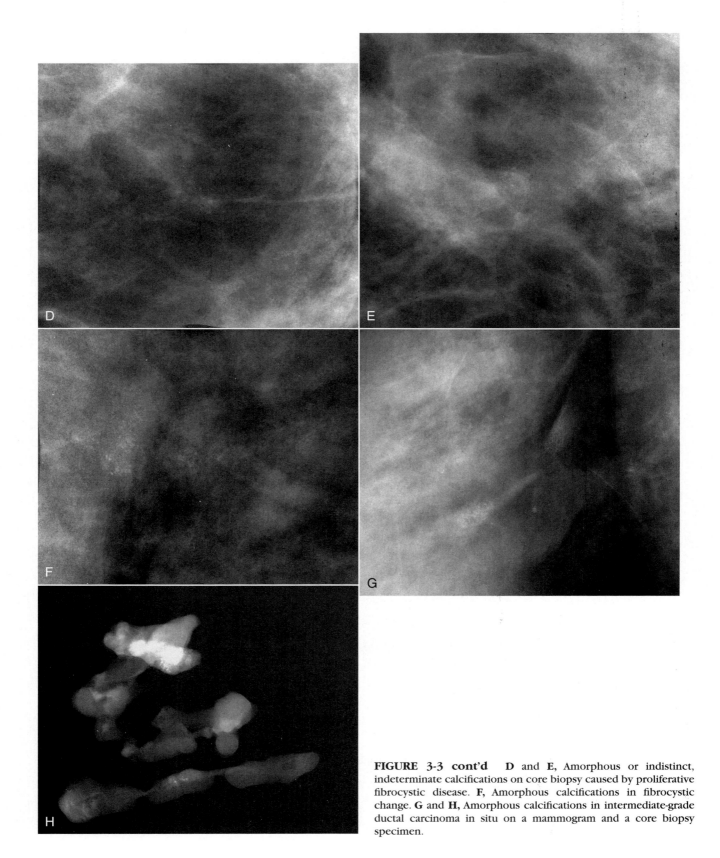

FIGURE 3-3 cont'd   D and **E,** Amorphous or indistinct, indeterminate calcifications on core biopsy caused by proliferative fibrocystic disease. **F,** Amorphous calcifications in fibrocystic change. **G** and **H,** Amorphous calcifications in intermediate-grade ductal carcinoma in situ on a mammogram and a core biopsy specimen.

Box 3-3	**Terms for Suspicious Calcifications**

INDIVIDUAL CALCIFICATION FORM	CALCIFICATION CLUSTER SHAPE
Pleomorphic, fine linear or branching	Clustered
Amorphous	Linear
Coarse or fine heterogeneous	Branching
Indistinct	Segmental

From American College of Radiology: ACR BI-RADS—Mammography, 4th ed. *In* ACR Breast Imaging Reporting and Data System, Breast Imaging Atlas. Reston, VA, American College of Radiology, 2003.

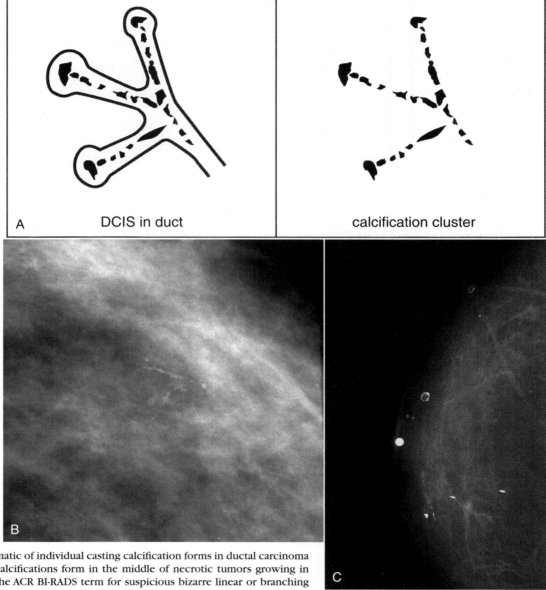

FIGURE 3-4   A, Schematic of individual casting calcification forms in ductal carcinoma in situ (DCIS). In DCIS, calcifications form in the middle of necrotic tumors growing in breast ducts *(left box).* The ACR BI-RADS term for suspicious bizarre linear or branching particle-shaped calcifications is "fine linear or fine linear branching (casting) calcifications" because the calcifications are in a line or form a cast of the duct. **B,** Photographic magnification of clustered pleomorphic calcifications in DCIS. Note the branching shape of the calcification in the uppermost part of the cluster. **C,** Benign linear calcifications in secretory disease are larger, denser, much more coarse, and more well defined than in DCIS, without additional tiny adjacent calcifications. Note the incidental oil cysts and a marker on the nipple.

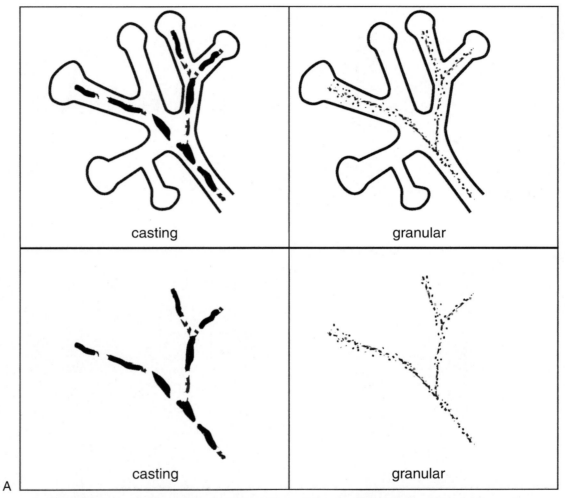

A

FIGURE 3-5   Schematic of Linear/Branching Calcifications versus Granular Calcifications. A, In ductal carcinoma in situ (DCIS), linear or branching calcifications form if the necrotic center extends along the duct *(left box).* Amorphous or granular calcifications in DCIS form in small pockets of DCIS and pack the duct with roundish, but irregular calcific particles *(right box).*

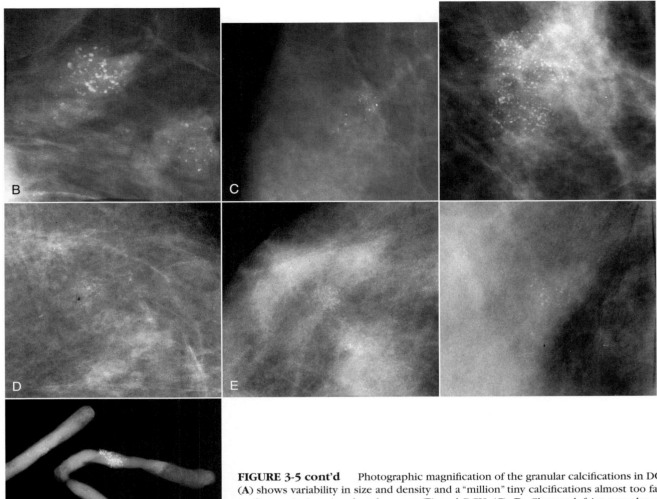

FIGURE 3-5 cont'd   Photographic magnification of the granular calcifications in DCIS (**A**) shows variability in size and density and a "million" tiny calcifications almost too faint to discern in invasive ductal cancer (**B**) and DCIS (**C**). **D,** Clustered, faint granular and amorphous calcification in DCIS. Amorphous or indistinct calcifications also can be present in benign sclerosing adenosis or fibrocystic change. In nonproliferative fibrocystic change, granular calcifications on mammography (**E**) and stereotactic core biopsy (**F**) show the overlap between benign and malignant calcifications.

calcifications may not exhibit casting or linear forms but should still be considered suspicious even in their absence. Although comedo-type DCIS calcifications are often "casting" and the calcifications in micropapillary and cribriform DCIS are often "granular," Stomper and Connolly showed that the calcification forms and DCIS architectural type can overlap. A particular calcification form predicts neither a specific DCIS histology nor a coexistent microinvasive or invasive cancer.

Because cancer calcifications vary enormously, it is important to analyze all the individual calcifications in a cluster. DCIS may grow into a lobule, in which case it is called cancerization of lobules, and result in some round or amorphous calcifications mixed with pleomorphic calcifications. The presence of some round calcifications

in a cluster does not exclude cancer; the radiologist bases the decision for biopsy on the worst-looking calcifications in the group.

Calcification Group Shape or Distribution

It is important to understand the anatomic structures forming the *shape* of the overall calcification cluster and their distribution because distributions requiring special attention are described by the ACR BI-RADS terms "clustered or grouped," "linear (calcifications in a line that may show branching)" (Fig. 3-6), and "segmental" (Fig. 3-7).

An isolated calcification cluster suggests an isolated disease process, perhaps DCIS or invasive cancer versus fibrocystic change, papilloma, or another benign entity.

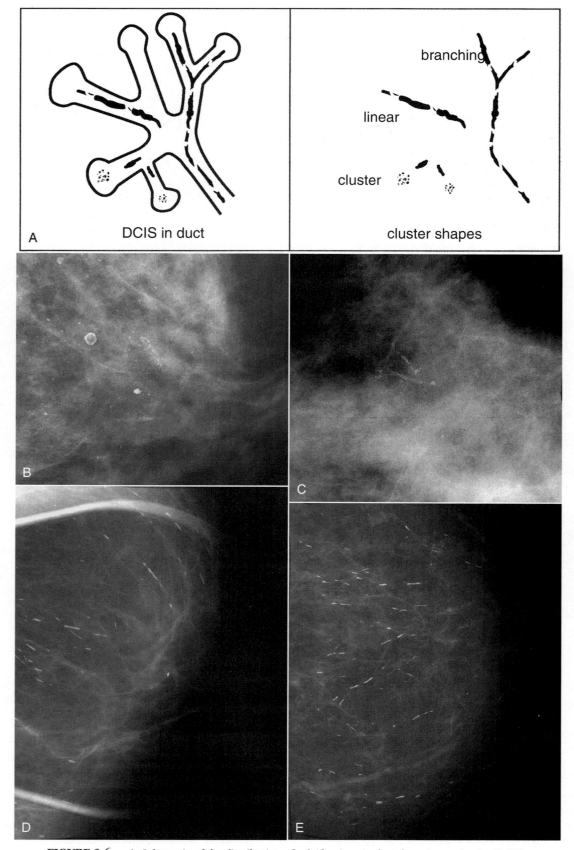

FIGURE 3-6   **A,** Schematic of the distribution of calcifications in ductal carcinoma in situ (DCIS). In DCIS, individual calcification forms are linear and branching, and the entire cluster can form a linear or branching shape by following the duct *(left box).* The resulting cluster distribution forms a cluster or a linear or branching pattern on the mammogram *(right box),* depending on where the tumor grows. **B,** Calcifications growing in a V-shaped linear pattern. Note the oil cyst and other nonspecific calcifications near the DCIS. **C,** DCIS calcifications growing in a branching pattern. Linear and branching patterns are seen in benign secretory disease on spot magnification **(D)** and craniocaudal **(E)** mammograms, but the calcifications are larger and rod-like and branch over a wider area than in DCIS shown in **B** and **C.**

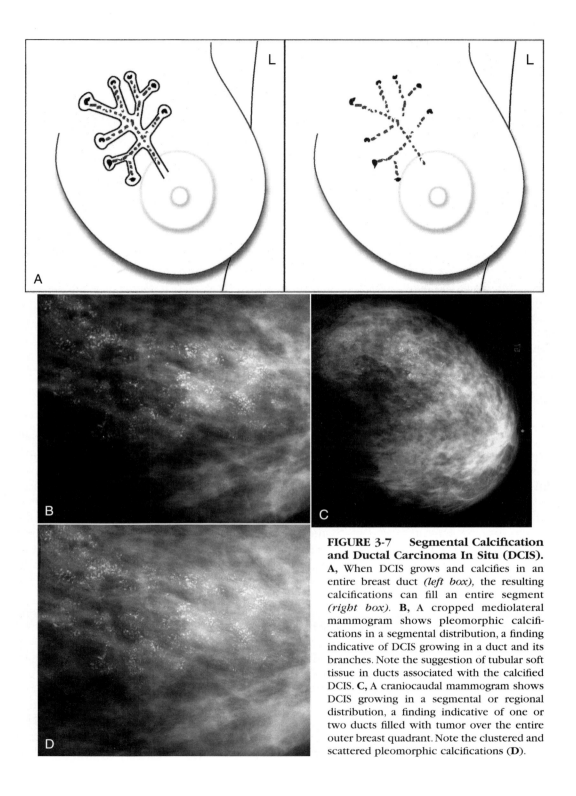

FIGURE 3-7   Segmental Calcification and Ductal Carcinoma In Situ (DCIS). **A,** When DCIS grows and calcifies in an entire breast duct *(left box),* the resulting calcifications can fill an entire segment *(right box).* **B,** A cropped mediolateral mammogram shows pleomorphic calcifications in a segmental distribution, a finding indicative of DCIS growing in a duct and its branches. Note the suggestion of tubular soft tissue in ducts associated with the calcified DCIS. **C,** A craniocaudal mammogram shows DCIS growing in a segmental or regional distribution, a finding indicative of one or two ducts filled with tumor over the entire outer breast quadrant. Note the clustered and scattered pleomorphic calcifications (**D**).

Box 3-4 Terms for Benign Calcifications	
INDIVIDUAL CALCIFICATION FORM	**CALCIFICATION CLUSTER SHAPE**
Round	Clustered
Punctate	Regional
	Multiple clusters
	Diffuse

Box 3-5   Typically Benign Calcifications
Artifacts (deodorant, hair, fingerprints)
Skin artifacts: antiperspirant, material in moles
Eggshell-type calcifications, radiolucent centers
Calcifying oil cysts
Intraparenchymal calcifications
Skin calcifications (obtain tangential views)
Fat necrosis (post-biopsy, post-trauma)
Vascular calcifications (tram-track appearance)
Fibroadenoma (mass with round, coarse peripheral calcifications)
Plasma cell mastitis or secretory disease (needle-like or sausage-shaped calcifications point toward the nipple; found in middle-aged women; benign entity, usually asymptomatic)
Milk of calcium (linear on the medial-lateral view, smudgy on the craniocaudal view)
Dystrophic calcifications (be alert for such calcifications in women after biopsy for cancer)
Suture calcifications (cat gut, post-radiation)
Calcifications in the fibrous implant capsule
Calcifications in polyurethane-type implant coverings
Silicon/paraffin injections
Dermatomyositis

For clusters, one analyzes the individual calcification forms and their stability over time, with irregular forms or increasing numbers of calcifications viewed as suspicious. Lanyi suggested that the overall cluster *shape* is especially suspicious if it has a "swallowtail" or "V" shape, which may be indicative of calcifying cancer in tightly branching tumor-packed ducts.

The ACR BI-RADS terms "linear" (branching) and "segmental" distribution of calcifications suggest a process within a duct and its branches. Although these distributions are seen in calcifying cancer-packed ducts, analysis of the individual calcification forms distinguishes cancer from benign secretory disease or other benign ductal processes. The term "linear" describes calcifications in a line, either tumor in a duct or a focal benign process. A "segmental" distribution is a suspicious finding because it suggests a process within a branch and its ducts and describes calcifications covering slightly less than a quadrant and extending in a triangular distribution with the apex pointing at the nipple.

BI-RADS terms suggesting benign calcification distributions include "regional" and "diffuse/scattered," or multiple similar-appearing calcification clusters widely dispersed over the breast. Benign processes are often spread widely throughout both breasts; they are usually due to fibrocystic change and reflect *calcifications with benign individual forms* in innumerable scattered and occasionally clustered distributions or in a "regional" location that extends over more than one ductal distribution (Box 3-4).

The decision to perform a biopsy or ignore the finding is based on the worst features of the individual calcification forms or distribution, change over time, the clinical scenario, and common sense.

BENIGN CALCIFICATIONS

The specific benign calcifying entities covered in the following subsections require no further work-up and *should prompt no further action* (Box 3-5).

Artifacts Simulating Calcifications

Artifacts may simulate breast calcifications. Such artifacts include radiopaque materials on the skin, such as deodorant and antiperspirant in the axilla, or radiopaque salves used on dermal skin tags or warts. The characteristic location of calcific particles over the axilla suggests radiopaque deodorant or antiperspirant, which should disappear on repeat films after the armpit has been washed (Fig. 3-8). Sometimes the deodorant or powder will produce dense particles in skin creases, thereby suggesting the diagnosis.

Dermal lesions may harbor residual radiopaque salves in their crevices, similar to calcifications in a mass. Some facilities use skin markers on moles or skin tags to distinguish dermal lesions from masses in the breast parenchyma (Fig. 3-9). To determine whether a calcified "mass" is a skin lesion, the radiologist reviews the patient's breast history sheet to see whether a skin lesion is marked on the breast diagram. Correlation between the diagram and the image should confirm the presence of a skin lesion. Otherwise, the radiologist performs a physical examination. If there are still questions about a skin lesion, the technologist places a radiopaque marker over the skin lesion and repeats the mammogram. The repeat mammogram should show the marker on the "mass" if it is the skin lesion.

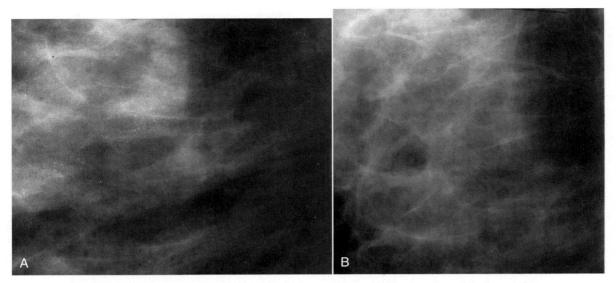

FIGURE 3-8   **A,** Powder on the skin simulating cancer. A magnification view of the breast shows round tiny calcific particles suggestive of DCIS, but they were not seen on the orthogonal view. **B, A** repeat mammogram after wiping the patient's skin off shows no particles, thereby confirming a skin artifact.

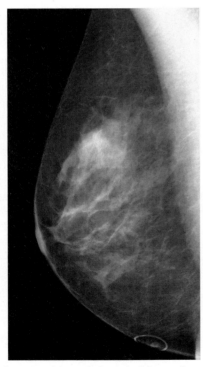

FIGURE 3-9   On the mediolateral oblique view, a skin mole covered by a radiopaque ring suggests a nodule. Visual inspection of the patient confirms its dermal location and eliminates the possibility of an intraparenchymal lesion.

Hair artifacts are thin, linear, strand-like opacities usually located near the chest wall (Fig. 3-10) that occur when patients with long hair lean forward for their mammogram. Long hair overlaps into the field of view along the chest wall and causes the artifact. A repeat mammogram with the patient's hair pulled away from the field of view will eliminate the strand-like artifacts on the mammogram.

Fingerprints have a characteristic whorled appearance and are caused by sticky fingers handling sensitive mammographic film (Fig. 3-11). Sometimes this artifact simulates the linear calcifications in DCIS. A repeat film in the same projection will have no fingerprint in the same location, thereby resolving the issue.

Round Calcifications (0.5 mm or Less Is Punctate)

Small, 2- to 4-mm round benign intraparenchymal breast calcifications can be seen in any location within the breast. Forming in the acini breast lobules, they are round in appearance, sharply marginated, and densely calcified, characteristics suggestive of a benign diagnosis, and they are often seen in fibrocystic change (Fig. 3-12).

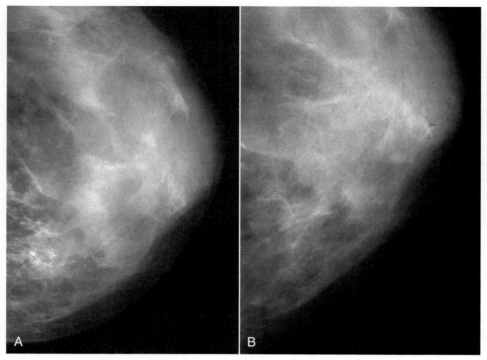

FIGURE 3-10   **A,** A craniocaudal mammogram shows a strand-like, curvilinear hair artifact near the chest wall over the pectoral muscle. **B,** After moving the patient's hair from the field of view, a repeat mammogram shows no hair artifact.

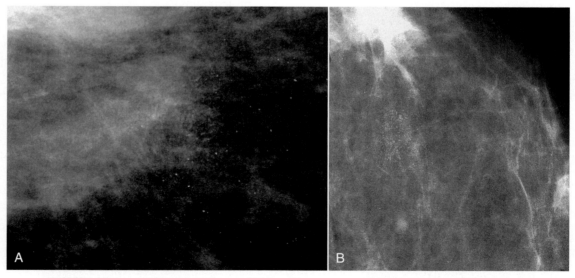

FIGURE 3-11   Whorled curvilinear whitish artifacts on two mammograms (**A** and **B**) from two different patients represent characteristic fingerprints caused by sticky fingers lifting the emulsion off sensitive mammography film.

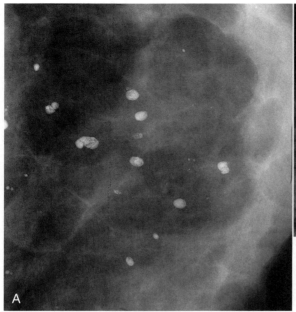

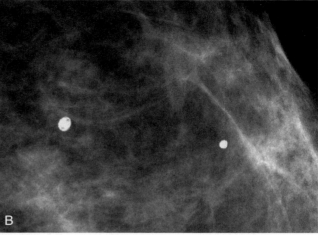

FIGURE 3-12   Craniocaudal Mammograms Showing Large Round Benign Calcifications. A, Rounded benign intraparenchymal calcifications scattered in the breast. **B,** Other eggshell-type calcifications may represent calcified dilated ductal structures, clearly uncharacteristic of malignancy.

Calcifications with Radiolucent Centers

Rim-like or eggshell-type calcifications with radiolucent centers are virtually always benign. They are usually round or oval and calcify along their edges, with the radiolucent center appearing darker than the rim. Small isolated calcifications with a radiolucent center can form around debris in ducts and are scattered in the breast tissue.

In patients who have sustained trauma or have previously undergone surgery, oil cysts with calcification around their edges may develop from fat necrosis. Rim-like calcifications surround a radiolucent center containing a fat- or oil-like substance (Fig. 3-13). The curvilinear portion of the oil cyst or fat necrosis can be seen at its edge, whereas amorphous sheet-like calcifications are seen en face. Calcified oil cysts distributed across the breast in a diagonal fashion may be due to blunt trauma from a seat belt or steering wheel injury sustained in an automobile accident.

Dermal Calcifications

Skin calcifications are quite small, about the size of skin pores seen in the axilla on the mammogram, are single or occasionally clustered, and often (but not always) have a calcific rim surrounding a radiolucent center (Fig. 3-14). This entity deserves special attention because dermal calcifications can occur as an isolated cluster and simulate grouped intraparenchymal calcifications, thereby prompting biopsy. One should suspect skin calcifications if the calcifications are in a peripheral location, are close to the skin surface in any projection when other skin calcifications are present, and occur at sites where skin touches skin, such as in the axilla, the inframammary fold, or the medial portion of the breast (Box 3-6).

Special tangential views confirm calcifications within the dermis and virtually exclude malignancy. To localize skin calcifications easily, a mammographic compression plate that contains perforations or an alphanumeric grid coordinate plate for preoperative needle localization should be used (Fig. 3-15). A key element for achieving success is to place the opening of the localizing device directly over the skin containing the calcifications as judged on orthogonal scout films. If the localizing device is placed over the *upper* part of the breast in the craniocaudal view and the calcifications are in the skin on the *under*side, the tangential view will not work.

While the patient is still in compression, determine the location of the calcifications in the aperture and superimpose a small radiopaque skin marker over the calcific particles. Repeat the mammogram to make sure that the marker is exactly over the calcifications; if the marker obscures the calcifications, it is in the right place. Take a view tangential to the skin marker. Dermal calcifications will be in the skin directly under the skin marker. Intraparenchymal calcifications will be within the breast tissue under the marker and not in the skin.

Milk of Calcium

Milk of calcium has a classic appearance consisting of sedimented calcifications within tiny benign cysts; this

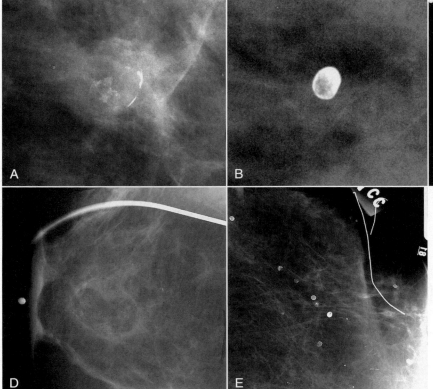
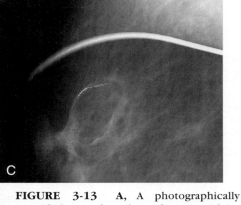
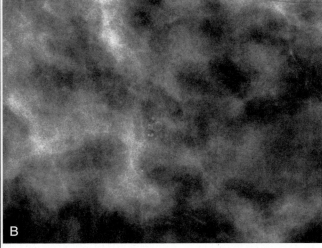

FIGURE 3-13   A, A photographically magnified view of an oil cyst shows partial rim calcification around a radiolucent center, with plaque-like calcifications seen en face in the cyst wall. Normal breast tissue can be seen through the oil cyst. **B,** This oil cyst is more completely calcified along its edge than the example in **A** is. Note that a discernible radiolucent center is still apparent. Lateral-medial (**C**) and craniocaudal (**D**) spot magnification mammograms show a thin rim of calcification around a mostly radiolucent oil cyst. **E,** This patient had previously undergone biopsy, as shown by a linear metallic skin scar marker, and has multiple eggshell-type calcified oil cysts in the biopsy site from surgical trauma. Note the incidental coarse linear secretory calcifications in the lower right-hand corner.

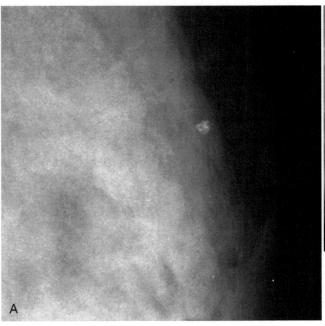

FIGURE 3-14   A, Photographic magnification shows a typical eggshell-type skin calcification around a radiolucent center near the periphery of the breast. **B,** Other skin calcifications with radiolucent centers.

appearance is pathognomonic on mediolateral and craniocaudal mammograms. The calcifications are not fixed to the cyst wall and can float around the cyst like fake snow in a winter scene paperweight. On the mediolateral mammogram, curvilinear, dependently layering milk of calcium settles to the bottom of tiny imperceptible cysts. The layering calcifications are dense, linear, or curvilinear in an upright patient (Fig. 3-16). On the craniocaudal projection, the calcifications will have a cloud-like or smudgy appearance like tea leaves in the bottom of a teacup (Fig. 3-17).

In *macro*cystic milk of calcium, lateral views with the x-ray beam directed horizontally will show typical layering semilunar, linear, or curvilinear calcifications *and* the cyst. Unlike milk of calcium in *macro*cysts, the

cysts in *micro*cystic milk of calcium are too small to be seen, and only the characteristic calcifications indicate their presence. Usually, the craniocaudal projection with the x-ray beam directed vertically will show cloud-like and smudgy calcifications. Occasionally, microcystic milk of calcium calcifications may not be seen on the craniocaudal projection at all, and only the linear or curvilinear calcifications will be displayed on mediolateral or mediolateral oblique views.

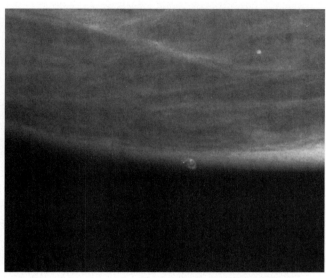

FIGURE 3-15 A view tangential to the calcification in Figure 3-14A confirms the dermal origin of the calcifications.

Box 3-6	Reasons to Suspect Skin Calcifications*

Peripheral location in the breast
Location close to the skin surface on one view
Location in the axilla, inframammary fold, or medial part of the breast
Size similar to skin pores
Other skin calcifications present

*A skin calcification study should be performed to exclude calcifications (see text).

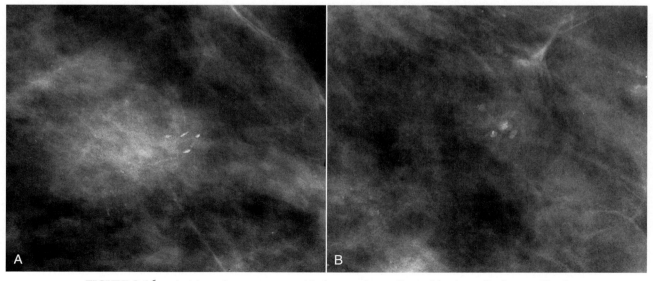

FIGURE 3-16 **A,** A lateral mammogram with the x-ray beam directed horizontally shows milk of calcium layering in the dependent aspect of a few microcysts and producing curvilinear lines *(arrow).* **B,** A craniocaudal view shows round smudgy calcifications representing the calcifications en face.

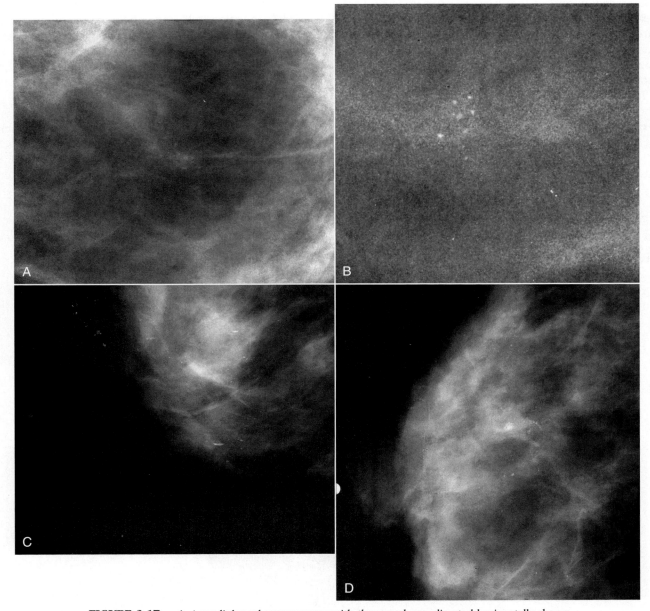

FIGURE 3-17 **A,** A mediolateral mammogram with the x-ray beam directed horizontally shows innumerable curvilinear calcifications representing calcium layering dependently in a multitude of tiny, invisible cysts. **B,** A craniocaudal view with the x-ray beam directed vertically shows round calcifications. In another example, milk of calcium is evident in the mediolateral (**C**) and craniocaudal (**D**) projections. These clusters could easily be mistaken for ductal carcinoma in situ without the two orthogonal views to confirm the diagnosis of milk of calcium.

DCIS producing linear calcifications can be distinguished from milk of calcium on the craniocaudal mammogram. Milk of calcium will be amorphous or smudgy on the craniocaudal projection, but DCIS will retain its linear form in all views (Table 3-1).

Even though the calcifications of milk of calcium are typically benign and should not undergo biopsy, unrecognized milk of calcium may be recommended for biopsy. In patients undergoing stereotactic core biopsy on a stereotactic table, the milk of calcium calcifications will layer dependently in the prone patient, thereby

Table 3-1 Milk of Calcium versus DCIS Calcifications		
	Milk of Calcium	**DCIS**
Lateral-medial mammogram	Linear	Linear
Craniocaudal mammogram	Smudgy	Linear

DCIS, ductal carcinoma in situ.

changing their position from the upright view and suggesting the diagnosis (Fig. 3-18).

Plasma Cell Mastitis, Secretory Disease, Duct Ectasia (Large Rod-like Calcifications)

The presence of calcified inspissated secretions within ectatic ducts in the subareolar region is the usual radiographic manifestation of plasma cell mastitis, an asymptomatic inflammation of the breast in older women. The inflammation is periductal or intraductal. Periductal inflammation results in dense, sausage-like calcifications with radiolucent centers oriented along the breast ducts and pointing at the nipple. Intraductal inflammation results in calcifications filling the ducts in a solid, large rod-like shape or a thinner, needle-like appearance (Fig. 3-19) along the long axis of the ducts; the calcifications are pointed toward the nipple. The calcifications are quite dense and have sharp margins, line up along the duct like cars in a train, and may be unilateral or bilateral. Unlike DCIS, secretory calcifications

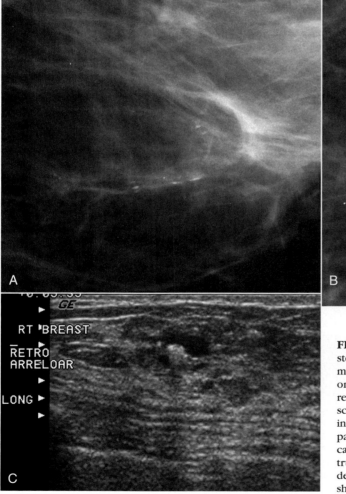

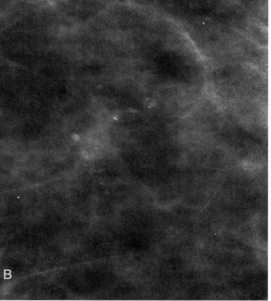

FIGURE 3-18 Microcalcifications recommended for stereotactic biopsy have a curvilinear shape on the mediolateral oblique projection (**A**) and are so smudgy on the craniocaudal view (**B**) that they are not recognized as milk of calcium. A stereotactic core biopsy scout film shows characteristic layering of calcifications in the dependent portion of the breast in a prone patient, which is suggestive of the diagnosis of milk of calcium. If a lateral scout view had been obtained, the true nature of the calcifications might have been detected and no biopsy recommended. Ultrasound shows milk of calcium in the tiny cysts (**C**).

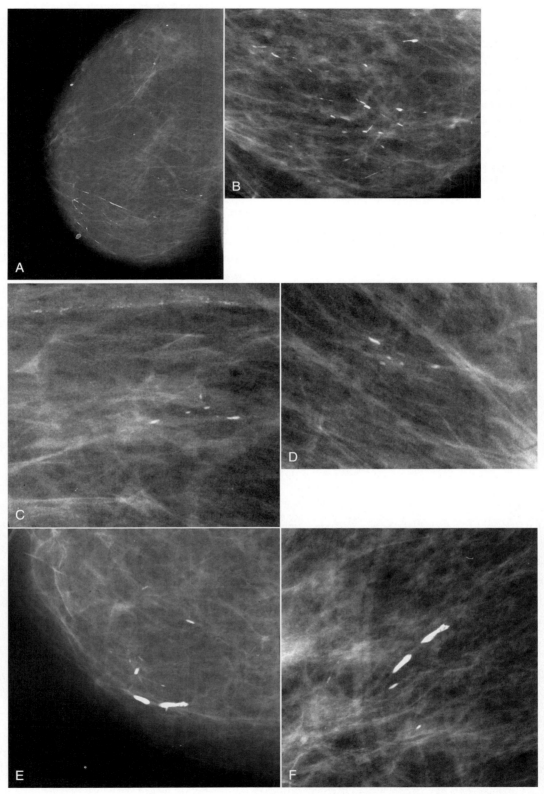

FIGURE 3-19 **A,** A craniocaudal mammogram demonstrates nonpalpable rod-like or needle-like and occasionally rounded calcifications in a ductal distribution pointing at the nipple, characteristic of plasma cell mastitis or secretory disease. The calcifications are coarse, quite dense, and easily seen and branch over a large portion of the breast. **B,** A magnification view of secretory disease shows typical large rod-like calcifications. Craniocaudal (**C**) and mediolateral oblique (**D**) mammograms show a linear form and coarse calcifications of early secretory disease. Unlike ductal carcinoma in situ, secretory disease does not usually show many smaller calcific particles associated with the larger calcifications on magnification views. Note the early vascular calcifications in the upper part of image **C. E** and **F,** Two views of secretory disease.

can usually be seen easily without a magnifier and are coarse; if they branch, they do so over many centimeters in the breast because they occur in larger ducts. DCIS, on the other hand, generally has very fine calcifications that branch many times over a small area because it occurs in smaller ducts (Table 3-2).

Clinically, the occasional subareolar inflammation from this entity may cause new nipple inversion and simulate carcinoma, thereby resulting in biopsy. How-

ever, in the absence of this clinical sign, the classic features of plasma cell mastitis or secretory disease on the mammogram should distinguish this entity from malignancy.

Calcifying Fibroadenomas (Coarse or "Popcorn-like")

Most commonly occurring between puberty and 30 years of age, benign fibroadenomas are oval or lobulated masses that are equal in density to breast tissue on the mammogram and occasionally calcify with coarse or "popcorn-like" features. Fibroadenomas are multiple in approximately 10% to 20% of cases and result from epithelial and intraductal proliferation of breast elements. Fibroadenomas can take two forms: intracanalicular and pericanalicular. These benign lesions are often well-circumscribed, low-density masses that are impossible to distinguish from cysts on the mammogram before they undergo calcific degeneration. Calcifications within a fibroadenoma usually start at its periphery and are large and dense, although at an early stage they may be somewhat irregular and small. Periodic mammography should show progression of the calcifications to a more classic appearance. Characteristically, early calcification progresses to a dense, popcorn-like appearance, with the fibroadenoma sometimes totally replaced by calcium (Fig. 3-20).

Table 3-2 Plasma Cell Mastitis versus DCIS Calcifications	
Plasma Cell Mastitis	**DCIS**
Lined up along ducts	Lined up along ducts
Point at nipple	Point at nipple
Linear, sometimes branching	Linear, sometimes branching, pleomorphic
Branches over a wide area	Branches many times over 1 cm (ducts are smaller)
No tiny additional calcifications	Magnification shows many more small calcifications
Big calcifications—can be seen without a magnifier	Big and small calcifications
Coarse, rod-like calcifications	Fine, linear calcifications
Sharply marginated	Indefinite margins

DCIS, ductal carcinoma in situ.

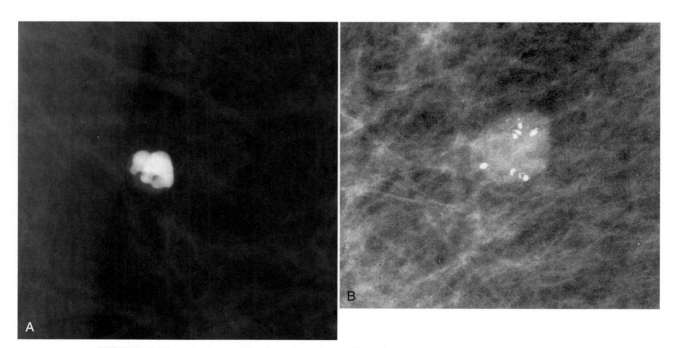

FIGURE 3-20   A, A magnification view shows fibroadenoma with complete replacement by calcification. **B,** In another patient, a fibroadenoma appears as dense round calcifications at the edges of the mass. Note the coarse appearance of the calcifications; such an appearance distinguishes fibroadenoma from invasive ductal carcinoma, which would contain fine or pleomorphic calcifications.

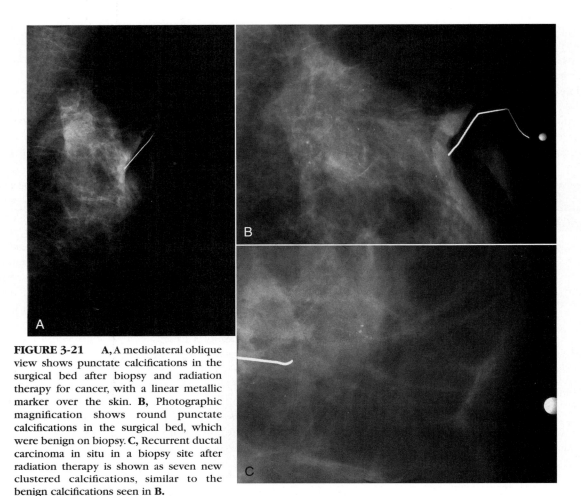

FIGURE 3-21 **A,** A mediolateral oblique view shows punctate calcifications in the surgical bed after biopsy and radiation therapy for cancer, with a linear metallic marker over the skin. **B,** Photographic magnification shows round punctate calcifications in the surgical bed, which were benign on biopsy. **C,** Recurrent ductal carcinoma in situ in a biopsy site after radiation therapy is shown as seven new clustered calcifications, similar to the benign calcifications seen in **B.**

Fibroadenomas with classic, characteristic calcifications should not be mistaken for malignancy. If the calcifications are not fully typical of fibroadenomas or if the mass shape or other features are not characteristic, consideration should be given to needle or surgical biopsy.

Dystrophic Calcifications

After breast biopsy, linear and amorphous calcifications can form in the surgical bed, occasionally accompanied by fat necrosis. This entity represents an inflammatory process that causes pleomorphic and bizarre calcifications in regions of previous biopsy or blunt breast trauma. A history of previous surgical biopsy or trauma, when correlated with a surgical scar, should identify the true nature of the calcifications (Fig. 3-21). Some facilities use a metallic scar marker to allow easier correlation of the surface skin scar with underlying post-biopsy scarring (Box 3-7). In fat necrosis, the calcifications will form around a radiolucent center; the previous mammogram

---

Box 3-7 Methods to Identify Post-traumatic Dystrophic Calcifications

Metallic scar marker to show the biopsy site
Look for fat on old films in the region where calcifications now project
Look at old films for biopsied lesions; correlate the scar site with the current location of calcifications

---

should be inspected for the previously radiolucent area to make this diagnosis.

Calcifications occurring in the operative site of a previously resected malignancy deserve special consideration and are much more difficult to assess. Calcifications in an irradiated breast can be due to

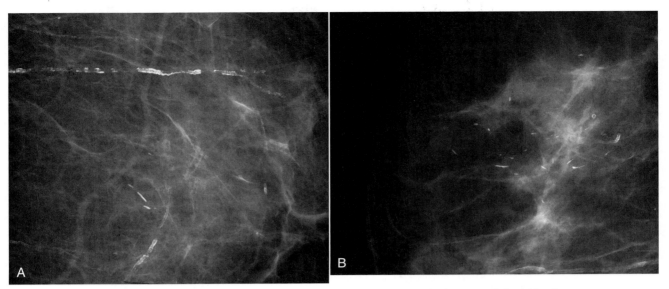

FIGURE 3-22   **A,** Photographic magnification of easily recognizable dense parallel calcifications along arterial walls. Calcification between the parallel calcific lines represents arterial wall calcifications seen en face. **B,** The tube-like vascular calcification on the right side of the image is easily distinguished from secretory disease and an early oil cyst.

calcifying sutures or benign fat necrosis, but they usually develop 2 years or later after surgery and radiation therapy. Dystrophic calcifications in this setting may be difficult to distinguish from cancer (see Fig. 3-21). Comparing the current study with the pre-biopsy, post-biopsy, and specimen mammograms can help determine whether the calcifications represent unresected tumor missed at the initial surgery, residual benign-appearing calcifications, or new calcifications. Fat necrosis calcifications will form around radiolucent areas in the biopsy site.

The differential diagnosis for new calcifications in an irradiated cancer biopsy site is fat necrosis or recurrent cancer. Radiation therapy fails at a rate of about 1% per year, thus resulting in failure rates of about 5% at 5 years and 10% to 15% after 10 years. If new calcifications are found in the biopsy site and they are fine, innumerable, pleomorphic, and increasing in number over time, biopsy should be performed to exclude recurrent tumor. Because of the problem of recurrent breast cancer in the cancer biopsy site, biopsy may be required more frequently for dystrophic calcifications to confirm or exclude the recurrence of carcinoma (versus post-surgical calcification).

Vascular Calcifications

Arterial calcification from atherosclerosis is characteristically imaged as two parallel lines of calcification in the arterial wall and is easily recognizable (Fig. 3-22). Early arterial calcification along vascular walls may simulate suspicious linear calcifications in DCIS.

Identification of a noncalcified vessel leading to the calcifications in question may establish the true diagnosis. Magnification views will show arterial tram-track–like calcifications in two parallel lines, with coarse calcifications en face in the vessel wall between them.

Calcifications from Foreign Bodies (Silicone Injections, Other)

Classically associated with the injection of silicone or a paraffin-like substance into the breast for purposes of augmentation, foreign-body granulomas have a characteristic eggshell-type appearance (see Fig. 9-64 on page 263). They are usually a few millimeters in size but can be larger because of fat necrosis or inflammation. They often cause a palpable mass and obscure the underlying breast on both mammography and ultrasound, thereby making it difficult to evaluate the breast by physical examination or imaging. Calcifications may form around the fibrous capsules surrounding breast implants and are characterized by dense, dystrophic calcifications in a rounded pattern (Fig. 3-23). Other foreign-body granulomas may sometimes be caused by objects inserted into the breast.

CALCIFICATIONS DEVELOPING IN MALIGNANCY

Calcifications that do not fulfill all the criteria for benign entities require further evaluation, and their shapes,

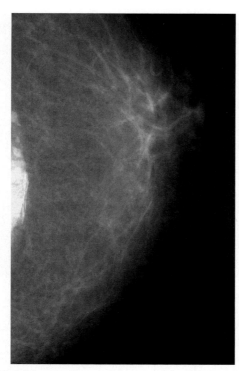

FIGURE 3-23 In Figure 9-6A on page 263, a craniocaudal mammogram shows multiple round tiny eggshell-type calcifications representing calcification around silicone injection granulomas. Silicone and other substances were injected directly into the breast for augmentation in Southeast Asia, but they cause dense calcifications. Direct injections of silicone are easily distinguished from dystrophic calcifications in the implant capsule after implant removal, shown here. When a breast implant is removed, the fibrous capsule that forms around the implant is often left in place. The dystrophic calcifications forming in the fibrous capsule are typically seen near the chest wall in the deflated capsule, as shown here.

Box 3-8   Benign Calcifications That Simulate Ductal Carcinoma In Situ

Skin calcifications
Scattered calcifications projecting as a group in one
    projection
Sclerosing adenosis
Fibrocystic change

---

location, and distribution must be analyzed carefully. Once skin calcifications are eliminated as a causative factor, orthogonal projections should be obtained to exclude simulated grouped calcifications caused by the superimposition of dispersed calcific particles (Box 3-8).

Box 3-9   Ductal Carcinoma In Situ

Beware of clusters containing
    A linear calcification
    Many more calcifications on magnification than
        initially suspected on the screening mammogram

Calcifications in malignancy are tightly clustered, vary in size and shape, and have bizarre branching irregular or linear forms consisting of at least five discrete particles smaller than 0.5 mm distributed over a 1 cm^3 region (Box 3-9). Calcifications that meet these criteria and do not have a characteristic benign appearance should be viewed with suspicion (Figs. 3-24 and 3-25).

Calcifications in malignancy are most commonly seen in invasive ductal carcinoma and DCIS. Calcifications are also seen in papillary carcinoma, but this is a rarer form of cancer. Calcifications are rarely seen in lobular carcinoma in situ (LCIS); typically, LCIS has no mammographic findings and is an incidental finding on a biopsy performed for another radiologic abnormality or patient symptom (Box 3-10). The extremely rare osteogenic sarcoma of the breast contains calcifications, but these sarcomas look like bone. Calcifications are not a feature of invasive lobular carcinoma.

DCIS is classified into high-, intermediate-, and low-grade forms. The descriptive histologic architecture of DCIS is also used in pathology reports. Comedocarcinoma extrudes thick tenacious material like a pimple and often calcifies centrally. The terms micropapillary, solid, and cribriform reflect the DCIS architecture in the duct. When suspicious calcifications are the only sign of malignancy, one may suspect DCIS, but the presence of frank invasion or microinvasion cannot be predicted, which is why percutaneous sampling of suspicious calcifications is preferred for optimal planning of surgical management. If breast conservation is desired, sentinel lymph node biopsy or axillary lymph node dissection is required for prognosis and planning of treatment, and general anesthesia is necessary. If the tumor contains only DCIS, axillary lymph node dissection is less commonly performed, and the patient may undergo only excisional biopsy under local anesthesia before radiation therapy.

Stability of Pleomorphic Calcifications

In general, calcifications in cancer are usually new or increasing over time. Occasionally, suspicious pleomorphic calcifications are stable, as shown by Lev-Toaff et al. In their study, calcifications in DCIS or invasive ductal cancer

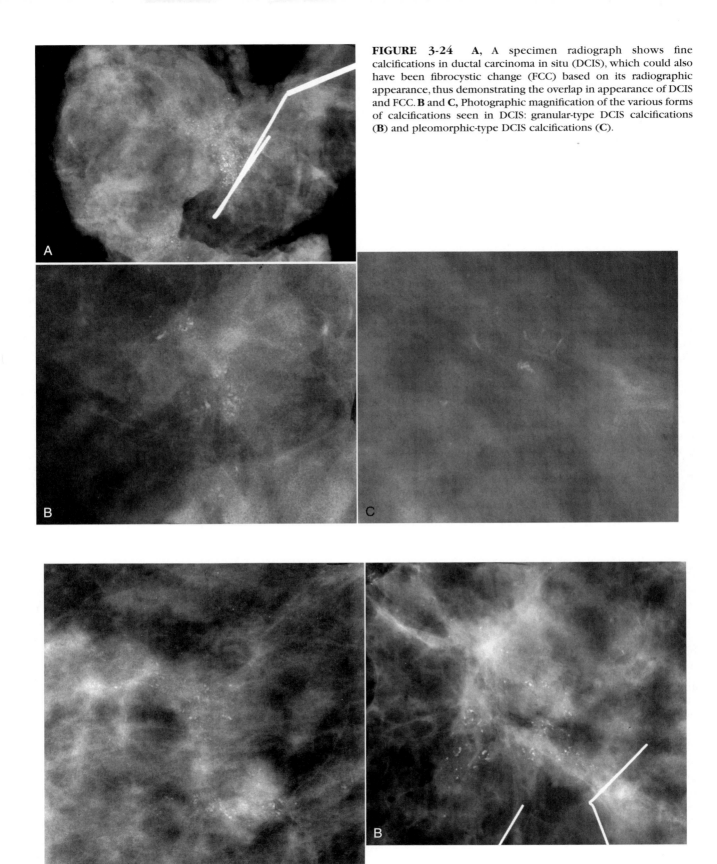

FIGURE 3-24 **A,** A specimen radiograph shows fine calcifications in ductal carcinoma in situ (DCIS), which could also have been fibrocystic change (FCC) based on its radiographic appearance, thus demonstrating the overlap in appearance of DCIS and FCC. **B** and **C,** Photographic magnification of the various forms of calcifications seen in DCIS: granular-type DCIS calcifications (**B**) and pleomorphic-type DCIS calcifications (**C**).

FIGURE 3-25 **A,** Grouped bizarre calcifications formed within an invasive ductal carcinoma as shown on magnification mammography. **B,** A specimen radiograph shows the hookwire and pleomorphic calcifications to greater advantage. Pleomorphic calcifications without an associated mass may represent invasive ductal cancer or DCIS and are indistinguishable.

were reviewed on previous examinations. Malignant-appearing calcifications were stable over a 6- to 50-month period, even when proved to represent DCIS at surgery. Changing pleomorphic calcifications were more likely to be associated with invasive cancer than with DCIS. These findings indicate that suspicious, pleomorphic calcifications may represent DCIS or invasive ductal cancer even if they are stable and that biopsy should be performed on suspicious pleomorphic calcifications.

INDETERMINATE CALCIFICATIONS AND MANAGEMENT

Even after careful analysis, some calcifications are indeterminate for malignancy (Figs. 3-26 to 3-28). At this point, either surgical biopsy, percutaneous biopsy, or periodic short-term mammographic follow-up may be recommended, depending on the clinical history and desires of the patient and referring physician. On the other hand, periodic mammographic follow-up to confirm stability is an accepted method of follow-up for probably benign lesions if the calcifications have less than a 2% chance of malignancy. Periodic follow-up at 6 months and then yearly for 2 to 3 years can be undertaken if the calcifications are round or punctate, have no malignant features, and are stable. New, increasing, or pleomorphic calcifications should be biopsied (Figs. 3-29 and 3-30). Specifically, short-term follow-up is an option only if the likelihood is high that the calcifications will *not* change. If this alternative is chosen, careful documentation of each follow-up visit is especially important in practices that accept self-referred women because in these cases, the radiologist becomes the "referring physician" and assumes primary care of the woman.

As regards biopsy of isolated clusters of tiny calcifications, a 20% to 30% true-positive biopsy rate for cancer is acceptable in the United States. It is to be expected that many benign biopsies will be obtained in the search for small carcinomas. Because some calcification clusters considered somewhat suspicious for malignancy ultimately prove to be benign, an audit of one's own practice is the only method to determine the local biopsy yield of cancer.

Ultrasound in Evaluation of Calcifications

Some preliminary scientific studies have shown that high-resolution ultrasound can detect calcifications in the breast. Though controversial, some investigators suggest that ultrasound scans in the region of calcification are helpful if the scan shows a suspicious mass representing invasive ductal cancer or if it pinpoints the calcifications for percutaneous biopsy (Fig. 3-31). Further studies and population-based studies would be needed to establish the scientific evidence to recommend this practice.

KEY ELEMENTS

Pleomorphic calcifications without a mass are important because they may represent DCIS or invasive ductal cancer.

Calcifications are not a feature of invasive lobular carcinoma.

Use a magnifier to view the mammogram; use magnification views to work up calcifications.

Recognize but do not biopsy dermal calcifications, milk of calcium, secretory disease (plasma cell mastitis), degenerating fibroadenomas, dystrophic calcifications, vascular calcifications, calcifying implant capsules, and silicone injection calcifications.

Tangential views are used to identify and diagnose skin calcifications.

Calcifications in malignancy occur in the parenchyma of the breast.

Carefully analyze individual calcification shapes in clustered, linear, and segmental calcification distributions.

Suggested Readings (*See page 88*)

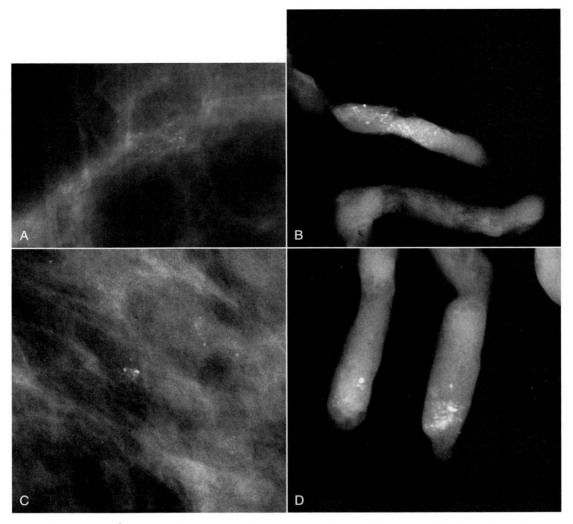

FIGURE 3-26   **A,** Isolated round punctate and amorphous calcifications grouped in the outer portion of the right breast on the craniocaudal view are of indeterminate suspicion for malignancy (20% to 30% likelihood of cancer). **B,** Calcifications contained within stereotactic core biopsy specimens represent fibrocystic change, sclerosing adenosis, and microcalcifications. **C,** Indeterminate round and amorphous calcifications in another patient. **D,** Stereotactic core biopsy specimens contain the calcifications, which proved to be due to nonproliferative fibrocystic change.

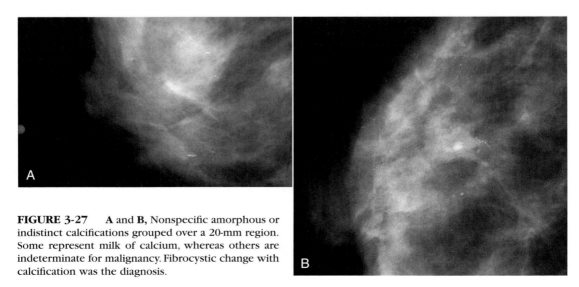

FIGURE 3-27   **A** and **B,** Nonspecific amorphous or indistinct calcifications grouped over a 20-mm region. Some represent milk of calcium, whereas others are indeterminate for malignancy. Fibrocystic change with calcification was the diagnosis.

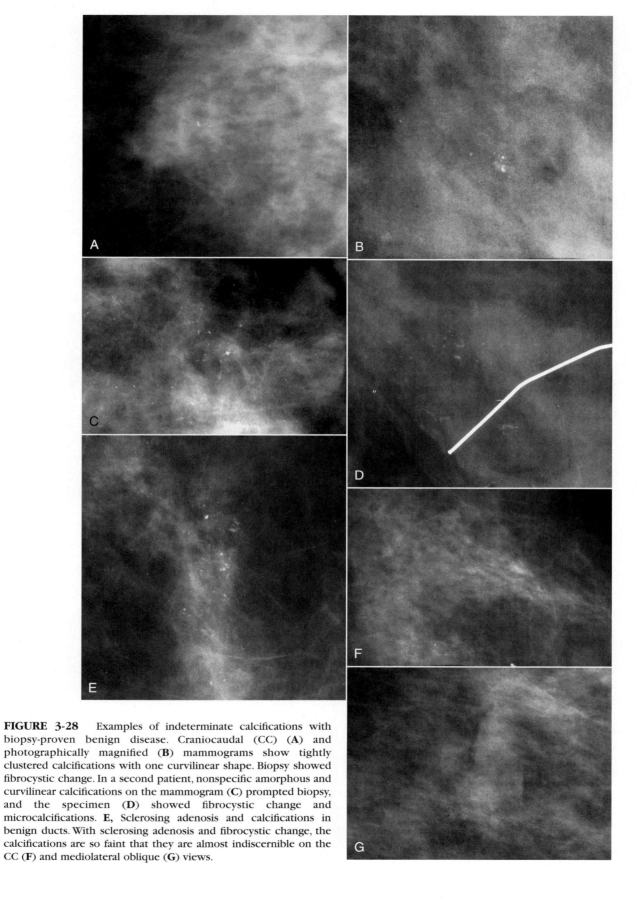

FIGURE 3-28   Examples of indeterminate calcifications with biopsy-proven benign disease. Craniocaudal (CC) (**A**) and photographically magnified (**B**) mammograms show tightly clustered calcifications with one curvilinear shape. Biopsy showed fibrocystic change. In a second patient, nonspecific amorphous and curvilinear calcifications on the mammogram (**C**) prompted biopsy, and the specimen (**D**) showed fibrocystic change and microcalcifications. **E,** Sclerosing adenosis and calcifications in benign ducts. With sclerosing adenosis and fibrocystic change, the calcifications are so faint that they are almost indiscernible on the CC (**F**) and mediolateral oblique (**G**) views.

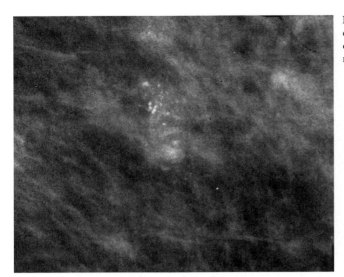

FIGURE 3-29 Round, clustered calcifications variable in size and density. Biopsy showed lobular carcinoma in situ (LCIS) with calcifications, a rare finding because LCIS does not usually have any mammographic features or calcifications.

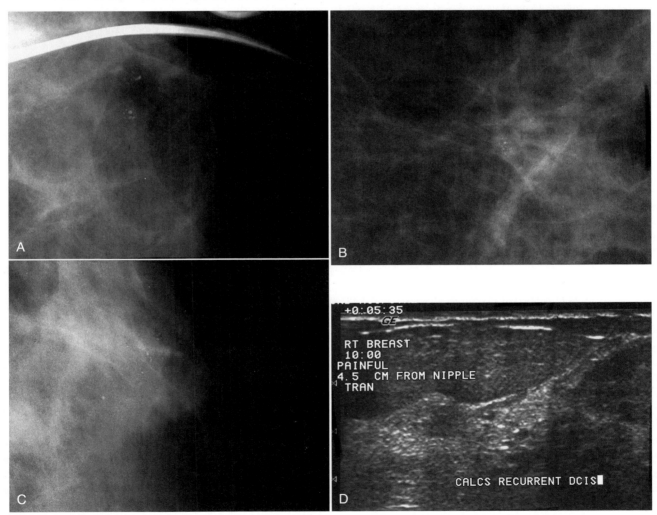

FIGURE 3-30   Ductal Carcinoma In Situ (DCIS) Manifested As Benign-Appearing, but New Calcifications. A, A tight cluster of round punctate calcifications was suspicious because they were not evident on the previous screening 12 months earlier. Stereotactic core biopsy showed ductal carcinoma in situ (DCIS). **B,** Faint tight cluster of round and granular calcifications in another patient. **C,** New, loosely grouped granular and amorphous calcifications. **D,** DCIS calcifications in **C** shown on ultrasound. Note that although calcifications can be seen, they might be difficult to detect without previous knowledge of their location.

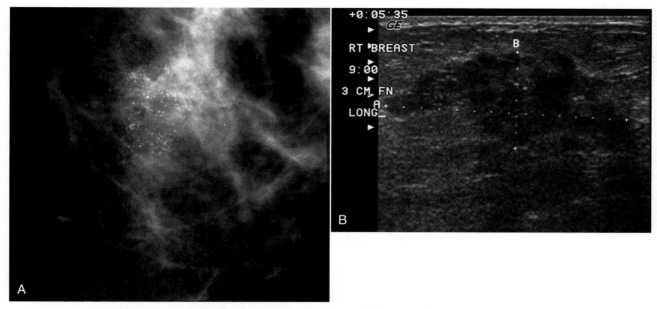

FIGURE 3-31   Calcifications on Ultrasound. The role of ultrasound in detecting calcifications is controversial, but it may be helpful if the scan shows a mass in a location known to have calcifications. **A,** Mammography shows suspicious clustered pleomorphic calcifications in a patient with Paget's disease of the nipple. **B,** Hypoechoic, irregular mass containing calcifications. Pathologic examination showed invasive lobular and ductal cancer and ductal carcinoma in situ with calcifications.

SUGGESTED READINGS

Adair FE, et al: Plasma cell mastitis—lesion simulating mammary carcinoma: Clinical and pathologic study with a report of 10 cases. Arch Surg 26:735-749, 1933.

Adair FE, et al: Fat necrosis of the female breast. Am J Surg 74:117-128, 1947.

Bassett LW, Gold RH, Mirra JM: Nonneoplastic breast calcifications in lipid cysts: Development after excision and primary irradiation. AJR Am J Roentgenol 138:335-338, 1982.

Berkowitz JE, Gatewood OM, Donovan GB, Gayler BW: Dermal breast calcifications: Localization with template-guided placement of skin marker. Radiology 163:282, 1987.

Black JW, Young B: A radiological and pathological study of the incidence of calcification in diseases of the breast and neoplasms of other tissues. Br J Radiol 38:596-598, 1965.

Brenner RJ, Sickles EA: Acceptability of periodic follow-up as an alternative to biopsy for mammographically detected lesions interpreted as probably benign. Radiology 171:645-646, 1989.

Coren GS, Libshitz HI, Patchefsky AS: Fat necrosis of the breast: Mammographic and thermographic findings. Br J Radiol 47:758-762, 1974.

Dershaw DD, Abramson A, Kinne DW: Ductal carcinoma in situ: Mammographic findings and clinical implications. Radiology 170:411-415, 1989.

Dershaw DD, Chaglassian TA: Mammography after prosthesis placement for augmentation or reconstructive mammoplasty. Radiology 170(Pt 1):69-74, 1989.

Dershaw DD, Shank B, Reisinger S: Mammographic findings after breast cancer treatment with local excision and definitive irradiation. Radiology 164:455-461, 1987.

DiPiro PJ, Meyer JE, Frenna TH, Denison CM: Seat belt injuries of the breast: Findings on mammography and sonography. AJR Am J Roentgenol 164:317-320, 1995.

D'Orsi CJ, Feldhaus L, Sonnenfeld M: Unusual lesions of the breast. Radiol Clin North Am 21:67-80, 1983.

Egan RL, McSweeney MB, Sewell CW: Intramammary calcifications without an associated mass in benign and malignant diseases. Radiology 137(Pt 1):1-7, 1980.

Evans AJ, Wilson AR, Burrell HC, et al: Mammographic features of ductal carcinoma in situ (DCIS) present on previous mammography. Clin Radiol 54: 644-646, 1999.

Gershon-Cohen J, Ingleby H, Hermel MB: Calcification in secretory disease of the breast. AJR Am J Roentgenol 76:132-135, 1956.

Harnist KS, Ikeda DM, Helvie MA: Abnormal mammogram after steering wheel injury. West J Med 159: 504-506, 1993.

Helvie MA, Baker DE, Adler DD, et al: Radiographically guided fine-needle aspiration of nonpalpable breast lesions. Radiology 174(Pt 1):657-661, 1990.

Helvie MA, Rebner M, Sickler EA, Oberman HA: Calcifications in metastatic breast carcinoma in axillary lymph nodes. AJR Am J Roentgenol 151:921-922, 1988.

Holland R, Hendriks JH: Microcalcifications associated with ductal carcinoma in situ: Mammographic-pathologic correlation. Semin Diagn Pathol 11:181-192, 1994.

Hunter TB, Roberts CC, Hunt KR, Fajardo LL: Occurrence of fibroadenomas in postmenopausal women referred for breast biopsy. J Am Geriatr Soc 44:61-64, 1996.

Ikeda DM, Sickles EA: Mammographic demonstration of pectoral muscle microcalcifications. AJR Am J Roentgenol 151:475-476, 1988.

Kopans DB, Meyer JE, Homer MJ, Grabbe J: Dermal deposits mistaken for breast calcifications. Radiology 149:592-594, 1983.

Kopans DB, Nguyen PL, Koerner FC, et al: Mixed form, diffusely scattered calcifications in breast cancer with apocrine features. Radiology 177:807-811, 1990.

Krishnamurthy R, Whitman GJ, Stelling CB, Kushwaha AC: Mammographic findings after breast conservation therapy. Radiographics 19(Spec No): S53-S62, quiz S262-S263, 1999.

Lanyi M: Diagnosis and Differential Diagnosis of Breast Calcifications. Springer-Verlag, 1988.

Lev-Toaff AS, Feig SA, Saitas VL, et al: Stability of malignant breast microcalcifications. Radiology 192(1):153-156, 1994.

Linden SS, Sickles EA: Sedimented calcium in benign breast cysts: The full spectrum of mammographic presentations. AJR Am J Roentgenol 152:967-971, 1989.

Mercado CL, Koenigsberg TC, Hamele-Bona D, Smith SJ: Calcifications associated with lactational changes of the breast: Mammographic findings with histologic correlation. AJR Am J Roentgenol 179:685-689, 2002.

Millis RR, Davis R, Stacey AJ: The detection and significance of calcifications in the breast: A radiological and pathological study. Br J Radiol 49:12-26, 1976.

Murphy WA, DeSchryver-Kecskemeti K: Isolated clustered microcalcifications in the breast: Radiologic-pathologic correlation. Radiology 127:335-341, 1978.

Orson LW, Cigtay OS: Fat necrosis of the breast: Characteristic xeromammographic appearance. Radiology 146:35-38, 1983.

Rebner M, Pennes DR, Adler DD, et al: Breast microcalcifications after lumpectomy and radiation therapy. Radiology 170(Pt 1): 691-693, 1989.

Ross BA, Ikeda DM, Jackman RJ, Nowels KW: Milk of calcium in the breast: Appearance on prone stereotactic imaging. Breast J 7:53-55, 2001.

Sickles EA: Further experience with microfocal spot magnification mammography in the assessment of clustered breast microcalcifications. Radiology 137(Pt 1):9-14, 1980.

Sickles EA: Mammographic detectability of breast microcalcifications. AJR Am J Roentgenol 139:913-918, 1982.

Sickles EA: Breast calcifications: Mammographic evaluation. Radiology 160:289-293, 1986.

Sickles EA: Mammography screening and the self-referred woman. Radiology 166(Pt 1):271-273, 1988.

Sickles EA, Abele JS: Milk of calcium within tiny benign breast cysts. Radiology 141:655-658, 1981.

Sigfusson BF, Andersson I, Aspegren K, et al: Clustered breast calcifications. Acta Radiol Diagn (Stockh) 24:273-281, 1983.

Spring DB, Kimbrell-Wilmot K: Evaluating the success of mammography at the local level: How to conduct an audit of your practice. Radiol Clin North Am 25:983-992, 1987.

Stomper PC, Connolly JL: Ductal carcinoma in situ of the breast: Correlation between mammographic calcification and tumor subtype. AJR Am J Roentgenol 159:483-485, 1992.

Stucker DT, Ikeda DM, Hartman AR, et al: New bilateral microcalcifications at mammography in a postlactational woman: Case report. Radiology 217:247-250, 2000.

Witten D: The Breast. An Atlas of Tumor Radiology. Chicago, Year Book, 1969.

CHAPTER 4

Mammographic and Ultrasound Analysis of Breast Masses

Introduction
Mammographic Technique and Analysis
Ultrasound Technique and Analysis
Masses with Spiculated Borders and Sclerosing Features
    Cancer
        Invasive Ductal Cancer
        Invasive Lobular Carcinoma
        Tubular Cancer
    Post-biopsy Scar
    Fat Necrosis, Sclerosing Adenosis, and Other Benign Breast Disease
    Radial Scar
Solid Masses with Rounded or Expansile Borders
    Malignant Tumors
        Invasive Ductal Cancer
        Medullary Cancer
        Mucinous (Colloid) Carcinoma
        Papillary Carcinoma
        Intracystic Carcinoma
        Breast Metastasis
    Benign Tumors
        Fibroadenoma
        Phyllodes Tumor
        Papilloma
        Lactating Adenoma
        Adenoid Cystic Carcinoma
Solid Masses with Indistinct Margins
    Invasive Ductal Cancer
    Invasive Lobular Carcinoma
    Sarcoma
    Lymphoma
    Pseudoangiomatous Stromal Hyperplasia
    Squamous Cell Carcinoma
Masses Containing Fat
    Lymph Nodes
    Hamartoma
    Oil Cyst
    Lipoma
    Liposarcoma
    Steatocystoma Multiplex
Fluid-Containing Masses
    Cyst
    Hematoma/Seroma
    Necrotic Cancer
    Intracystic Carcinoma
    Intracystic Papilloma
    Abscess
    Sebaceous and Epidermal Inclusion Cysts
    Galactocele
Key Elements

INTRODUCTION

The American College of Radiology (ACR) Breast Imaging Reporting and Database System (BI-RADS) lexicon defines a breast mass as a three-dimensional space-occupying lesion that is seen on at least two mammographic projections. Otherwise, the finding should be called an asymmetry. Benign masses do not invade or traverse tissue margins and will usually have pushing or round borders. Because breast cancers invade the basement membrane and extend into the surrounding glandular tissue, in general, cancers produce an irregularly shaped mass with indistinct or spiculated margins, with a few exceptions. Thus, analysis of breast masses on mammography involves determination of the shape and margins of the mass and change over time.

Ultrasound evaluation of masses goes hand in hand with mammographic mass evaluation and is key to determining whether the mass is a cyst or a solid mass. The shape, border, and internal characteristics of solid masses on ultrasound lend important clues to the diagnosis of cancer or benign findings. This chapter will discuss the mammographic and ultrasound analysis of breast masses.

MAMMOGRAPHIC TECHNIQUE AND ANALYSIS

On mammograms, a true mass is about the same size, shape, and density in two projections, thereby confirming that it is a three-dimensional object rather than overlapping normal breast tissue. Fine-detail views such as spot compression or spot magnification mammograms assess the shape and margins of the mass. Mass shapes and borders are easiest to assess when displayed against a fatty background; thus, spot magnification views are most optimal in a projection in which the mass overlies

Table 4-1	ACR BI-RADS Mass Descriptors	
Shape	**Margin**	**Density**
Round	Circumscribed	High
Oval	Microlobulated	Equal
Lobular	Obscured	Low
Irregular	Indistinct	Fat containing
	Spiculated	

From ACR Breast Imaging Reporting and Data System (BI-RADS)—Mammography, 4th ed. Reston, VA, American College of Radiology, 2003.

fat. A lateral medial view triangulates the location of the mass and provides an orthogonal view for planning biopsies.

The ACR BI-RADS lexicon (Table 4-1) defines mass shapes as round, oval, lobular, or irregular, and as the shape of the mass becomes more irregular, the probability of cancer increases (Fig. 4-1). Once the shape of the mass has been established, it is important to evaluate the margins of the mass because a spiculated or ill-defined margin is significant for cancer.

The ACR BI-RADS lexicon describes mass margins as circumscribed (well defined or sharply defined), microlobulated, obscured by surrounding glandular tissue, indistinct, or spiculated. Masses that have well-circumscribed borders are likely to be benign, and less than 10% of cancers are smooth. Microlobulated masses have small undulations, like petals on a flower, and are more worrisome for cancer than are smooth masses. An obscured mass has a border hidden by overlapping adjacent fibroglandular tissue and cannot be assessed. An indistinct mass is worrisome for carcinoma because it suggests that the surrounding glandular tissue may be infiltrated by malignancy. Finally, spiculated masses are characterized by thin lines radiating from the central portion of the mass and are especially worrisome for cancer. Spiculations may be produced either by productive tumor fibrosis or by growth of tumor into the surrounding glandular tissue.

Mass density is important because high-density masses are especially worrisome for cancer. Dense masses contain

MASSES

FIGURE 4-1   Illustration of ACR BI-RADS Mass Shapes and Margins. The probability of cancer increases as mass shape progresses from round to irregular or as mass margin progresses from circumscribed to spiculated.

Box 4-1   ACR BI-RADS
Associated Findings

Skin retraction
Nipple retraction
Skin thickening
Trabecular thickening
Skin lesion
Axillary adenopathy
Architectural distortion
Calcifications

From ACR Breast Imaging Reporting and Data System (BI-RADS)—Mammography, 4th ed. Reston, VA, American College of Radiology, 2003.

Box 4-2   Masses and Microcalcifications

Beware of pleomorphic calcifications adjacent to a suspicious breast mass. Both the mass and the calcifications should undergo biopsy because the calcifications may represent ductal carcinoma in situ.

cells with a higher atomic number than do normal glandular tissue and fat. Low-density masses and masses with density equal to that of surrounding fibroglandular tissue are less worrisome for cancer. However, low-density cancers do exist, such as mucinous cancers. Fat-containing masses are almost always benign, except for the rare liposarcoma.

Associated findings are also important and should be reported (Box 4-1). In particular, calcifications in or around a suspicious mass are important for two reasons. First, calcifications around a breast cancer may represent ductal carcinoma in situ (DCIS). If the mass is cancer, subsequent excisional biopsy must remove both the mass and all surrounding suspicious calcifications to excise the entire malignancy (Box 4-2). Knowing the extent of the suspicious calcifications helps plan surgery (Fig. 4-2). Second, suspicious calcifications inside a mass may be an important indicator of malignancy and the need for biopsy. At histology, greater than 25% DCIS associated with invasive ductal cancer is known as an "extensive intraductal component" (EIC) and is called EIC+ (positive). Because EIC+ tumors have an increased risk of local recurrence, breast-conserving surgery is less successful.

Other important associated mammographic findings include skin thickening, which may indicate breast edema or focal tumor invasion; skin retraction or nipple retraction as a result of focal tumor tethering; axillary lymph node metastases; or architectural distortion.

ULTRASOUND TECHNIQUE AND ANALYSIS

The ACR BI-RADS ultrasound lexicon describes terms and features of breast masses that are key for the diagnosis of cancer (Table 4-2). Stavros and colleagues described other features that are often used in evaluating

breast masses (Box 4-3). Evaluation of a breast mass on ultrasound includes determining whether the mass is cystic or solid, along with careful analysis of the shape and borders of the mass by scanning in more than one plane. The analysis also includes evaluation of the boundary, internal echo pattern, and acoustic features of the mass; its effect on surrounding breast tissue; and the presence and location of calcifications. Ultrasound labeling includes the left or right breast, position of the mass in terms of clock face and/or quadrant, location in centimeters from the nipple, scan angle (radial or anti-radial, transverse or longitudinal), and imaging of lesion without and with calipers (Box 4-4). It is helpful to indicate whether the mass is palpable or nonpalpable.

By combining terms from the ACR BI-RADS ultrasound lexicon and the study of Stavros and colleagues, ultrasound findings suggestive of cancer include an irregular shape, noncircumscribed margins, a thick echogenic rim or halo, duct extension or other effect on surrounding breast tissue, microcalcifications, taller-than-wide configuration, and acoustic spiculation or acoustic shadowing. Benign ultrasound findings include no malignant features, a circumscribed border, intense homogeneous hyperechogenicity, fewer than four gentle lobulations, wider-than-tall configuration, and a thin echogenic capsule. Because benign and malignant features in solid masses overlap, common sense should play a major part of patient management in clinical practice.

It is often necessary to correlate palpable findings with ultrasound findings. To accomplish this task, an examining finger placed directly on the physical finding directs the scan. The sonographer scans over the finger palpating the mass to generate a ring-down shadow. Subsequent removal of the finger from under the probe produces a scan of the palpable finding and thus leaves no doubt that the palpable finding has been interrogated. A skin marker over the palpable finding and a repeat mammogram will show that the palpable, mammographic, and ultrasound findings correlate with each other.

To correlate *nonpalpable* ultrasound findings with mammographic findings, the sonographer identifies the ultrasound finding and places a finger, cotton-tipped swab, or large unwound paper clip under the transducer so that a ring-down shadow is superimposed over the

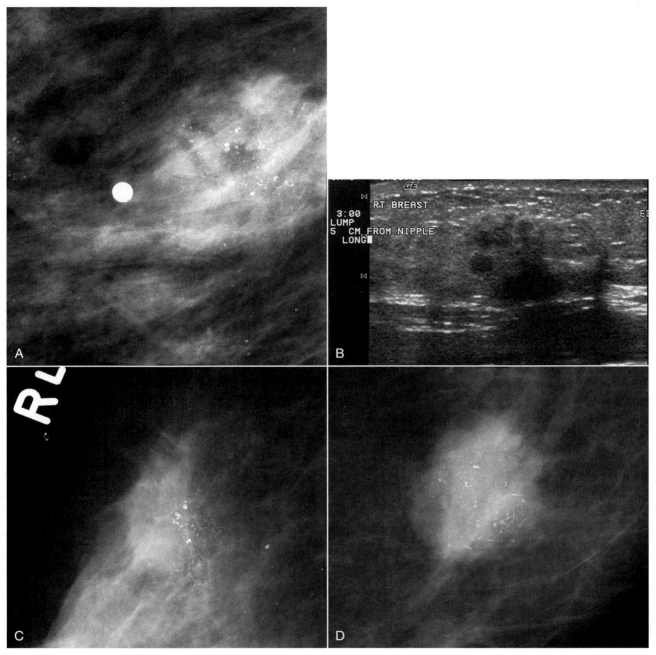

FIGURE 4-2   Relationship of Suspicious Masses and Calcifications. The mammogram shows a suspicious dense mass containing calcifications, as well as surrounding pleomorphic calcifications that represent invasive ductal cancer (the mass) and ductal carcinoma in situ (DCIS, the calcifications) (**A**). The radiologist reports both the mass and the extent of calcifications to ensure that all suspicious findings are removed at surgery. Ultrasound of this mass shows a microlobulated hypoechoic suspicious mass, but the calcifications are hard to see because of the speckles of surrounding normal breast tissue (**B**). A lateral medial mammogram in another patient shows a spiculated cancer with pleomorphic calcifications and adjacent microcalcifications near but not in the mass; biopsy showed invasive ductal cancer and DCIS with calcifications (**C**). Another patient with grade II invasive ductal cancer and DCIS has a suspicious irregular mass containing pleomorphic calcifications on the mammogram (**D**).

Table 4-2   ACR BI-RADS Ultrasound Lexicon Descriptors

Shape	Margin	Boundary	Echo Pattern	Posterior Acoustic Features
Oval	Circumscribed	Abrupt interface	Anechoic	No posterior acoustic features
Round	Angular	Echogenic halo	Hyperechoic	Enhancement
Irregular	Indistinct		Complex	Shadowing
	Microlobulated		Isoechoic	Combined
	Spiculated		Hypoechoic	

Effect on surrounding tissue: No effect, duct changes, Cooper's ligament changes, edema, architectural distortion, skin thickening, skin retraction/irregularity.
Calcifications: none, macrocalcifications (>0.5 mm), microcalcifications in or out of a mass.
From ACR Breast Imaging Reporting and Data System (BI-RADS)—Ultrasound. Reston, VA, American College of Radiology, 2003.

Box 4-3   Ultrasound Features of Solid Breast Masses

Malignant	Benign
Very hypoechoic	Intense homogeneous hyperechogenicity
Angulated margins	Four or fewer gentle lobulations
Acoustic shadowing	Thin echogenic pseudocapsule/ellipsoid shape
Microcalcifications	No malignant characteristics
Duct extension	
Taller than wide	
Spiculation	
Branch pattern	

From Stavros AT, Thickman D, Rapp CL, et al: Solid breast nodules: Use of sonography to distinguish between benign and malignant lesions. Radiology 196:123-134, 1995.

Box 4-4   Ultrasound Labeling

Right or left breast
Mass position in terms of clock face and/or quadrant
Location in centimeters from nipple
Scan angle (radial/antiradial, transverse/long)
Lesion without and with calipers

finding. The sonographer removes the transducer and marks this location on the skin with an indelible ink marker. A technologist places a metallic skin marker, such as a BB, on the ink spot and takes orthogonal mammographic views. The skin marker over the ultrasound finding should be in the same location as the mammographic finding on the films. It should be expected that the mammographic finding might be 1 cm or more away from the skin marker on the films because the metallic skin marker will be compressed away from the ultrasound finding on the mammogram.

If it is still uncertain whether an ultrasound and mammographic finding are one and the same and the patient agrees to an invasive procedure to make this determination, a metallic marker may be placed into the mass through an ultrasound-guided, percutaneously placed needle (Fig. 4-3). Repeat mammograms should show the marker in the mass if the two findings are one and the same. Alternatively, a retractable hookwire may be placed in the mass, a mammogram obtained to show

that the ultrasound finding and the mammographic finding are the same thing, with subsequent removal of the retractable hookwire once this determination is established.

The mammography and ultrasound report for a breast mass should describe the size, shape, margin, and density of the mass; its location and associated findings; and any change if previous examinations are available. The report should also include the ultrasound finding and whether it correlates with the mammographic finding. Finally, each report including a mammogram should be assigned an ACR BI-RADS code indicating the level of suspicion for cancer and follow-up management recommendations (Box 4-5).

MASSES WITH SPICULATED BORDERS AND SCLEROSING FEATURES (Box 4-6)

Cancer

Invasive Ductal Cancer

Invasive ductal carcinoma is the most common breast cancer and accounts for about 90% of all cancers. Also known as invasive ductal carcinoma not otherwise specified (NOS), ductal cancer usually grows as a hard irregular mass (Fig. 4-4). A classic appearance of invasive ductal cancer is a dense irregular or spiculated mass that

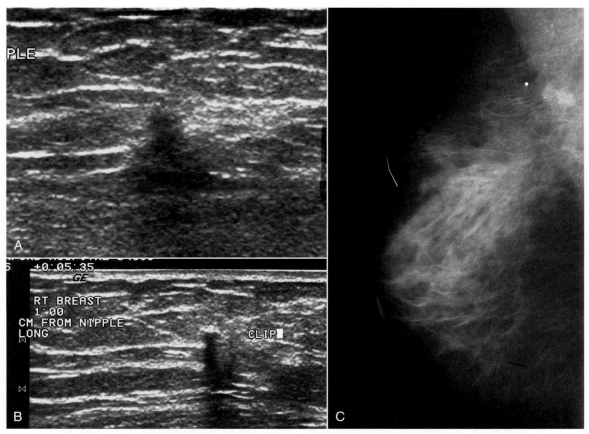

FIGURE 4-3   Ultrasound-Guided Marker Placement to Correlate Ultrasound and Mammography Findings. A patient with a mass seen on only the mediolateral oblique (MLO) view underwent ultrasound showing an ill-defined round mass with an echogenic rim and acoustic shadowing (**A**). Under ultrasound guidance a marker was placed in the mass (**B**), and a skin marker (BB) was placed over the position where ultrasound detected the mass. An MLO view shows the marker in the mass and the BB over the mass, thus proving that the ultrasound-detected finding represents the abnormality on mammography (**C**). This mass proved to be invasive ductal cancer.

Box 4-5   ACR BI-RADS Mass Reporting
Size and location
Mass type and modifiers (shape, margin, density)
Associated calcifications
Associated findings
How changed if previously present
Summary and BI-RADS code (0 to 6)

From ACR Breast Imaging Reporting and Data System (BI-RADS)—Mammography, 4th ed. Reston, VA, American College of Radiology, 2003.

Box 4-6   Differential Diagnosis of Spiculated Masses
Invasive ductal carcinoma
Invasive lobular carcinoma
Tubular cancer
Post-biopsy scar
Radial scar
Fat necrosis (atypical)
Sclerosing adenosis

occasionally contains pleomorphic calcifications and may have adjacent pleomorphic calcifications representing DCIS. On the mammogram, the mass is about the same size and density on two orthogonal mammographic views. Spot compression magnification views may show

unsuspected calcifications in or around the mass. Spiculated masses on the mammogram may be round, irregular, or spiculated on ultrasound and commonly produce acoustic shadowing as a result of either productive fibrosis or tumor extension, but shadowing is not

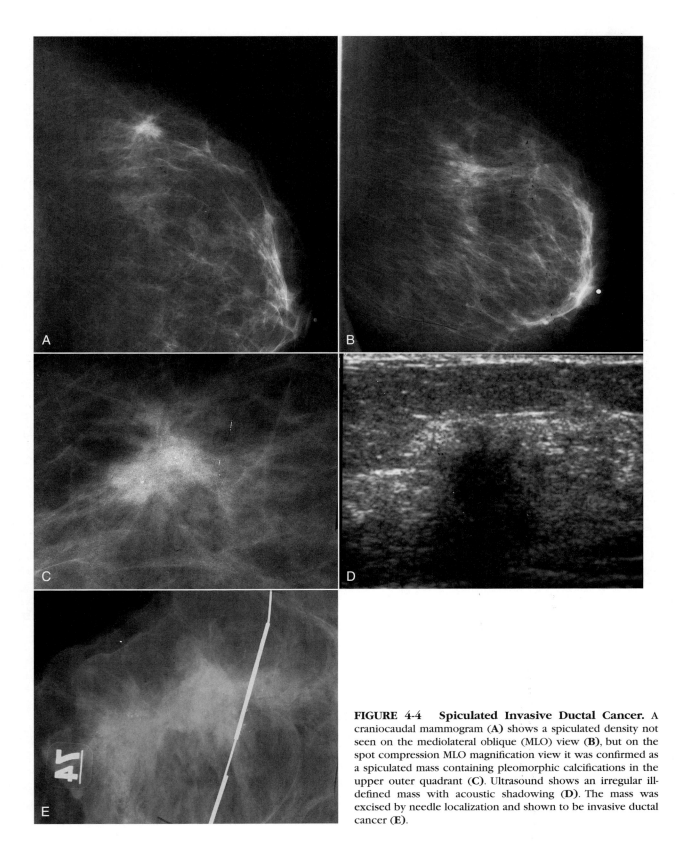

FIGURE 4-4   Spiculated Invasive Ductal Cancer. A craniocaudal mammogram (**A**) shows a spiculated density not seen on the mediolateral oblique (MLO) view (**B**), but on the spot compression MLO magnification view it was confirmed as a spiculated mass containing pleomorphic calcifications in the upper outer quadrant (**C**). Ultrasound shows an irregular ill-defined mass with acoustic shadowing (**D**). The mass was excised by needle localization and shown to be invasive ductal cancer (**E**).

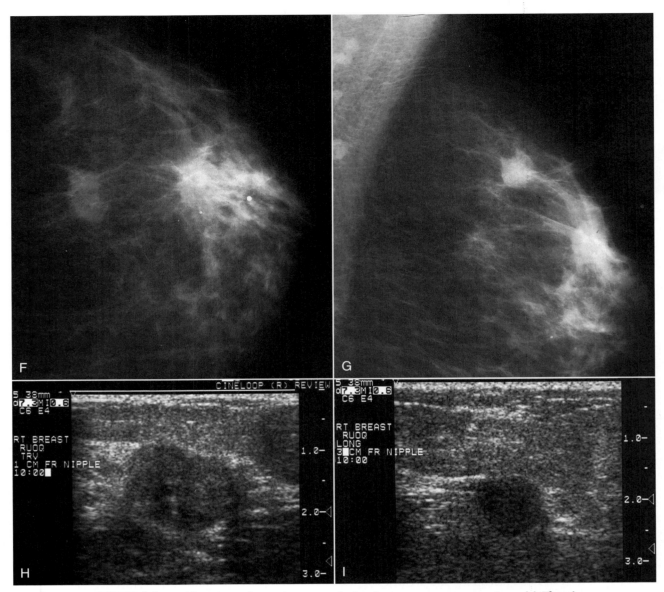

FIGURE 4-4 cont'd   In another patient, two spiculated masses are seen on craniocaudal (**F**) and MLO (**G**) views. Ultrasound of the spiculated masses shows an irregular mass (**H**) and a round mass (**I**) without sonographic spiculation. Invasive ductal cancers.

always present. When present, acoustic spiculation is seen as thin radiating lines extending from the tumor into surrounding breast structures. In a dense breast, the spicules are dark. In a fatty breast, the spicules appear white against the dark fatty background. On magnetic resonance imaging (MRI), the usual appearance of invasive ductal cancer is a brightly enhancing mass with or without spiculation; enhancement is rapid initially with a late-phase plateau or washout curve. Rim enhancement or enhancing internal septations are also a worrisome sign for invasive ductal cancer on MRI.

Invasive Lobular Carcinoma

Invasive lobular carcinoma is most commonly seen as an equal- or high-density noncalcified mass with spiculation or ill-defined borders. It has a higher rate of bilaterality and multifocality than does invasive ductal cancer. Invasive lobular carcinoma accounts for less than 10% of all invasive cancers, but it is historically the most difficult breast cancer to see on mammograms (Box 4-7). Classically, the tumor grows in single lines of tumor cells and infiltrates the surrounding glandular tissue, thus rendering it difficult to see by mammography and difficult to feel by physical examination. Invasive lobular carcinoma usually does *not* contain microcalcifications, is often seen on only one view, and may cause subtle distortion of the surrounding glandular tissue. When apparent on the mammogram, invasive lobular cancer masses are often of equal or higher density than fibroglandular tissue and are detected by visualization of the mass itself or by its effect on surrounding tissue, such as architectural distortion and straightening of Cooper's ligaments. Distortion is most easily seen in locations where ligaments extend out into surrounding fat from normal fibroglandular tissue and cause tenting of normal, scalloped fibroglandular tissue at the edge of the glandular tissue cone or in retroglandular fat (Fig. 4-5).

On ultrasound, invasive lobular cancer is a hypoechoic irregular spiculated or ill-defined mass that may or may not have acoustic shadowing. When invasive lobular carcinoma becomes very large, only the acoustic shadowing may be apparent and the mass itself is difficult to discern because of its large size. On MRI, it is detected to greater advantage than on mammography, with some limitations. Unfortunately, invasive lobular carcinoma has variable enhancing patterns, some similar to invasive ductal cancer and others resembling segmental nodular regions, or its enhancement may be difficult to distinguish from normal breast tissue and can thus be a cause of false-negative MRI examinations.

Tubular Cancer

Tubular carcinoma is a generally slow-growing tumor with a bilateral incidence of 12% to 40%. On mammog-

---

Box 4-7	Features of Invasive Lobular Cancer

Ten percent of all breast cancers
Grows in single-cell files
Hardest tumor to see on mammography
Often seen on one view
Causes mass or architectural distortion
Calcifications not a feature

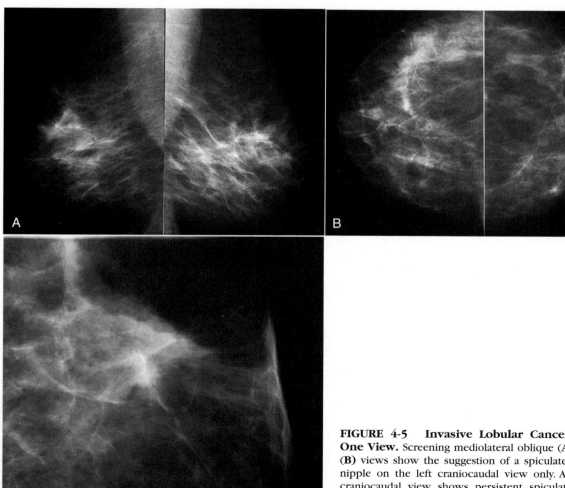

FIGURE 4-5 Invasive Lobular Cancer Seen on Only One View. Screening mediolateral oblique (**A**) and craniocaudal (**B**) views show the suggestion of a spiculated mass behind the nipple on the left craniocaudal view only. A spot compression craniocaudal view shows persistent spiculation and distortion caused by the invasive lobular carcinoma behind the nipple on the left (**C**). The straight lines extending from the tumor into subcutaneous tissue are indicative of its presence.

raphy, tubular cancer is a dense or equal-density spiculated mass with occasional microcalcifications, and on occasion it may be apparent on the previous mammogram because of its slow growth. Though controversial, some pathologists believe that radial scars may be a precursor to tubular carcinoma. In general, tubular carcinoma has a good prognosis and a lower incidence of metastases than does invasive ductal cancer. On ultrasound, tubular cancers are hypoechoic, irregular masses that occasionally produce acoustic shadowing (Fig. 4-6).

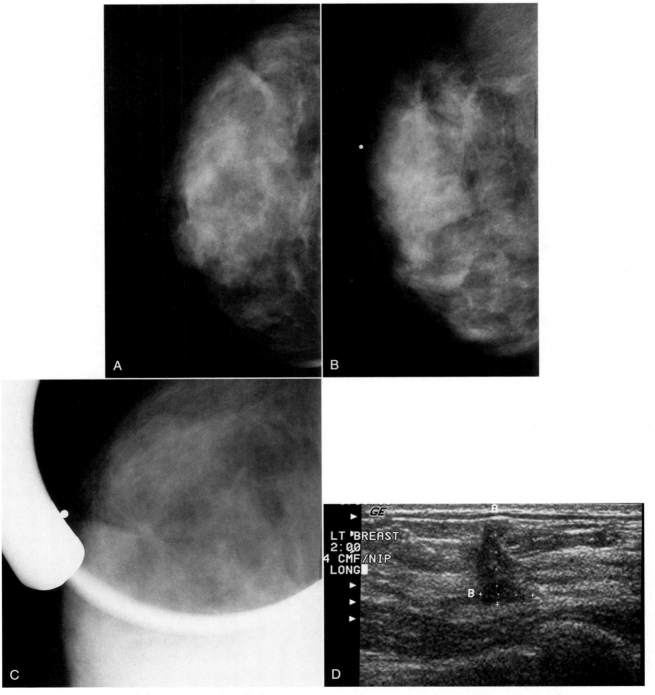

FIGURE 4-6   Spiculated Tubular Cancer. Craniocaudal (**A**) and mediolateral oblique (**B**) mammograms show a palpable spiculated mass in the upper outer quadrant of the right breast. Spot compression confirms the presence of the spiculated mass (**C**). Ultrasound shows a spiculated irregular mass that is taller than wide (**D**).   *Continued*

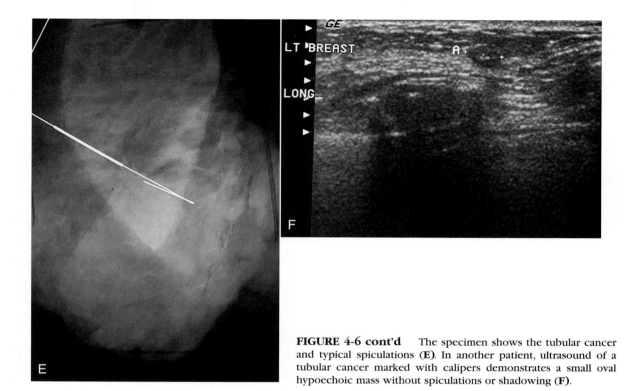

FIGURE 4-6 cont'd   The specimen shows the tubular cancer and typical spiculations (**E**). In another patient, ultrasound of a tubular cancer marked with calipers demonstrates a small oval hypoechoic mass without spiculations or shadowing (**F**).

Box 4-8

To determine whether a spiculated mass is a post-biopsy scar, look for a linear scar marker showing the location of the previous biopsy or correlate with old pre-biopsy mammograms.

Post-biopsy Scar

Initially, mammograms of post-biopsy scars obtained in the immediate postoperative period show air and fluid at the biopsy site. Later, the air and fluid are absorbed and the surrounding glandular tissue is drawn to a central dense nidus of scar tissue. As a result, the mammogram shows a centrally dense spiculated mass with straightening of the surrounding Cooper ligaments and indrawing of normal glandular tissue, findings simulating those of breast cancer. In some patients, no dense central nidus occurs, and the scar appears as a focal architectural distortion. On ultrasound, a post-biopsy scar is a hypo-echoic mass with acoustic spiculation and shadowing, similar to cancer. There should be distortion of sub-cutaneous tissue extending from the scar on the patient's skin in the plane of the incision down to the spiculated mass representing the post-biopsy scar.

A post-biopsy scar looks like spiculated cancer on both mammography and ultrasound but is not of concern for cancer if it can be shown to occupy a surgical site (Box 4-8). To distinguish post-biopsy scars from cancer, one correlates the location of the finding with previous biopsy locations on the breast history form. Review of older films will confirm that the presumed scar is located at the site of the removed finding. Some facilities place a radiopaque linear metallic scar marker on the skin scar to show the scar's location on the mammogram (Fig. 4-7A-D). Correlation of the metallic linear skin scar marker with the underlying spiculated finding and review of the pre-biopsy mammogram distinguish post-biopsy scars from other spiculated masses (Fig. 4-7E and F). Spiculated masses not corresponding to a post-biopsy scar should be considered suspicious and undergo histologic diagnosis.

Fat Necrosis, Sclerosing Adenosis, and Other Benign Breast Disease

Fat necrosis is due to saponification of fat from previous trauma, usually surgery or blunt trauma such as injury from a steering wheel or seat belt in an auto-mobile accident. On mammography, fat necrosis typically contains a fatty lipid center and is round in shape, but it

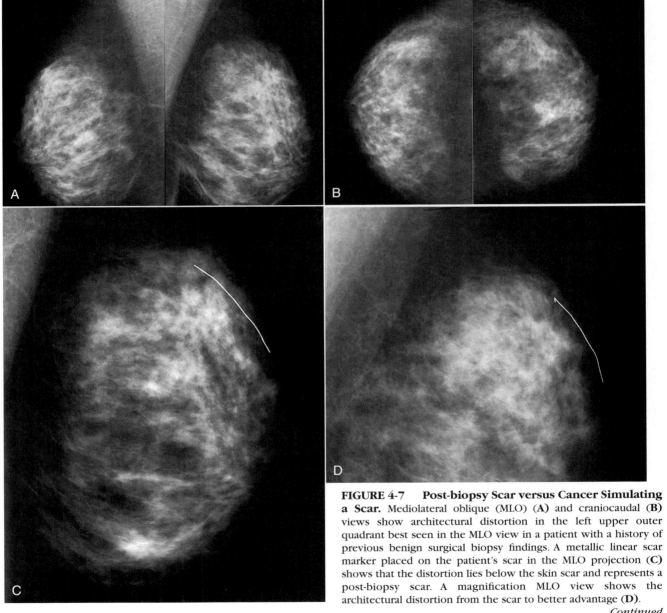

FIGURE 4-7   Post-biopsy Scar versus Cancer Simulating a Scar. Mediolateral oblique (MLO) (**A**) and craniocaudal (**B**) views show architectural distortion in the left upper outer quadrant best seen in the MLO view in a patient with a history of previous benign surgical biopsy findings. A metallic linear scar marker placed on the patient's scar in the MLO projection (**C**) shows that the distortion lies below the skin scar and represents a post-biopsy scar. A magnification MLO view shows the architectural distortion from the scar to better advantage (**D**).

Continued

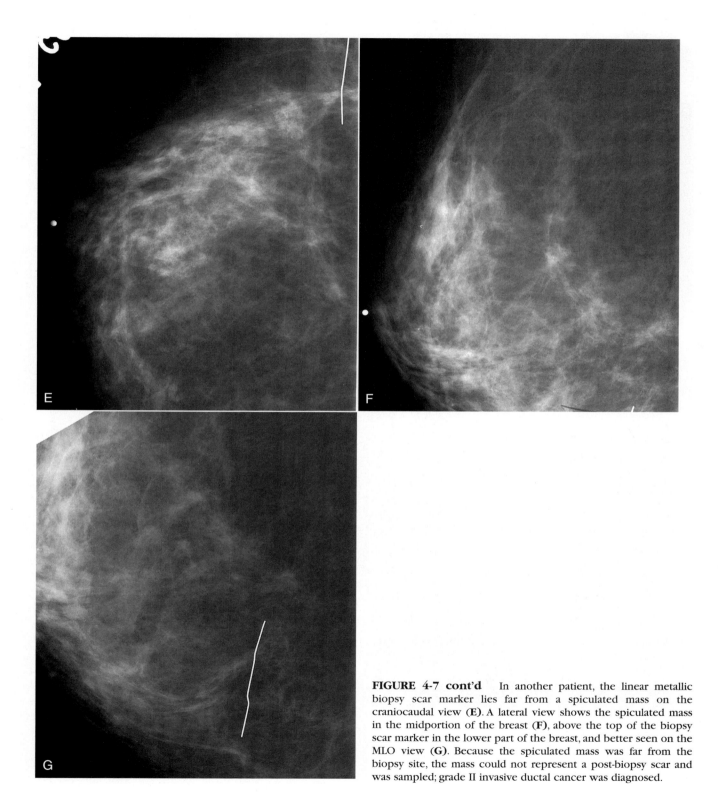

FIGURE 4-7 cont'd   In another patient, the linear metallic biopsy scar marker lies far from a spiculated mass on the craniocaudal view (**E**). A lateral view shows the spiculated mass in the midportion of the breast (**F**), above the top of the biopsy scar marker in the lower part of the breast, and better seen on the MLO view (**G**). Because the spiculated mass was far from the biopsy site, the mass could not represent a post-biopsy scar and was sampled; grade II invasive ductal cancer was diagnosed.

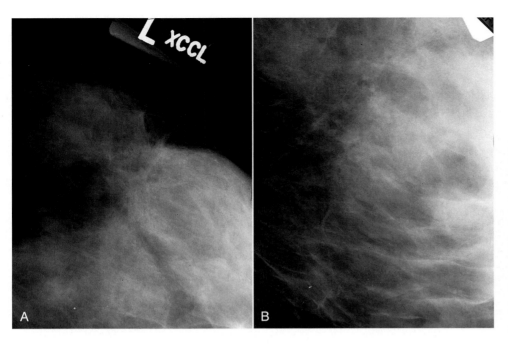

FIGURE 4-8 Proliferative Fibrocystic Change Appearing as Architectural Distortion. A magnification exaggerated craniocaudal view (**A**) shows architectural distortion that is very hard to see on the corresponding magnification mediolateral view (**B**) in the upper outer quadrant of the left breast. Excisional biopsy showed proliferative fibrocystic change and calcifications in benign ducts—a very unusual appearance of proliferative fibrocystic change.

occasionally has a spiculated appearance. The diagnosis may be established when eliciting a history of blunt trauma or previous surgery. On occasion, fat necrosis contains a dense or equal-density central nidus with radiating folds extending from its center, similar to cancer and thereby prompting biopsy.

Sclerosing adenosis is a proliferative benign lesion resulting from mammary lobular hyperplasia; it is characterized by the formation of fibrous tissue that distorts and envelops the glandular tissue. The resulting process produces sclerosis of the surrounding tissue, and small duct lumens may contain microcalcifications. On mammography, the spiculations associated with sclerosis can be difficult to distinguish from invasive cancer, and the microcalcifications can be difficult to distinguish from DCIS, thereby resulting in biopsy. There are almost no ultrasound studies of sclerosing adenosis.

Both sclerosing adenosis and proliferative fibrocystic change may have a slightly spiculated appearance on mammography, and they occasionally also contain calcifications. Spiculated fat necrosis, sclerosing adenosis, and benign breast disease that is spiculated cannot be distinguished from cancer and are therefore an indication for biopsy (Fig. 4-8).

Radial Scar

A radial scar is a benign proliferative breast lesion that has nothing to do with a post-biopsy scar. Both radial scars and their larger variants called complex sclerosing lesions may include adenosis and hyperplasia. In autopsy series, small radial scars are common on histologic examination but are not apparent mammographically. A radial scar has a central portion that undergoes atrophy, thereby resulting in a scar-like formation; pulling in of the surrounding glandular tissue produces a spiculated mass. On occasion, because of entrapment of breast ductules, the scar may be difficult for pathologists to distinguish from infiltrating ductal carcinoma. However, detection of both epithelial and myoepithelial cells in benign radial scar ductules by pathologic analysis will distinguish it from the single-cell population seen in breast cancer. Radial scars may contain or be associated with atypical ductal hyperplasia or low-grade DCIS and should be excised surgically, although the need for surgical excision after the diagnosis of a radial scar by core biopsy is controversial. Also controversial, some pathologists believe that a radial scar may be a precursor to tubular carcinoma and should be excised for this reason.

On mammography, a radial scar is a spiculated mass with either a dark or white central area that may or may not have associated microcalcifications (Fig. 4-9). It is a myth that radial scars have dark centers in the mass on mammography (Fig. 4-10) whereas breast cancers have white-centered masses. Such differentiation has been disproved by scientific studies showing that radial scars cannot be distinguished from breast cancer on mammograms on this basis, and it is therefore suggested that all spiculated masses not representing a post-biopsy scar be sampled histologically (Box 4-9). On ultrasound, a radial scar is a hypoechoic mass, with or without acoustic shadowing.

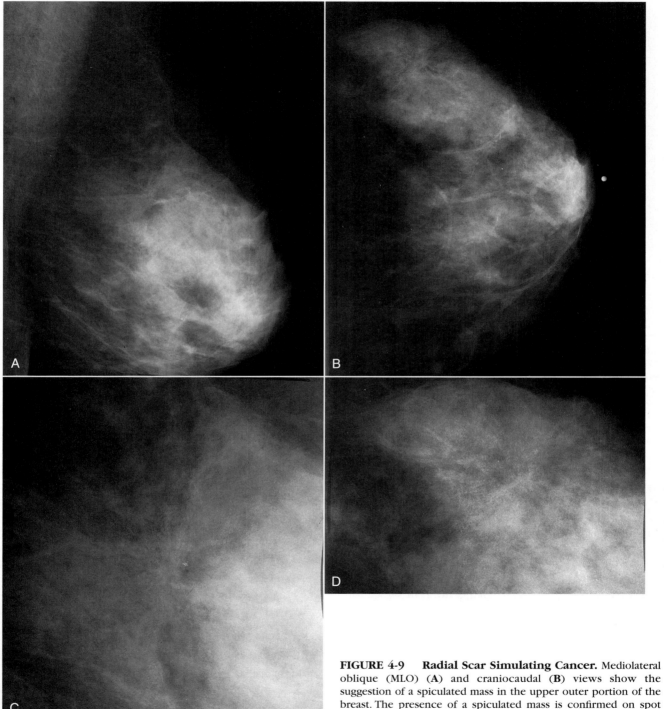

FIGURE 4-9   Radial Scar Simulating Cancer. Mediolateral oblique (MLO) (**A**) and craniocaudal (**B**) views show the suggestion of a spiculated mass in the upper outer portion of the breast. The presence of a spiculated mass is confirmed on spot magnification MLO (**C**) and craniocaudal (**D**) views.

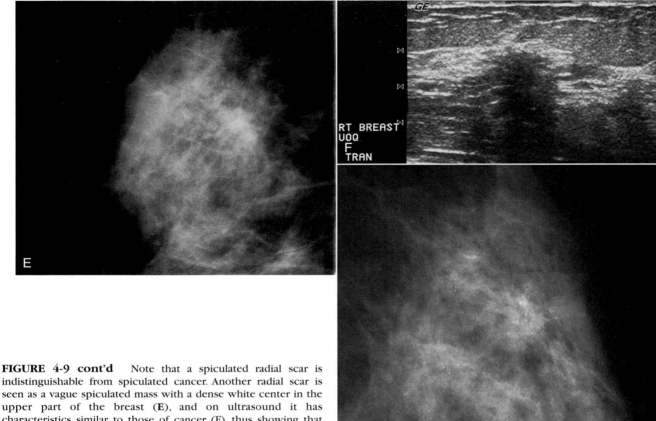

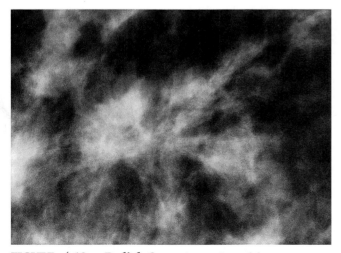

FIGURE 4-9 cont'd   Note that a spiculated radial scar is indistinguishable from spiculated cancer. Another radial scar is seen as a vague spiculated mass with a dense white center in the upper part of the breast (**E**), and on ultrasound it has characteristics similar to those of cancer (**F**), thus showing that radial scars can be indistinguishable from cancer on imaging. A radial scar in a third patient appears as a spiculated mass with associated calcifications and on biopsy contained high-grade ductal carcinoma in situ, fibrocystic change, and calcifications (**G**).

FIGURE 4-10   Radial Scar. A craniocaudal mammogram shows a dense spiculated mass suggestive of cancer. Spot compression magnification shows that the central dense portion of the mass is less dense but the architectural distortion remains. Cancer can look exactly the same.

Box 4-9

Radial scars cannot be distinguished from cancer on mammography. Spiculated masses not representing post-biopsy scar tissue require a histologic diagnosis.

SOLID MASSES WITH ROUNDED OR EXPANSILE BORDERS (Box 4-10)

Malignant Tumors

Invasive Ductal Cancer

Invasive ductal cancer is the most common round breast cancer (Fig. 4-11). Although the classic invasive ductal cancer is a dense spiculated or irregular mass on mammography, the less common round forms of invasive

---

Box 4-10   Differential Diagnosis of Round Masses

Cyst
Fibroadenoma
Invasive ductal cancer not otherwise specified (most common round cancer)
Medullary cancer
Mucinous (colloid) carcinoma
Papillary carcinoma
Intracystic carcinoma
Metastasis
Phyllodes tumor
Papilloma
Lactating adenoma
Adenoid cystic carcinoma
Sebaceous cyst (near skin)
Epidermal inclusion cyst (near skin or in breast after biopsy)

---

ductal cancer may grow so rapidly that spiculated margins are not produced. Because invasive ductal cancer represents about 90% of all invasive breast cancers, this uncommon form of the most frequent breast cancer is the most common histologic type of round cancer (Box 4-11).

On screening mammography, round invasive ductal cancer may appear to have a smooth border. However, magnification views may show irregular, microlobulated, or indistinct borders, thus suggesting invasion of surrounding tissue and the true diagnosis. On ultrasound, a round mass shape that is "taller than wide" is suspicious, particularly if the borders are not smooth and a thick echogenic rim is present. "Taller than wide" also describes a mass that has invaded through the normal horizontal tissue planes as defined by the thin echogenic Cooper ligaments. "Taller" means that the tumor extends up toward the skin and is violating normal tissue planes rather than growing horizontally between Cooper's ligaments like benign tumors. This ultrasonographic sign is important in the diagnosis of breast cancer.

Medullary Cancer

Medullary cancer is a variant of invasive ductal cancer that most commonly grows with a rounded or pushing border. On pathologic examination, medullary cancers occasionally display a surrounding lymphoid infiltrate and have a better prognosis than infiltrating ductal cancer (NOS) does. Atypical medullary cancers have the same prognosis as infiltrating ductal cancer. On screening mammography, medullary cancer appears as a high- or equal-density round mass whose margins may appear well circumscribed, suggestive of a cyst or fibroadenoma (Fig. 4-12). On ultrasound, medullary cancers are round, solid, and homogeneous and contain homogeneous tumor cells that may occasionally cause posterior acoustic enhancement. Because medullary cancer may simulate a breast cyst in terms of acoustic enhancement, careful attention to technical details during scanning will show that the internal features are hypoechoic rather than anechoic. Color or power Doppler may show internal vascularity, unlike an anechoic simple cyst. The pushing expansile growth of medullary cancer may produce well-circumscribed borders, similar to fibroadenoma, and is a cause for misdiagnosis.

Mucinous (Colloid) Carcinoma

This rare, round or oval tumor contains malignant tumor cells that float in mucin within a solid rim. The mucinous portion can have fibrovascular bands segregating the mucinous compartments that comprise most of the tumor, and a low-density round mass that can suggest a cyst or fibroadenoma is seen on mammography. On ultrasound, the tumor mass is round, occasionally contains fluid-filled hypoechoic spaces, and may have posterior acoustic enhancement (Fig. 4-13). The mass may simulate a cyst but will not be entirely anechoic. Thus, new round masses on a mammogram that do not have all the specific criteria for a simple cyst on ultrasound should be considered for biopsy.

Papillary Carcinoma

This rare tumor accounts for only 1% to 2% of all cancers and is the malignant form of benign intraductal papilloma. Papillary cancers may be single or multiple (Box 4-12), and DCIS is sometimes seen in surrounding breast tissue. Classically, these masses are round, oval, or lobulated on mammography, sometimes containing calcifications, and are solid on ultrasound. If associated with nipple discharge and detected by ultrasound, papillary cancers are solid intraductal masses outlined by a fluid-filled structure and difficult to distinguish from a benign intraductal papilloma (Fig. 4-14).

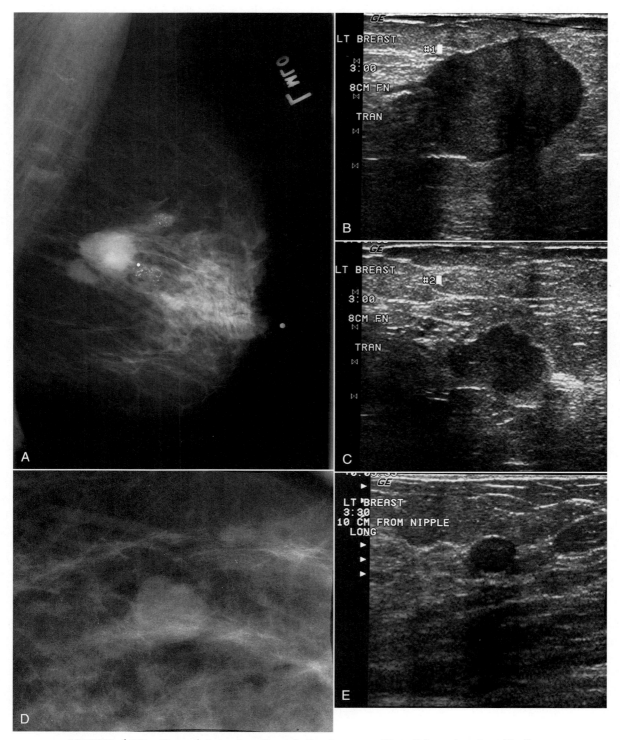

FIGURE 4-11   Round Invasive Ductal Carcinomas (Not Otherwise Specified). A mediolateral oblique mammogram shows a round dense mass with associated pleomorphic calcifications and a suggestion of smaller round masses adjacent to it **(A)**. Ultrasound shows an oval hypoechoic irregular mass **(B)** and a multilobulated mass **(C)**, both representing invasive ductal cancer. In another patient, a slightly lobulated, circumscribed, round equal-density mass on mammography **(D)** simulates a fibroadenoma; on ultrasound it has a benign circumscribed oval shape **(E)**. Biopsy showed invasive ductal cancer.

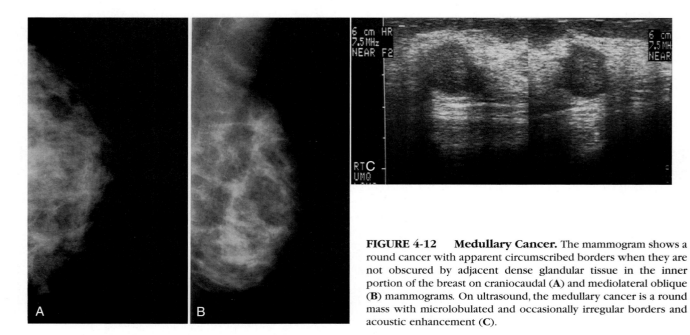

FIGURE 4-12   Medullary Cancer. The mammogram shows a round cancer with apparent circumscribed borders when they are not obscured by adjacent dense glandular tissue in the inner portion of the breast on craniocaudal (**A**) and mediolateral oblique (**B**) mammograms. On ultrasound, the medullary cancer is a round mass with microlobulated and occasionally irregular borders and acoustic enhancement (**C**).

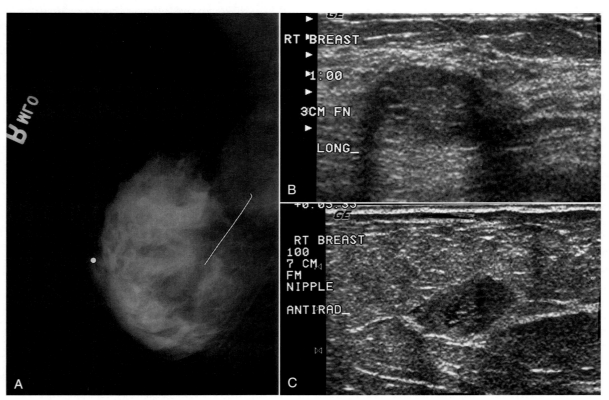

FIGURE 4-13   Mucinous Cancer. A mediolateral oblique mammogram shows dense tissue and a metallic scar marker over a previous benign biopsy site (**A**), and the palpable mass is not seen. Ultrasound shows an oval solid heterogeneous mass representing the mucinous cancer (**B**). Ultrasound of another patient with mucinous cancer (**C**) shows an oval heterogeneous mass containing fluid-filled spaces.

Cysts
Fibroadenomas
Multiple round invasive breast cancers
Metastases—vary in size, nonductal growth pattern
Papillomas—may grow in a ductal pattern
False masses: skin lesions

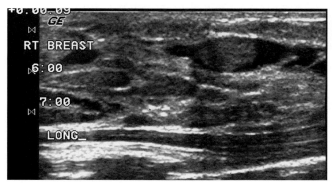

FIGURE 4-14   Papillary Carcinoma. Ultrasound of a papillary cancer shows a fluid-filled dilated duct with a solid oval intraductal solid mass that cannot be distinguished from a benign intraductal papilloma on the scan.

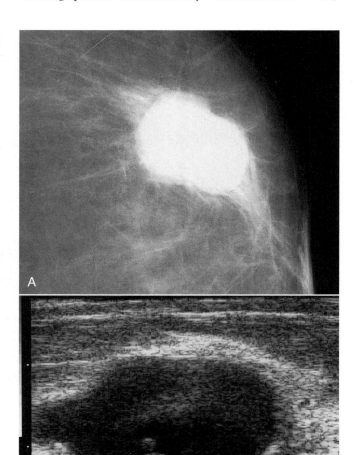

FIGURE 4-15   Intracystic Carcinoma. A mammogram shows a dense oval mass (**A**). Ultrasound shows a fluid-filled cyst with an irregular mural mass (**B**). Although this mass was an intracystic carcinoma, the differential diagnosis is papilloma or debris in a benign cyst.

Intracystic Carcinoma

This extremely rare tumor produces a solid mass in a cyst wall, and the mass looks like a cyst on mammography. Because the tumor is mostly fluid, the mammographic mass is low density unless it has a denser solid component or bleeding into the cystic portion that produces a dense mass (Fig. 4-15A). On ultrasound, an intracystic carcinoma is a solid mural mass surrounded by cystic fluid that yields fresh or old blood on aspiration (Fig. 4-15B). On pneumocystography, the air inside the cyst wall will outline a solid mass along the border of the cyst wall. Intracystic carcinomas must be excised, just as all other cancers are excised. The differential diagnosis for a solid intracystic mass is intracystic carcinoma, intracystic papilloma, and a cyst with debris adherent to the cyst wall.

Breast Metastasis

Metastasis to the breast can occur from breast cancer, lymphoma, or other malignancy spreading to an intramammary lymph node, or it may represent hematologic metastasis of cancer from breast or another primary tumor. On mammography, metastasis to an intramammary or axillary lymph node changes the normal benign lymph node shape and configuration from an oval or lobular shape with a central radiolucency and a defined rim to a rounder, bigger, and denser mass with loss of the fatty hilum (Fig. 4-16).

Hematologically spread metastases are single or multiple, round, usually circumscribed, and very dense, and they can vary in size as a result of the various lengths of time that the metastases have had to grow in breast tissue. Typically, the appearance of multiple new solid masses is worrisome for hematologic spread of carcinoma from a primary site other than in the breast, and they are displayed as new solid masses appearing all over the breast in a nonductal pattern, similar to pulmonary metastases. Melanoma and renal cell carcinoma have been noted to metastasize to the breast in this manner.

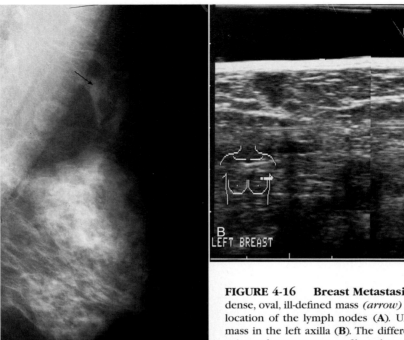

FIGURE 4-16   Breast Metastasis. A left lateral view shows a dense, oval, ill-defined mass *(arrow)* in the axilla in the expected location of the lymph nodes (**A**). Ultrasound shows a solid oval mass in the left axilla (**B**). The differential diagnosis is metastasis, primary breast cancer, or fibroadenoma. Biopsy showed metastatic renal cell carcinoma.

The differential diagnosis of multiple breast masses includes multiple fibroadenomas or papillomas.

Benign Tumors

Fibroadenoma

This most common solid benign tumor in young women is thought to arise from the terminal ductal lobular unit via localized hypertrophy. Fibroadenomas can be single or multiple. A fibroadenoma contains structures suggesting breast ductules and also has stromal tissue, which can be quite cellular in young women. Fibroadenomas may also undergo adenosis or hyperplasia and proliferation and may contain fibrous bands or septations. DuPont et al. suggest that fibroadenomas containing such proliferation or cysts be called "complex fibroadenomas." Giant fibroadenomas are fibroadenomas that are 8 cm or larger. Juvenile fibroadenomas occur in adolescents and can grow rapidly, stretch the skin, and become huge. Because juvenile fibroadenomas may grow to such a large size, they may be called giant fibroadenomas, but not all giant fibroadenomas are juvenile fibroadenomas.

On mammograms, the classic fibroadenoma is an oval or lobular equal-density mass with smooth margins, and in young patients, it is very cellular. As the fibroadenoma ages, it may become sclerotic and less cellular, and popcorn-like calcifications subsequently develop at the periphery of the mass. Subsequently, the entire mass may

be replaced by dense calcification. On ultrasound, fibroadenomas are oval, well-circumscribed homogeneous masses, usually wider than tall, with up to four gentle lobulations. They are hypoechoic but may occasionally contain cystic spaces. Posterior acoustic enhancement is increased, equal, or shadowing (Fig. 4-17). Fibroadenomas occasionally display irregular borders or heterogeneous internal characteristics, so biopsy is necessary to distinguish atypical fibroadenomas from cancer.

Because fibroadenomas contain ductal elements, rare cases of ductal or lobular carcinoma in situ occurring in fibroadenomas have been reported. Any suspicious change in a fibroadenoma should prompt biopsy for this reason.

On MRI, fibroadenomas have the classic appearance of an enhancing oval or lobulated mass with well-circumscribed borders, and they contain dark internal septations with a gradual initial enhancement rate and a late persistent enhancement curve. In premenopausal women, the initial enhancement may be as rapid as cancer *just before menses*, but unlike cancer, which shows late plateau or washout curves, the late enhancement curve is still persistent in fibroadenoma. In *the week or two after the onset of menses*, the initial enhancement curves will revert back to normal and show a gradual initial enhancement curve.

Phyllodes Tumor

Phyllodes tumors used to be called "cystosarcoma phyllodes," which is a misnomer because most of these

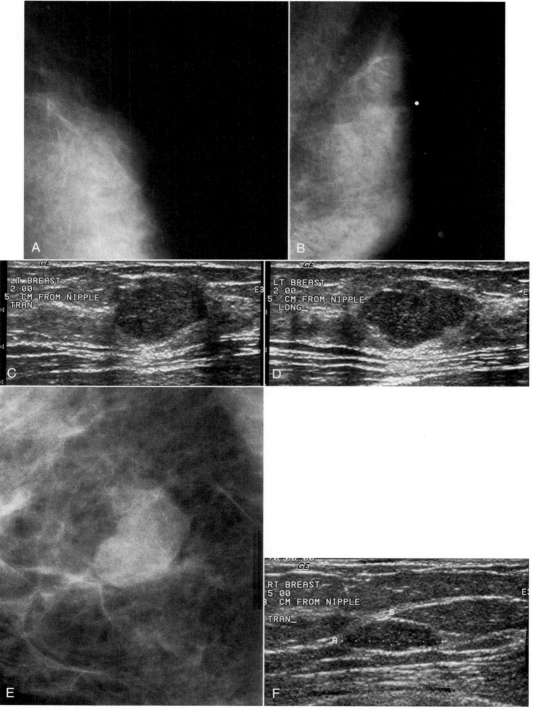

FIGURE 4-17   Biopsy-Proven Fibroadenomas. Magnification craniocaudal (**A**) and medio-lateral oblique (**B**) views show an equal-density, circumscribed oval mass in a young woman that is hard to see against the dense tissue. Ultrasound shows an oval, lobulated, well-circumscribed homogeneous mass on transverse (**C**) and longitudinal (**D**) scans. In another patient, the mammogram shows a lobular well-circumscribed mass whose borders are partly obscured (**E**). Ultrasound shows an oval well-circumscribed homogeneous mass (**F**).   *Continued*

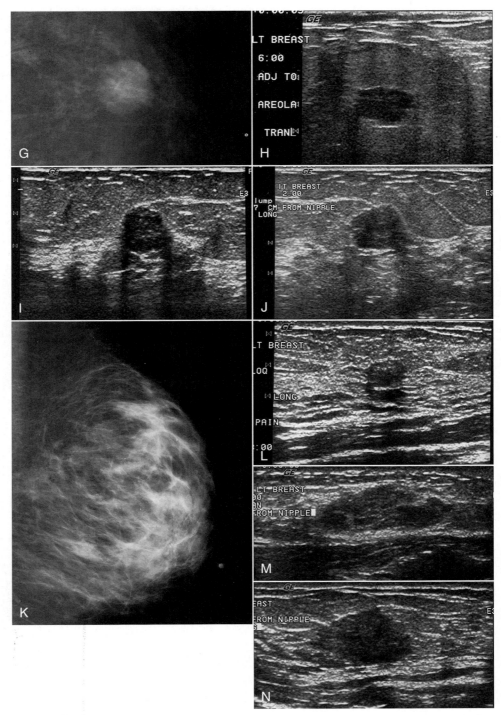

FIGURE 4-17 cont'd   Another patient has a round equal-density mass on a mammogram (**G**), but on ultrasound the mass is multilobulated and very hypoechoic (**H**), similar to cancer. Ultrasound of another atypical biopsy-proven fibroadenoma shows a taller than wide multilobulated mass with internal speckles (**I, J**). Ultrasound of another atypical palpable biopsy-proven microlobulated fibroadenoma (**L**); seen on the mammogram in the lower part of the breast in **K**. Other various atypical appearances of biopsy-proven fibroadenoma on ultrasound (**M** and **N**).

uncommon tumors are benign. Classically, the tumor occurs in women in their fifth decade and can be quite large, up to 5 cm in size when first detected. Most often women seek advice for a rapidly growing palpable mass. A phyllodes tumor has both stromal and epithelial elements, in contrast to fibroadenoma, as well as fluid-like spaces containing solid growth of cellular stroma and epithelium in a leaf-like configuration from which the tumor gets its name. Incomplete excision of either benign or malignant phyllodes tumors may result in local recurrence, and they may be excised again and again, only to grow back. About 10% of phyllodes tumors are malignant (range, 5% to 25%) and may metastasize to the lung. No distinguishing imaging features can be used to differentiate malignant phyllodes tumors from the more common benign form. On mammography, a phyllodes tumor is a dense round, oval, or lobulated noncalcified mass with smooth borders. On ultrasound, a phyllodes tumor is a smoothly marginated inhomogeneous mass that occasionally contains cystic spaces producing acoustic posterior enhancement, and it can be mistaken for a fibroadenoma or circumscribed cancer (Fig. 4-18). Treatment includes wide excisional biopsy.

Papilloma

Papillomas are either solitary or multiple and in young patients are called juvenile papillomas. Solitary papillomas

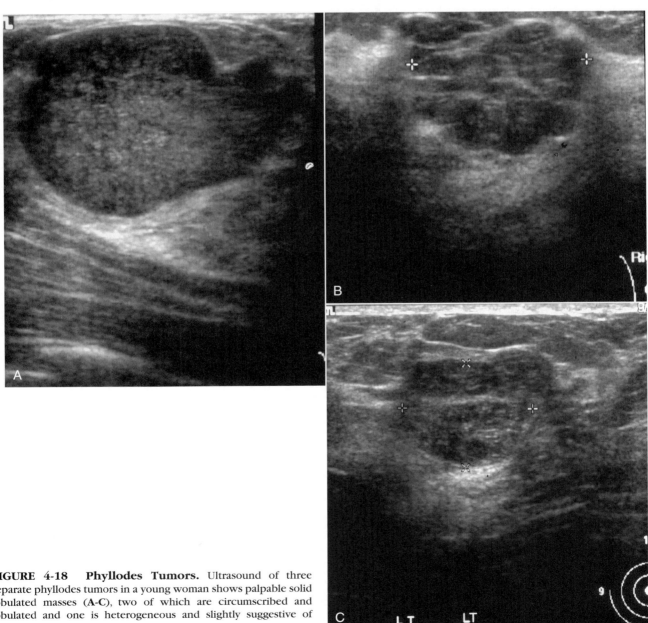

FIGURE 4-18   Phyllodes Tumors. Ultrasound of three separate phyllodes tumors in a young woman shows palpable solid lobulated masses (**A-C**), two of which are circumscribed and lobulated and one is heterogeneous and slightly suggestive of cancer.

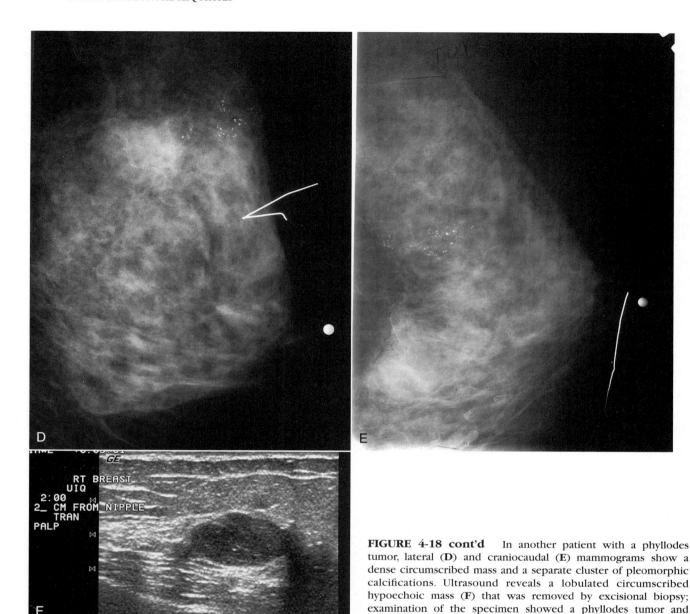

FIGURE 4-18 cont'd   In another patient with a phyllodes tumor, lateral (**D**) and craniocaudal (**E**) mammograms show a dense circumscribed mass and a separate cluster of pleomorphic calcifications. Ultrasound reveals a lobulated circumscribed hypoechoic mass (**F**) that was removed by excisional biopsy; examination of the specimen showed a phyllodes tumor and calcifications in benign ducts.

are central or peripheral, originate in the ductal epithelium, and are often seen in the subareolar region or in subareolar ducts. Multiple papillomas are usually in a more peripheral location in younger women. Juvenile papillomatosis occurs in young women but may be associated with the fibrocystic changes more often seen in much older women. Tumors starting in the terminal ducts further from the nipple are called peripheral papillomas and are considered a risk factor for breast cancer. Papillomas grow on fibrovascular stalks, which can twist and lead to ischemia, necrosis, and blood extending into the duct and result in the classic symptom of bloody nipple discharge, similar to the symptoms of

DCIS. Clinically, papillomas can also cause a spontaneous clear discharge, symptoms for which the patient seeks advice. Papillomas are usually excised to exclude the presence of DCIS.

On mammography, papillomas are round, well-circumscribed, equal-density masses that may contain calcifications; they are usually located in the subareolar region but can be multiple and peripheral in papillomatosis (Fig. 4-19). Often, papillomas are not seen on mammography or ultrasound at all. When seen on ultrasound, papillomas are solid round, oval, or microlobulated hypoechoic masses. Small internal cystic spaces are seen occasionally in juvenile papillomatosis. In patients with

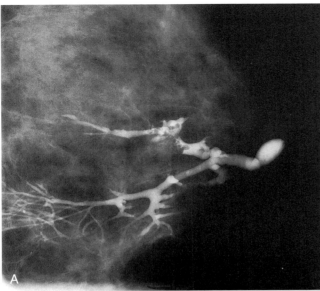

FIGURE 4-19 Papillomas. Craniocaudal **(A)** and mediolateral **(B)** magnification views of a galactogram show an irregular microlobulated filling defect from a papilloma. A galactogram in another patient shows a papilloma as a smooth filling defect obstructing a dilated duct **(C)**. A mammogram in another patient shows a palpable round irregular mass with calcifications **(D)**. Ultrasound shows a circumscribed oval homogeneous mass **(E)**. Biopsy revealed intraductal papilloma with apocrine atypia.

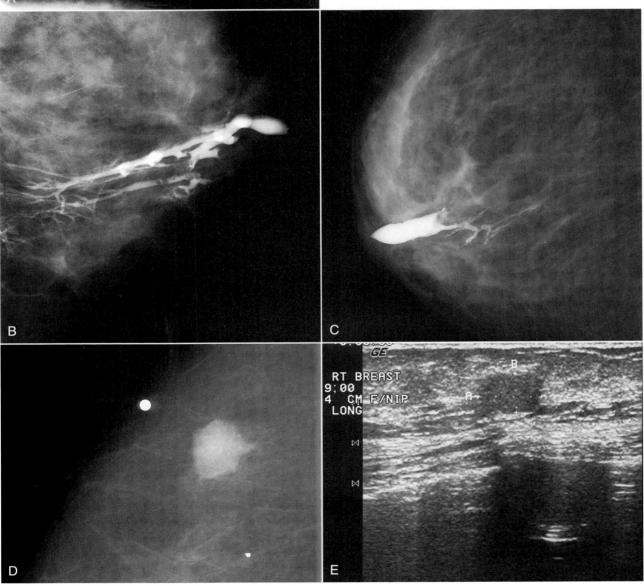

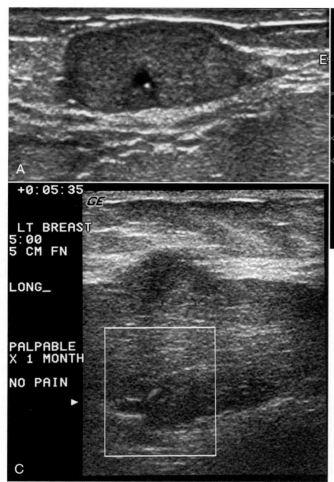

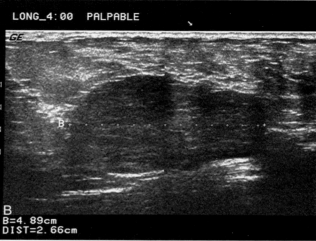

FIGURE 4-20   Lactating Adenoma. A periareolar, well-circumscribed mass containing one calcification in a 7-month-pregnant woman grew in the last few weeks (**A**) and was confirmed to be a lactating adenoma on biopsy. A 4.8-cm heterogeneous lobulated oval mass in another pregnant patient (**B**) is seen to contain blood vessels within the lactating adenoma on Doppler ultrasonography (**C**).

nipple discharge, ultrasound may show papilloma as a solid mass in a fluid-filled subareolar duct. On galactography, papilloma produces an intraductal or intraluminal filling defect.

Treatment is usually surgical. Follow-up for papillomas diagnosed by core biopsy is controversial, with surgical excisional biopsy universally advised for papillomas with papillary carcinoma, atypia, or nonconcordant imaging findings. Surgical excisional biopsy for all papillomas diagnosed by core biopsy is conservative; follow-up imaging alone for papillomas diagnosed by core biopsy is controversial.

Lactating Adenoma

Occurring in young pregnant patients in the second or third trimester, lactating adenomas are solid well-circumscribed masses that can enlarge rapidly during pregnancy. Patients seek clinical evaluation because of a palpable mass. On ultrasound, a lactating adenoma is oval or lobular and smoothly marginated and can contain cystic or necrotic spaces (Fig. 4-20). The mass may regress in size in the postpartum period.

Adenoid Cystic Carcinoma

A very rare tumor that is clinically manifested as a palpable firm mass, adenoid cystic carcinoma has a mixture of glandular and stromal elements that infiltrate the normal fibroglandular tissue in about 50% of cases. The tumor has a good prognosis if completely resected; however, recurrence is possible if the mass is not entirely excised. Imaging characteristics vary because of the rarity of reported cases and range from a well-circumscribed lobulated mass to ill-defined masses or focal asymmetric densities.

SOLID MASSES WITH INDISTINCT MARGINS (Box 4-13)

Invasive Ductal Cancer

On mammography, the indistinct margins of invasive ductal cancer are due to infiltration of the surrounding glandular tissue by tumor. The margin of the mass appears unsharp or smudged, similar to a line partially erased by a pencil eraser. The indistinct margin is best seen on spot magnification views against a fatty background. On ultrasound, the mass occasionally has an echogenic rim or halo that suggests the diagnosis (Fig. 4-21).

Invasive Lobular Carcinoma

Often seen on only one view, lobular carcinoma may appear as an indistinct mass without microcalcifications. A more typical appearance of invasive lobular carcinoma is a spiculated mass or architectural distortion without calcifications.

Box 4-13	Solid Masses with Indistinct Margins

Invasive ductal cancer
Invasive lobular cancer
Primary or secondary non-Hodgkin's lymphoma
Breast sarcoma
Squamous cell carcinoma
Focal fibrosis
Pseudoangiomatous stromal hyperplasia (PASH)

Sarcoma

Breast sarcomas are rare. Typically, they contain malignant stromal elements but, on occasion, may contain fibrous elements seen in the rare fibrosarcoma or osseous elements and bone. As in invasive ductal cancer, these tumors are usually solid masses with ill-defined margins on both mammography and ultrasound.

Lymphoma

Lymphoma can involve breast lymph nodes as a manifestation of lymphoma elsewhere in the body or can occur as a primary or secondary site in the breast parenchyma. Lymphadenopathy is the most common appearance of lymphoma involving the breast and is seen on the mammogram as large dense lymph nodes in the axilla that have lost their fatty hila and become bigger and round (Fig. 4-22A). Primary or secondary breast lymphoma is usually caused by non-Hodgkin's lymphomatous infiltration into breast tissue and not into a lymph node. It is a rare cause of an ill-defined mass that looks just like invasive ductal cancer on mammography (Fig. 4-22B-F). Its mass borders are indistinct because of lymphomatous infiltration into the surrounding glandular tissue, but it can occasionally be well circumscribed or lobulated. On ultrasound, primary or secondary breast lymphomas appear as hypoechoic masses.

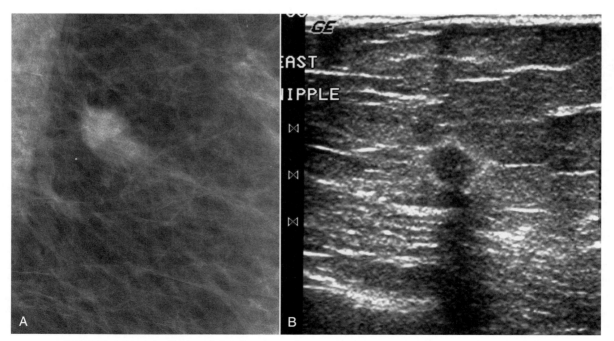

FIGURE 4-21   Indistinct Invasive Ductal Cancer. A mammogram shows a round mass with indistinct margins and an upper partly spiculated border displayed against a fatty background (**A**). Ultrasound shows a round, irregular mass with a thick echogenic halo (**B**).

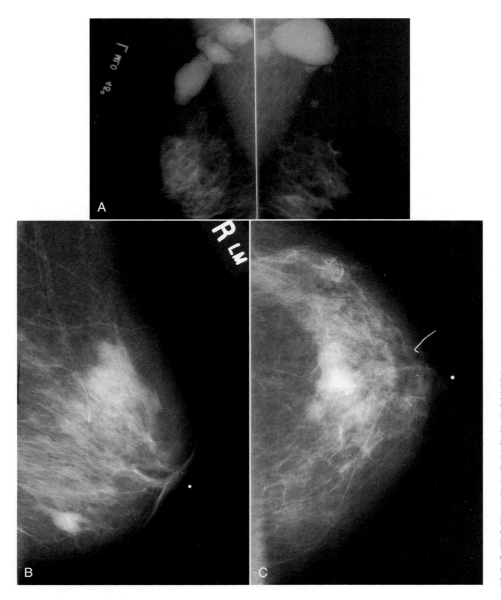

FIGURE 4-22   Breast Lymphoma Involving the Axillary Lymph Nodes. Bilateral mediolateral oblique mammograms show large dense masses in each axilla representing lymphadenopathy from lymphoma (**A**). Bilateral lymphadenopathy suggests systemic disease such as lymphoma, leukemia, metastatic disease, systemic infection, or collagen vascular disease. Primary breast lymphoma in another patient appears as an equal-density, ill-defined mass in the lower part of the breast on lateral medial (**B**) and craniocaudal mammograms (**C**) in breast tissue that is indistinguishable from breast cancer.

Without a diagnosis of lymphoma elsewhere in the body, the diagnosis of primary breast lymphoma is often unsuspected until percutaneous biopsy is performed. Primary breast lymphoma is treated by chemotherapy and radiation therapy, not by surgical excisional biopsy, thus distinguishing its treatment from that for breast cancer. If a patient has a primary diagnosis of lymphoma elsewhere in the body and a new ill-defined breast mass, the first and foremost diagnosis should be primary breast cancer, with a secondary but important differential diagnosis of secondary lymphoma of the breast. Because breast cancer and lymphoma of the breast are treated differently, fine-needle or core biopsy should be considered in appropriate cases to determine the diagnosis and patient management.

Pseudoangiomatous Stromal Hyperplasia

Pseudoangiomatous stromal hyperplasia (PASH) is a rare benign cause of a growing ill-defined noncalcified round or oval mass in premenopausal women or in postmenopausal women receiving exogenous hormone therapy (Fig. 4-23). Occasionally, the mass may be well circumscribed. This entity is of unknown etiology and is composed of stromal and epithelial proliferation; it occasionally shows rapid growth on mammography and requires biopsy. It is thought that there is a hormonal influence on its development, and PASH is more often seen in premenopausal women or postmenopausal women receiving hormone therapy. Fine-needle aspiration can be inconclusive, as can core biopsy. Because low-grade

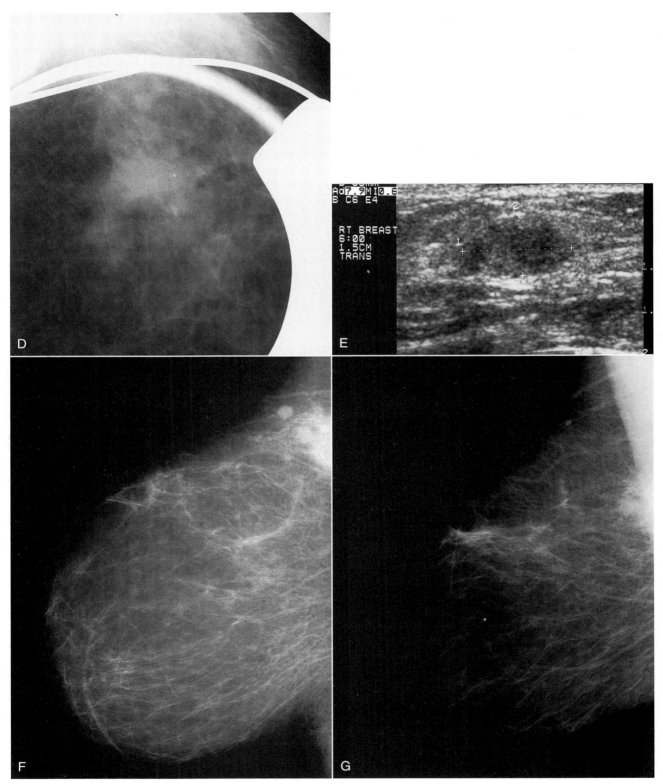

FIGURE 4-22 cont'd   Craniocaudal spot compression shows that the mass persists (**D**). Ultrasound reveals a hypoechoic mass (**E**). Primary breast lymphoma in another patient appearing as an ill-defined mass near the chest wall on craniocaudal (**F**) and mediolateral (**G**) mammograms is less distinct and less dense than the lymphoma that appears more mass-like in **B** to **D**.

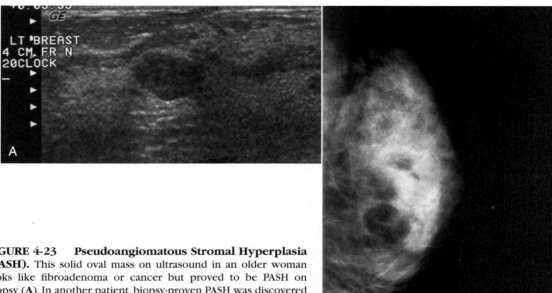

FIGURE 4-23   Pseudoangiomatous Stromal Hyperplasia (PASH). This solid oval mass on ultrasound in an older woman looks like fibroadenoma or cancer but proved to be PASH on biopsy (**A**). In another patient, biopsy-proven PASH was discovered on the mammogram as a dense, partly obscured mass in the mid-portion of the breast, and a biopsy of the mass was performed (**B**).

angiosarcoma can mimic PASH on core biopsy, excisional biopsy is recommended if the mass grows.

Squamous Cell Carcinoma

Squamous cell tumors are even more rare than adenoid cystic carcinoma and produce a large, round, noncalcified ill-defined mass. Other reports describe well-defined masses. On ultrasound, the masses are hypoechoic, with some reports describing central cystic spaces. They are located in breast tissue and are not found near the skin. The diagnosis should be established after the exclusion of either a primary skin lesion or a metastasis to the breast from a distant site such as cervical carcinoma.

MASSES CONTAINING FAT (Box 4-14)

Lymph Nodes

The lymph nodes typically seen in the axilla may be round or oval and contain a radiolucent fatty center. Benign lymph nodes may be of any size, have a thin or varyingly thick rim, and contain a fatty hilum (Fig. 4-24). An intramammary lymph node has the same appearance as lymph nodes in the axilla and is often located in the upper outer quadrant of the breast along blood vessels and should not be mistaken for a malignancy. In questionable cases, spot magnification views demonstrate a well-circumscribed oval or lobulated mass and,

Box 4-14   Masses Containing Fat

Lymph node
Hamartoma
Oil cyst
Lipoma
Liposarcoma
Steatocystoma multiplex

importantly, its fatty hilum. On breast ultrasound, the lymph node is hypoechoic and bean shaped and contains a fatty center. On color Doppler, the lymph node hilum or fatty center will contain a pulsating blood vessel (Fig. 4-24D). On MRI, the lymph node may show rapid initial enhancement with late washout, similar to cancer. However, its typical appearance on MRI, the fatty hilum, and high signal on T2-weighted images should distinguish it from cancer, which commonly has low signal on T2-weighted images.

Hamartoma

This entity is also known as fibroadenolipoma, a benign mass that contains fat and other elements found in the breast. On physical examination, a hamartoma may not be felt distinctly if it contains mostly fat and glandular tissue. The classic appearance is that of an oval mass

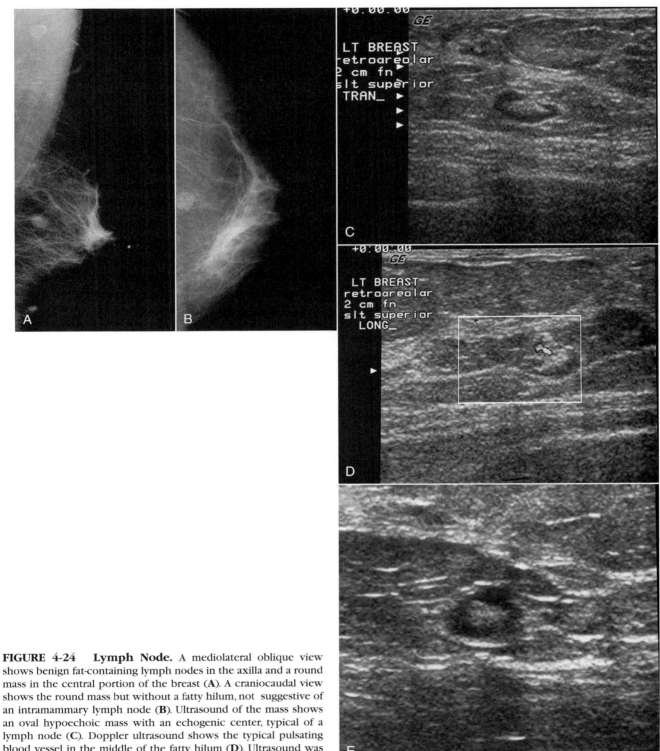

FIGURE 4-24   Lymph Node. A mediolateral oblique view shows benign fat-containing lymph nodes in the axilla and a round mass in the central portion of the breast (**A**). A craniocaudal view shows the round mass but without a fatty hilum, not suggestive of an intramammary lymph node (**B**). Ultrasound of the mass shows an oval hypoechoic mass with an echogenic center, typical of a lymph node (**C**). Doppler ultrasound shows the typical pulsating blood vessel in the middle of the fatty hilum (**D**). Ultrasound was performed on another lymph node in the axilla of same breast (**E**).

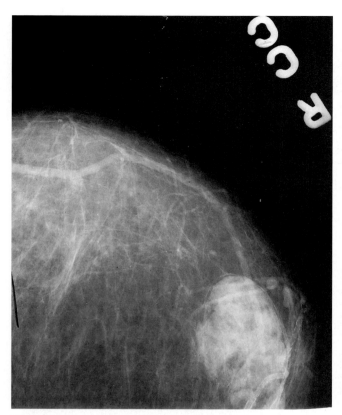

FIGURE 4-25   Typical Hamartoma. A mammogram shows an oval mass containing fat and fibroglandular elements typical of a hamartoma. On breast physical examination, the mass was difficult to feel despite its large size.

containing fat and fibroglandular tissue with a thin capsule or rim, the "breast within a breast" appearance (Fig. 4-25). Breast hamartomas have a variable appearance, depending on the amount of fat and stromal elements contained within. On occasion, a hamartoma may have mostly stromal and glandular elements and appear as a dense mass rather than one containing mostly fat and glandular elements (Fig. 4-26). Because cancer can develop in breast elements and ducts, cancer can develop in hamartomas, biopsy should be performed on any new mass or suspicious microcalcifications developing in a hamartoma. Otherwise, a classic hamartoma is benign and should be left alone.

Oil Cyst

An oil cyst is a sequela of fat necrosis after blunt trauma or surgery. A benign oil cyst is a radiolucent oval or round mass containing fatty fluid and a thin radiodense rim (Fig. 4-27). Oil cysts may subsequently calcify and result in eggshell-type calcifications. On ultrasound, oil cysts are round or oval and contain liquefied fat that is usually hypoechoic or isoechoic.

Lipoma

Breast lipomas are similar to lipomas elsewhere in the body, and they produce a soft mass or a mass that may not be felt at all. A lipoma is a fatty mass containing a radiolucent center that may or may not have a distinguishable thin discrete rim separating it from the surrounding glandular tissue. Unlike a post-traumatic oil cyst, a lipoma never calcifies. Typically, a lipoma is discovered because the patient feels a mass. A skin marker is placed over the mass, and a spot compression view of the mass shows only fat (Fig. 4-28). Ultrasound of a lipoma shows only fatty tissue in a well-circumscribed oval or round mass.

Liposarcoma

Liposarcoma is the only fat-containing malignancy and is extremely rare. Detection of a fat-containing, but rapidly growing mass should raise suspicion of the rare liposarcoma.

Steatocystoma Multiplex

This rare, autosomal dominantly inherited condition is characterized by multiple and extensive intradermal oil cysts bilaterally that may be palpable. Mammography shows extensive bilateral well-circumscribed radiolucent masses with a typical appearance of oil cysts, but unlike post-traumatic intraparenchymal oil cysts, the oil cysts in steatocystoma multiplex are intradermal in location, innumerable, and bilateral without a history of trauma, and affected patients have a typical family history of steatocystoma multiplex that confirms the diagnosis.

FLUID-CONTAINING MASSES (Box 4-15)

Cyst

A simple cyst occurs in 10% of all women and is frequently seen in women receiving exogenous hormone therapy. Caused by obstruction and dilatation of the terminal ducts with fluid trapped within them, a cyst can enlarge with the patient's menstrual cycle and decrease after the onset of menses. Cysts may be asymptomatic or become painful and produce a palpable lump, they may be single or multiple, and they can regress or grow spontaneously and rapidly. On mammography, cysts are round or oval, are well circumscribed, and have a density that ranges from lower to the same as that of fibroglandular tissue. Spot compression magnification will show an equal-density or low-density mass with a sharply marginated border when it is not obscured by adjacent dense glandular tissue. Breast ultrasound shows

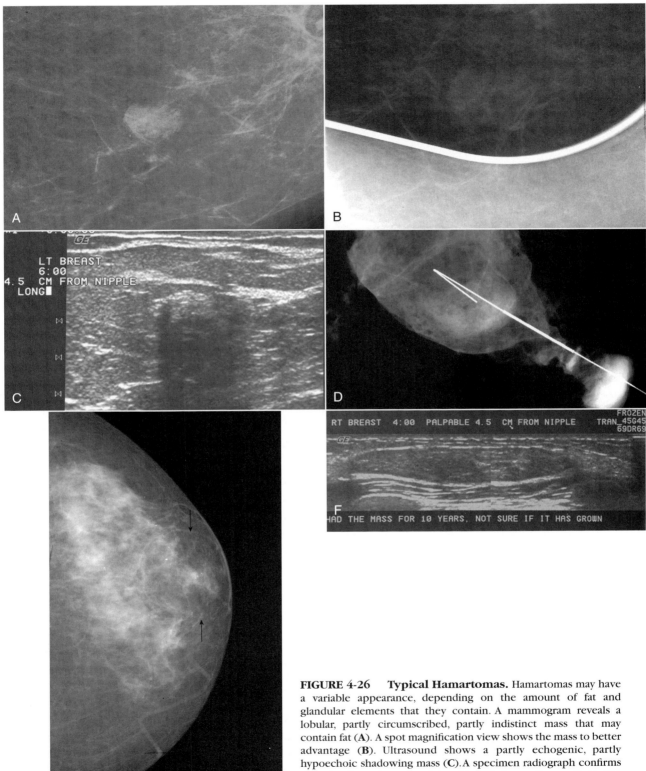

FIGURE 4-26   Typical Hamartomas. Hamartomas may have a variable appearance, depending on the amount of fat and glandular elements that they contain. A mammogram reveals a lobular, partly circumscribed, partly indistinct mass that may contain fat (**A**). A spot magnification view shows the mass to better advantage (**B**). Ultrasound shows a partly echogenic, partly hypoechoic shadowing mass (**C**). A specimen radiograph confirms that the hamartoma contains fat (**D**). In another patient, the hamartoma is an oval mass containing fat and fibroglandular elements with a thin capsule near the anterior portion of the breast *(arrows)* (**E**); it has an oval shape on ultrasound (**F**).

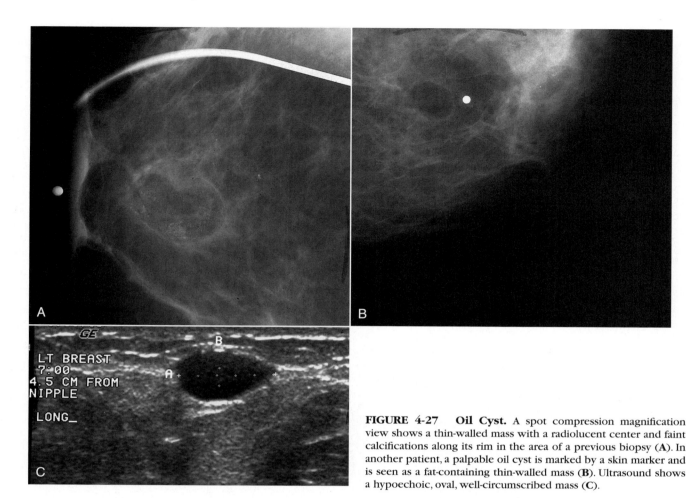

FIGURE 4-27   Oil Cyst. A spot compression magnification view shows a thin-walled mass with a radiolucent center and faint calcifications along its rim in the area of a previous biopsy (**A**). In another patient, a palpable oil cyst is marked by a skin marker and is seen as a fat-containing thin-walled mass (**B**). Ultrasound shows a hypoechoic, oval, well-circumscribed mass (**C**).

an anechoic mass with imperceptible walls, a sharp back wall, and enhanced posterior transmission of sound (Fig. 4-29). Cysts may have internal echoes as a result of debris. Cysts may be left alone (Box 4-16) or can be aspirated by palpation or under ultrasound guidance if symptomatic, but they have no malignant potential. If a cyst is causing the palpable mass, the palpable finding should resolve after aspiration.

Hematoma/Seroma

Breast hematomas and seromas occur after biopsy or trauma, and their diagnosis is established by correlating the finding to the clinical history. On mammography, a hematoma has an irregular or ill-defined border and may be of high or equal density (Fig. 4-30). In the acute phase, surrounding hemorrhage may obscure hematomas. A hematoma will become smaller with time as the hematoma is resorbed and can thus be distinguished from other masses. Initially on ultrasound, a hematoma is a fluid-filled mass. Later, as the hematoma evolves,

ultrasound shows that the previously hypoechoic blood-filled mass changes to serous fluid. Subsequently, the seroma may contain thin movable septa that move on real-time ultrasound, and it may contain debris or fluid/fluid levels.

Necrotic Cancer

Round necrotic cancer may contain fluid but in general will usually have a thicker tumor rim, thus distinguishing it from a thin-walled simple or complex cyst.

Intracystic Carcinoma

See the section "Solid Masses with Rounded or Expansile Borders."

Intracystic Papilloma

This tumor is also rare and appears as a round mass on mammography. On ultrasound, an intracystic papilloma

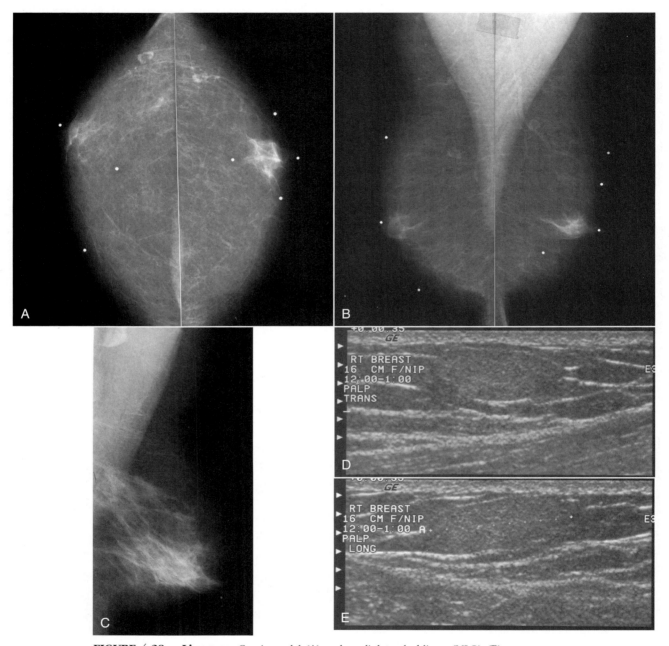

FIGURE 4-28   Lipomas. Craniocaudal (**A**) and mediolateral oblique (MLO) (**B**) mammograms show markers over palpable masses where only fat is present. In another patient, the palpable lipoma is not seen high in the breast on the MLO view where only fat is present (**C**), but ultrasound shows a hypoechoic fatty mass corresponding to the palpable finding that proved to be a lipoma on excisional biopsy (**D** and **E**). Note that the lipoma blends into the surrounding fat and is only seen with the calipers.

is a solid mural nodule or mass in a round fluid-filled mass.

Abscess

A breast abscess occurs after mastitis usually caused by *Staphylococcus* or *Streptococcus*. In a nursing mother, the infection develops as a result of bacterial entry through a cracked nipple. In teenagers, infection may occur during sexual contact. In older women, those who are diabetic or immunocompromised are especially at risk. Typically, an abscess is painful mass that is tender to touch, with overlying red, edematous skin and surrounding cellulitis. On mammography, an abscess is usually subareolar, appears as a dense or equal-density non-calcified irregular mass with focal or diffuse skin

thickening, and may be obscured by surrounding breast edema. On ultrasound, an abscess is an irregular fluid-filled mass occasionally containing debris or septations (Fig. 4-31). The surrounding edema blurs the normal adjacent breast structures, and the skin is thickened. Bright echoes or specular reflectors may indicate air in the abscess, but this finding is usually seen after attempted drainage. Treatment involves antibiotic therapy and drainage of the abscess by either percutaneous or surgical methods. Percutaneous needle aspiration without catheter placement is usually unsuccessful as the only method of drainage if the abscess is large (>2.4 to 3.0 cm), septated, and not completely drained or if pockets of infection are

---

Box 4-15   Fluid-Containing Masses

Cyst
Necrotic cancer
Hematoma
Intracystic carcinoma
Intracystic papilloma
Abscess
Galactocele
Seroma

Box 4-16   Benign Masses That Should Be Left Alone

Simple cyst
Benign post-biopsy scar
Lymph node
Hamartoma
Oil cyst
Lipoma
Hematoma
Seroma
Sebaceous and epidermal inclusion cysts
Galactocele

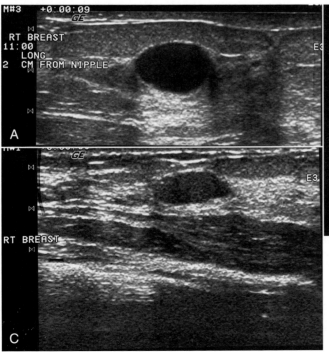

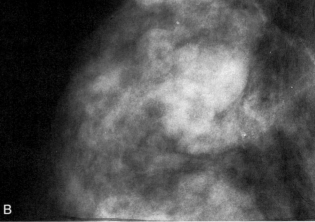

FIGURE 4-29   Cyst on Ultrasound. A well-circumscribed anechoic mass with an imperceptible back wall and enhanced transmission of sound is a simple cyst and needs no further follow-up unless it is symptomatic (**A**). In another patient, a mammogram shows multiple round circumscribed, partly obscured, equal-density masses representing cysts (**B**). Notice on the ultrasound that this complex cyst had debris within it and cannot be distinguished from a solid mass until aspiration (**C**).

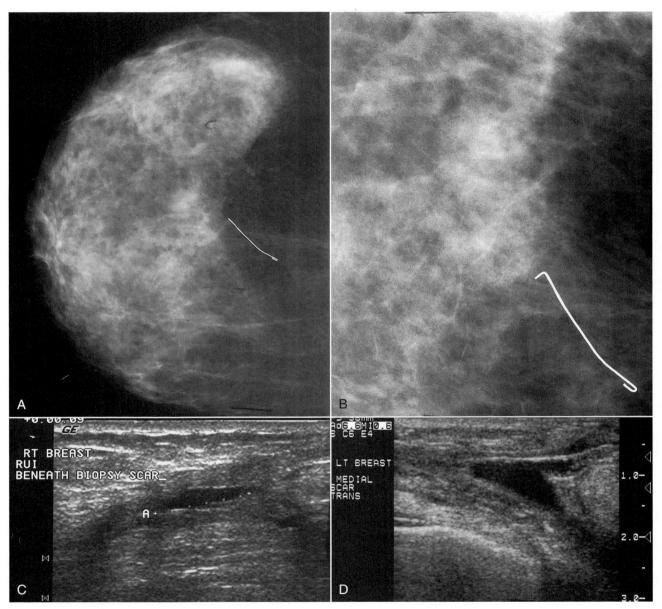

FIGURE 4-30   Hematoma/Seroma. A mammogram shows a density near a linear metallic scar marker 5 months after biopsy of a benign tumor that is hard to see on the craniocaudal mammogram (**A**) but easier to see on the magnification (**B**) view. Ultrasound shows a fluid-filled biopsy cavity (**C**) with healing hypoechoic breast tissue surrounding it. Ultrasound of another biopsy cavity (**D**) shows a V-shaped fluid-filled cavity, with the upper portion of the "V" representing fluid tracking along the incision toward the skin.

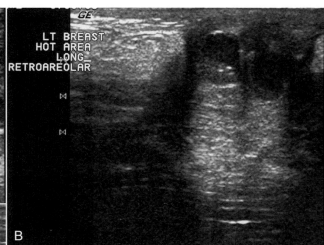

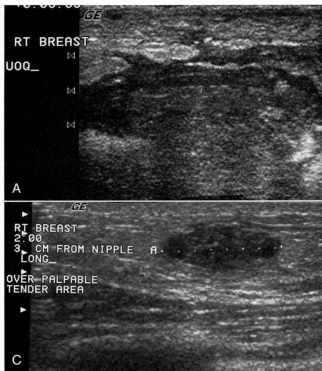

FIGURE 4-31   **Abscesses.** Ultrasound shows an irregular heterogeneous mass with extensions of fluid into tissue. Notice the thickened skin and indistinctness of the surrounding breast tissue structures from cellulitis (**A**). In another patient, two hot retroareolar, painful, round, well-organized fluid-filled abscesses were surrounded by a less well organized infection (**B**). In a third patient, the abscess is well formed and encapsulated and appears as an oval mass with septated fluid collections within it (**C**).

left undrained in the surrounding breast tissue. In these cases, percutaneous needle drainage without an indwelling catheter may be palliative. Women with a chronic subareolar abscess caused by chronic duct obstruction are in a special category and require duct excision as well as abscess treatment.

Sebaceous and Epidermal Inclusion Cysts

These entities are not cysts at all, but keratin accumulation in plugged glands. Sebaceous cysts have an epithelial cell lining, whereas epidermal cysts have a true epidermal cell lining and no sebaceous glands. Because they have almost no malignant potential, biopsy is not required unless the patient desires removal.

Clinically, these entities can produce a palpable mass, a "blackhead" that when squeezed will yield cheesy yellow or white material. On mammography, sebaceous and epidermal inclusion cysts are identical, with subcutaneous oval or round well-defined masses that are often overexposed because of their location near the skin surface and, occasionally, calcifications within them (Fig. 4-32A-C). Ultrasound shows an oval, well-circumscribed, hypoechoic or anechoic mass in a subcutaneous location with a little tail extending into the skin representing the dilated hair follicle (Fig. 4-32D-F).

In the case of epidermal inclusion cysts caused by displacement of epidermal fragments from the skin surface to locations deep within the breast parenchyma after percutaneous biopsy or surgery, the mass may be located within breast tissue far away from the skin surface. These epidermal inclusion cysts produce a growing mass on the mammogram as a result of accumulating inspissated material within them and often require biopsy to exclude cancer.

Galactocele

Typically seen in lactating women, a galactocele represents a focal collection of breast milk. On mammography, a galactocele is a low- or equal-density, oval or round, well-circumscribed mass (Fig. 4-33A and C), but it can be of higher density, depending on resorption of its fluid contents. On an upright mammogram, a classic, but rarely seen finding of a fat/fluid level in the mass represents fat rising to the top of the galactocele while the other milk components layer dependently below. On ultrasound, a galactocele may look like a well-defined hypoechoic cyst-like mass or may contain more solid elements and simulate a solid mass that occasionally displays posterior acoustic shadowing (Fig. 4-33B and D). On aspiration, milky fluid will be obtained.

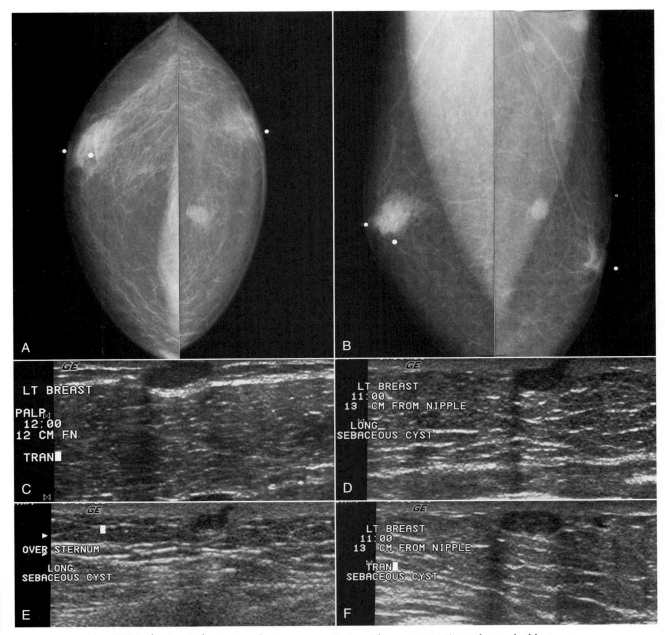

FIGURE 4-32   Sebaceous Cyst. In a patient with gynecomastia and a palpable mass, craniocaudal (**A**) and mediolateral oblique (**B**) views show bilateral subareolar breast tissue that is palpable on the left and marked by a skin marker, as well as a separate discrete upper inner quadrant mass that was detected in the skin on physical examination. Ultrasound of the sebaceous cyst (**C**) shows an oval, hypoechoic, well-circumscribed mass in the skin that correlates with the physical finding. In another patient, ultrasound scans of two sebaceous cysts show oval hypoechoic sebaceous cysts at the junction of the skin surface and subcutaneous fat, with the typical thin tail extending into the skin from the cyst (**D** and **E**). Note that on the transverse scan (**F**) the sebaceous cyst in **D** is seen as an oval mass without the "tail." The "tail" is seen only with careful scanning and attention to the skin surface in masses suspected of being a sebaceous cyst.

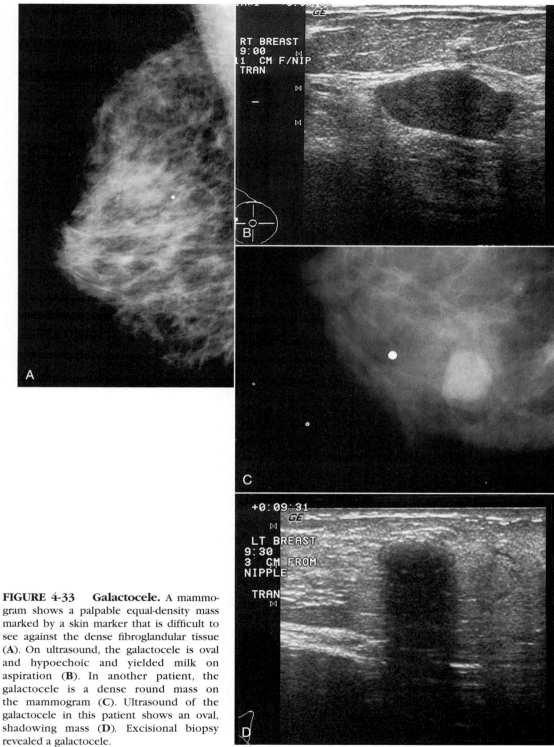

FIGURE 4-33   Galactocele. A mammogram shows a palpable equal-density mass marked by a skin marker that is difficult to see against the dense fibroglandular tissue (**A**). On ultrasound, the galactocele is oval and hypoechoic and yielded milk on aspiration (**B**). In another patient, the galactocele is a dense round mass on the mammogram (**C**). Ultrasound of the galactocele in this patient shows an oval, shadowing mass (**D**). Excisional biopsy revealed a galactocele.

KEY ELEMENTS

A mass is a three-dimensional object seen on at least two mammographic projections.

On mammography, analysis of masses includes a description of the shape, margins, density, location, associated findings, and how changed if previously present.

Mass shapes are round, oval, lobular, and irregular, with the probability of cancer increasing with increasing irregularity of the shape.

In order of suspicion for cancer, mass margins are circumscribed, microlobulated, obscured, indistinct, or spiculated.

Fat-containing masses are almost never malignant.

In order of suspicion for cancer, mass density is lower, equal to, or higher than an equal amount of fibroglandular tissue.

The differential diagnosis for spiculated masses is invasive ductal cancer, invasive lobular cancer, tubular cancer, post-biopsy scar, radial scar, fat necrosis, and sclerosing adenosis.

To determine whether a spiculated mass represents a post-biopsy scar, correlate the post-biopsy mammogram with the pre-biopsy study.

Spiculated masses that do not represent post-biopsy scars should undergo biopsy.

Because radial scars cannot be distinguished from spiculated breast cancer on mammography, biopsy should be performed.

Invasive lobular cancer accounts for about 10% of all cancers but is one of the hardest to see on mammography because of its single-file growth pattern.

The differential diagnosis for solid masses with round or expansile borders is fibroadenoma, cancer, phyllodes tumor, papilloma, lactating adenoma, and tubular adenoma.

The most common round cancer is invasive ductal cancer.

Medullary and mucinous breast cancers are commonly round in shape, but they are much more rare than invasive ductal cancer.

Fat-containing masses include lymph nodes, hamartoma, oil cyst, lipoma, and the rare liposarcoma.

Normal lymph nodes are oval and have an echogenic fatty hilum that may contain a pulsating blood vessel on color or power Doppler ultrasound.

Fluid-containing masses include cysts, hematoma/seroma, necrotic cancer, intracystic carcinoma, intracystic papilloma, abscess, and galactocele.

Hamartomas look like a "breast within a breast" and should be left alone.

Galactoceles may show a fat/fluid level on upright mammographic views.

Know the typical appearance of benign lymph nodes, hamartomas, oil cysts, lipomas, galactoceles, cysts, and post-biopsy scars.

SUGGESTED READINGS

Adler DD, Helvie MA, Oberman HA, et al: Radial sclerosing lesion of the breast: Mammographic features. Radiology 176:737-740, 1990.

Adler DD, Hyde DL, Ikeda DM: Quantitative sonographic parameters as a means of distinguishing breast cancers from benign solid breast masses. J Ultrasound Med 10:505-508, 1991.

American College of Radiology: Illustrated Breast Imaging Reporting and Data System (BI-RADS), 3rd ed. Reston, VA, American College of Radiology, 1998.

Baker JA, Soo MS: Breast US: Assessment of technical quality and image interpretation. Radiology 223:229-238, 2002.

Baker TP, Lenert JT, Parker J, et al: Lactating adenoma: A diagnosis of exclusion. Breast J 7:354-735, 2001.

Bilgen IG, Ustun EE, Memis A: Fat necrosis of the breast: Clinical, mammographic and sonographic features. Eur J Radiol 39:92-99, 2001.

Castro CY, Whitman GJ, Sahin AA: Pseudoangiomatous stromal hyperplasia of the breast. Am J Clin Oncol 25:213-216, 2002.

Cawson JN, Law EM, Kavanagh AM: Invasive lobular carcinoma: Sonographic features of cancers detected in a BreastScreen Program. Australas Radiol 45:25-30, 2001.

Chao TC, Lo YF, Chen SC, Chen MF: Sonographic features of phyllodes tumors of the breast. Ultrasound Obstet Gynecol 20:64-71, 2002.

Chapellier C, Balu-Maestro C, Bleuse A, et al: Ultrasonography of invasive lobular carcinoma of the breast: Sonographic patterns and diagnostic value: Report of 102 cases. Clin Imaging 24:333-336, 2000.

Cheung YC, Wan YL, Chen SC, et al: Sonographic evaluation of mammographically detected microcalcifications without a mass prior to stereotactic core needle biopsy. J Clin Ultrasound 30:323-331, 2002.

Chopra S, Evans AJ, Pinder SE, et al: Pure mucinous breast cancer—mammographic and ultrasound findings. Clin Radiol 51:421-424, 1996.

Cohen MA, Morris EA, Rosen PP, et al: Pseudoangiomatous stromal hyperplasia: Mammographic, sonographic, and clinical patterns. Radiology 198:117-120, 1996.

Cole-Beuglet C, Soriano RZ, Kurtz AB, Goldberg BB: Fibroadenoma of the breast: Sonomammography correlated with pathology in 122 patients. AJR Am J Roentgenol 140:369-375, 1983.

Conant EF, Dillon RL, Palazzo J, et al: Imaging findings in mucin-containing carcinomas of the breast: Correlation with pathologic features. AJR Am J Roentgenol 163:821-824, 1994.

Darling ML, Smith DN, Rhei E, et al: Lactating adenoma: Sonographic features. Breast J 6:252-256, 2000.

Denison CM, Ward VL, Lester SC, et al: Epidermal inclusion cysts of the breast: Three lesions with calcifications. Radiology 204:493-496, 1997.

Domchek SM, Hecht JL, Fleming MD, et al: Lymphomas of the breast: Primary and secondary involvement. Cancer 94:6-13, 2002.

Dupont WD, Page DL, Pari FF, et al: Long-term risk of breast cancer in women with fibroadenoma. N Engl J Med 351(1):10-15, 1994.

Elson BC, Helvie MA, Frank TS, et al: Tubular carcinoma of the breast: Mode of presentation, mammographic appearance, and frequency of nodal metastases. AJR Am J Roentgenol 161:1173-1176, 1993.

Elson BC, Ikeda DM, Andersson I, Wattsgard C: Fibrosarcoma of the breast: Mammographic findings in five cases. AJR Am J Roentgenol 158:993-995, 1992.

Estabrook A, Asch T, Gump F, et al: Mammographic features of intracystic papillary lesions. Surg Gynecol Obstet 170:113-116, 1990.

Fornage BD, Lorigan JG, Andry E: Fibroadenoma of the breast: Sonographic appearance. Radiology 172:671-675, 1989.

Gordon PB, Goldenberg SL: Malignant breast masses detected only by ultrasound. A retrospective review. Cancer 76:626-630, 1995.

Gunhan-Bilgen I, Memis A, Ustun EE: Metastatic intramammary lymph nodes: Mammographic and ultrasonographic features. Eur J Radiol 40:24-29, 2001.

Gunhan-Bilgen I, Zekioglu O, Ustun EE, et al: Invasive micro-papillary carcinoma of the breast: Clinical, mammographic, and sonographic findings with histopathologic correlation. AJR Am J Roentgenol 179:927-931, 2002.

Harnist KS, Ikeda DM, Helvie MA: Abnormal mammogram after steering wheel injury. West J Med 159:504-506, 1993.

Harvey JA, Moran RE, Maurer EJ, DeAngelis GA: Sonographic features of mammary oil cysts. J Ultrasound Med 16:719-724, 1997.

Hashimoto BE, Kramer DJ, Picozzi VJ: High detection rate of breast ductal carcinoma in situ calcifications on mammo-graphically directed high-resolution sonography. J Ultrasound Med 20:501-508, 2001.

Hilton SV, Leopold GR, Olson LK, Willson SA: Real-time breast sonography: Application in 300 consecutive patients. AJR Am J Roentgenol 147:479-486, 1986.

Homer MJ: Proper placement of a metallic marker on an area of concern in the breast. AJR Am J Roentgenol 167:390-391, 1996.

Jorge Blanco A, Vargas Serrano B, Rodriguez Romero R, Martinez Cendejas E: Phyllodes tumors of the breast. Eur Radiol 9:356-360, 1999.

Lee CH, Giurescu ME, Philpotts LE, et al: Clinical importance of unilaterally enlarging lymph nodes on otherwise normal mammograms. Radiology 203:329-334, 1997.

Lindfors KK, Kopans DB, Googe PB, et al: Breast cancer metastasis to intramammary lymph nodes. AJR Am J Roentgenol 146:133-136, 1986.

Memis A, Ozdemir N, Parildar M, et al: Mucinous (colloid) breast cancer: Mammographic and US features with histologic correlation. Eur J Radiol 35:39-43, 2000.

Meyer JE, Amin E, Lindfors KK, et al: Medullary carcinoma of the breast: Mammographic and US appearance. Radiology 170:79-82, 1989.

Paramagul CP, Helvie MA, Adler DD: Invasive lobular carcinoma: Sonographic appearance and role of sonography in improving diagnostic sensitivity. Radiology 195:231-234, 1995.

Rosen EL, Soo MS, Bentley RC: Focal fibrosis: A common breast lesion diagnosed at imaging-guided core biopsy. AJR Am J Roentgenol 173:1657-1662, 1999.

Salvador R, Salvador M, Jimenez JA, et al: Galactocele of the breast: Radiologic and ultrasonographic findings. Br J Radiol 63:140-142, 1990.

Samardar P, de Paredes ES, Grimes MM, Wilson JD: Focal asymmetric densities seen at mammography: US and pathologic correlation. Radiographics 22:19-33, 2002.

Schneider JA: Invasive papillary breast carcinoma: Mammo-graphic and sonographic appearance. Radiology 171:377-379, 1989.

Sheppard DG, Whitman GJ, Huynh PT, et al: Tubular carcinoma of the breast: Mammographic and sonographic features. AJR Am J Roentgenol 174:253-257, 2000.

Sickles EA: Mammographic features of 300 consecutive nonpalpable breast cancers. AJR Am J Roentgenol 146:661-663, 1986.

Sickles E: Practical solutions to common mammographic problems: Tailoring the examination. AJR 151:31-39, 1988.

Sickles EA, Herzog KA: Intramammary scar tissue: A mimic of the mammographic appearance of carcinoma. AJR Am J Roentgenol 135:349-352, 1980.

Soo MS, Dash N, Bentley R, et al: Tubular adenomas of the breast: Imaging findings with histologic correlation. AJR Am J Roentgenol 174:757-761, 2000.

Sperber F, Blank A, Metser U: Adenoid cystic carcinoma of the breast: Mammographic, sonographic, and pathological correlation. Breast J 8:53-54, 2002.

Stavros AT, Thickman D, Rapp CL, et al: Solid breast nodules: Use of sonography to distinguish between benign and malignant lesions. Radiology 196:123-134, 1995.

Sumkin JH, Perrone AM, Harris KM, et al: Lactating adenoma: US features and literature review. Radiology 206:271-274, 1998.

Tabar L, Pentek Z, Dean PB: The diagnostic and therapeutic value of breast cyst puncture and pneumocystography. Radiology 141:659-663, 1981.

Venta LA, Wiley EL, Gabriel H, Adler YT: Imaging features of focal breast fibrosis: Mammographic-pathologic correlation of non-calcified breast lesions. AJR Am J Roentgenol 173:309-316, 1999.

Wahner-Roedler DL, Sebo TJ, Gisvold JJ: Hamartomas of the breast: Clinical, radiologic, and pathologic manifestations. Breast J 7:101-105, 2001.

Walsh R, Kornguth PJ, Soo MS, et al: Axillary lymph nodes: Mammographic, pathologic, and clinical correlation. AJR Am J Roentgenol 168:33-38, 1997.

Weigel RJ, Ikeda DM, Nowels KW: Primary squamous cell carcinoma of the breast. South Med J 89:511-515, 1996.

Woods ER, Helvie MA, Ikeda DM, et al: Solitary breast papilloma: Comparison of mammographic, galactographic, and pathologic findings. AJR Am J Roentgenol 159:487-491, 1992.

Breast Ultrasound

Introduction

Technical Considerations

Normal Sonographic Breast Anatomy

Evaluation of Mammographically Detected Findings

    Breast Cysts, Intracystic Tumors, and Cystic-Appearing Masses

    Benign Solid Masses—Fibroadenoma and Fatty Pseudolesions

    Malignant Solid Masses

    Breast Calcifications

Palpable or Mammographically Detected Findings

Undetected by Ultrasound

Young Patients and Palpable Findings in Dense Breasts

Correlating Mammographic Findings with Ultrasound

Findings

Breast Edema

Breast Abscess

Breast Biopsy Scars

Cancers Undergoing Neoadjuvant Chemotherapy

Post-biopsy Breast Markers and Core Biopsy Sites

Color Doppler, Power Doppler, Ultrasound Contrast

Agents, and Three-Dimensional Imaging

Breast Cancer Screening with Ultrasound

Key Elements

INTRODUCTION

Ultrasound is a useful adjunct to mammography for the diagnosis and management of benign and malignant breast disease. Technical advances have resulted in high spatial resolution, and most practices use high-resolution hand-held real-time scanners. Scientific evidence and clinical experience support the use of hand-held real-time breast ultrasound to distinguish cysts from solid masses, determine the sonographic characteristics of solid masses, evaluate palpable lumps in young women, and provide guidance for percutaneous biopsy. Given the improvement in image quality and data processing, preliminary studies suggest possible roles of breast ultrasound in breast cancer screening or evaluation of breast calcifications identified on mammography. This chapter will explore these and other indications for breast ultrasound.

TECHNICAL CONSIDERATIONS

Real-time hand-held scanners provide easy and rapid direct visualization of breast lesions for diagnosis or ultrasound-directed breast biopsy. Hand-held units should include a linear-array, high-frequency transducer operating at a frequency of 7.5 to 10 MHz or greater, which provides good tissue penetration to 4 or 5 cm. The unit should include a marking system to document and annotate the scanned region of the breast.

Technical factors have an impact on sonographic image quality. Superficial lesions in the near field of the transducer may be distorted, but they can be imaged by using a soft rubber or fluid offset or a high-frequency transducer. The heterogeneity of breast tissue results in absorption of the ultrasound beam with increasing distance, and extensive diffraction of the ultrasound beam may lead to beam defocusing. Accurate diagnosis of cysts and deep lesions depends on appropriate power, gain, and focal zone settings. Improper adjustments of any of these parameters may lead to suboptimal images and produce artifactual echoes within simple cysts that can result in misdiagnosis. Routine calibration of the unit and evaluation of the unit's performance with a breast phantom help prevent technical errors.

The amount of shadowing at normal breast tissue interfaces depends on the transducer's diameter and the distance of the tissue from the transducer. Proper positioning flattens the breast tissue in the quadrant of interest, decreases the amount of tissue to be penetrated by the ultrasound beam, and diminishes edge artifacts by straightening Cooper's ligaments parallel to the transducer.

Non-flattening of breast tissue allows Cooper's ligaments and normal breast structures to angle up toward the skin and the transducer, thereby causing artificial shadowing and false masses. To flatten the breast tissue in the upper outer quadrant, the patient is scanned supine with her hand behind her head in a posterior oblique position and her back supported by a wedge, such as the sponge wedges used for positioning posterior oblique lumbar spine radiographs. For medial lesions, the patient lies flat on her back, which flattens the medial breast tissue. Using the transducer to produce moderate compression during scanning further decreases the amount of tissue to be scanned, reduces beam absorption and defocusing, allows better penetration, and decreases shadowing from ligaments and glandular elements.

To ensure that the field of view includes all the breast tissue from the skin surface to the chest wall, the operator should see the pectoralis muscle and chest wall at the bottom of the screen. The time-compensated gain (TCG) curve should be adjusted so that fat is uniformly gray from the subcutaneous tissues to the chest wall. Such adjustment enables accurate evaluation of masses as cystic or solid; incorrect settings that make the fat look anechoic may make a solid mass look like an anechoic cyst.

Once an area of interest or a mass is identified, the image should be large enough to fill the monitor or screen to evaluate important border and internal characteristics. The focal zone, TCG curve, and depth-compensated gain (DCG) curve are reset on the lesion to evaluate the internal characteristics to greatest advantage.

When scanning a patient with palpable findings, the patient is asked to identify the mass or symptomatic area of the breast so that the region prompting investigation is evaluated. If the patient is unsure of the location of the mass, the quadrant or area requested by the referring physician on the order or requisition is evaluated. If the mass is palpable, the operator can ensure that the palpable finding is scanned by placing an examining finger over the mass, scanning the finger on the mass, and then removing the finger so that only the palpable finding is scanned. Alternatively, the palpable finding can be trapped between two fingers and scanned so that the mass does not roll out of the field of view from under the transducer. The location of the palpable mass is clearly documented on the ultrasound film.

For image labeling, each finding should be labeled regarding right or left breast, quadrant or clock position, scan plane (radial or antiradial, longitudinal or transverse), and number of centimeters from the nipple (Box 5-1). An image of the mass with and without measuring calipers may also be taken, as clinically indicated. Any other pertinent clinical information, such as whether the lesion is palpable, may also be helpful.

The ACR has recommended specific descriptors for breast masses. For example, mass shapes are reported as oval, round, or irregular (Table 5-1). Mass margins are circumscribed, angular, indistinct, microlobulated, or spiculated. The boundary between the mass and the surrounding tissue is described as an abrupt interface or containing an echogenic halo. The internal echo pattern is described as anechoic, hyperechoic, complex, isoechoic, or hypoechoic. Acoustic features are

---

Box 5-1   Ultrasound Labeling

Breast side (left or right)
Quadrant or clock position
Scan plane (radial or antiradial, transverse or longitudinal)
Number of centimeters from the nipple
Image of pertinent findings, with and without measuring
  calipers

Table 5-1   American College of Radiology BI-RADS Ultrasound Lexicon Descriptors

Shape	Margin	Boundary	Echo Pattern	Posterior Acoustic Features
Oval	Circumscribed	Abrupt interface	Anechoic	No posterior acoustic features
Round	Angular	Echogenic halo	Hyperechoic	Enhancement
Irregular	Indistinct		Complex	Shadowing
	Microlobulated		Isoechoic	Combined
			Hypoechoic	

Effect on surrounding tissue: No effect, duct changes, Cooper's ligament changes, edema, architectural distortion, skin thickening, skin retraction/irregularity.
Calcifications: none, macrocalcifications (>0.5 mm), microcalcifications in or out of a mass.
From American College of Radiology (ACR): ACR BI-RADS—Ultrasound. Breast Imaging Reporting and Data System—Breast Imaging Atlas. Reston, VA, American College of Radiology, 2003.

described as no posterior acoustic features, enhancement, shadowing, or a combined pattern. Calcifications are described as no calcifications, macrocalcifications larger than 0.5 mm, microcalcifications within the mass, or microcalcifications outside the mass. Any effect of the mass on surrounding breast tissue should also be described as no effect, duct changes, changes in Cooper's ligaments, edema, architectural distortion, skin thickening, skin retraction, or skin irregularity.

NORMAL SONOGRAPHIC BREAST ANATOMY

The breast is composed of fibrous connective tissue (Cooper's ligaments) arranged in a honeycomb-like structure surrounding the breast ducts and fat (Fig. 5-1A). The proportion of supporting stroma to glandular tissue varies widely in the normal population and depends on

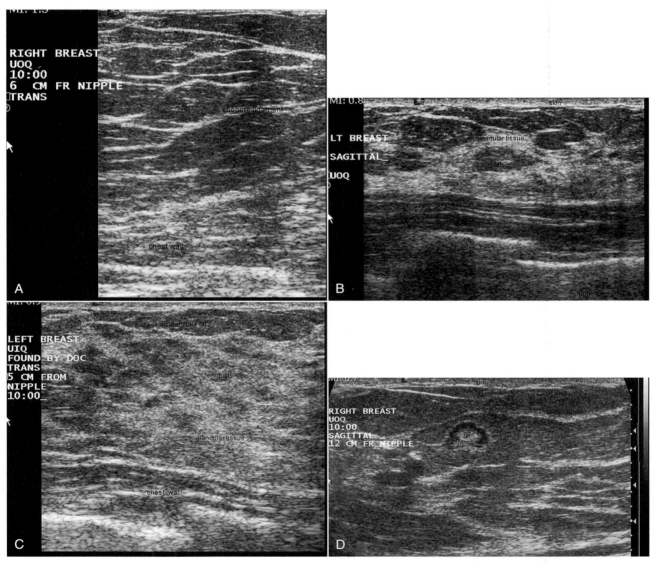

FIGURE 5-1   Normal Breast Ultrasound Scans. A, Ultrasound of a normal fatty breast shows sharp thin Cooper's ligaments interspersed with hypoechoic fat. Note that the fat is uniformly gray throughout the image. **B,** Ultrasound of normal fibroglandular and fatty breast tissue shows echogenic glandular tissue interspersed with islands of hypoechoic fat. Note how the fatty islands might be mistaken for a breast mass. **C,** Ultrasound of normal dense breast tissue shows mostly glandular tissue with scant amounts of fat and hypoechoic ducts over an area of thickening in a young patient. **D,** Ultrasound of a normal lymph node shows a lobulated hypoechoic mass with an echogenic center that represents the fatty hilum seen on mammography.

**Box 5-2   Normal Ultrasound
Appearance of Breast Tissue**

Skin: 2- to 3-mm echogenic superficial line
Fat: hypoechoic (exception: fatty hilum in lymph nodes)
Glandular tissue: echogenic
Breast ducts: hypoechoic tubular structures, oval in
     cross section
Nipple: hypoechoic, can shadow intensely
Cooper's ligaments: thin echogenic lines
Ribs: hypoechoic, periodic at the chest wall

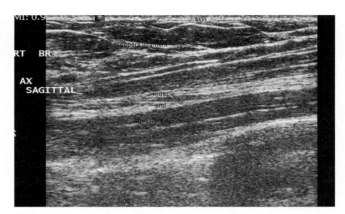

FIGURE 5-2   Normal breast ultrasound showing the thin echogenic skin line at the top of the image; thin, gently curving Cooper's ligaments coursing through the fat; and the thin, parallel, tightly packed lines of muscle just above the chest wall and the rib.

the patient's age, parity, and hormonal status. In young women, breast tissue is composed of mostly dense fibroglandular tissue (Fig. 5-1B and C). With age, the dense tissue turns into fat.

The echogenic skin line is immediately under the transducer in the near field, is normally about 2 to 3 mm thick, and has a hypoechoic layer of subcutaneous fat immediately beneath it (Box 5-2). Unlike echogenic or white-appearing fat around the superior mesenteric artery in the abdomen, fat in the breast appears dark or hypoechoic (Fig. 5-1D). The only exception to hypoechoic fat in the breast is echogenic fat in the middle of a lymph node. Breast parenchyma and connective tissue are echogenic or white. The latter has the highest acoustic impedance, fat has the lowest, and glandular parenchyma is of intermediate echogenicity. The retromammary fascia and Cooper ligaments are thin, sharply defined linear structures that support the surrounding fat and glandular elements (Fig. 5-2). The thin lines of Cooper's ligaments are best seen in a fatty breast as gently curving lines surrounding hypoechoic fat. Normally, Cooper's ligaments are thin and sharply demarcated. In breast edema, the fat becomes gray and the normally sharp Cooper ligaments become blurred.

The nipple is a hypoechoic structure that may produce an acoustic shadow as a result of the dense connective tissue within it (Fig. 5-3A). Because of the retroareolar ducts and blood vessels, there may be marked vascularity in the retroareolar region on color or power Doppler imaging. Newcomers to breast ultrasound may mistake the nipple for a breast mass because of its hypoechoic appearance, shadowing, and the intense vascularity beneath it. In children, the breast bud may produce a lump that can be asymmetric and mistaken for a mass rather than a normal developing structure (Fig. 5-3B and C). This normal structure should be left alone because surgical removal of the breast bud results in no breast formation on the ipsilateral side.

Subareolar ducts are hypoechoic tubular structures leading to the nipple. The glandular tissue elements are echogenic and may contain hypoechoic ducts that appear tubular when imaged along their long axis. In cross section, the ducts are hypoechoic, round or oval circles seen against the white echogenic normal glandular tissue.

The pectoral muscle is a hypoechoic structure of varying thickness that contains thin lines of supporting stroma coursing along the long axis of the muscle. The pectoral muscle abuts the intercostal muscles and fascia of the chest wall (Fig. 5-4). Ribs contained in the intercostal muscles are round or oval in cross section, shadow intensely, and are seen at regular intervals along the chest wall. High-resolution transducers may display calcifications in the anterior portions of the cartilaginous elements of the ribs.

EVALUATION OF MAMMOGRAPHICALLY DETECTED FINDINGS

Breast Cysts, Intracystic Tumors, and Cystic-Appearing Masses

The most frequent clinical application of breast ultrasonography is to characterize a mass initially detected by mammography as cystic or solid. Cysts are the most common breast mass and occur in an estimated 7% to 10% of all women. Cysts are lined either by apocrine cells that actively secrete material, thereby predisposing these types of cysts to recurrence after aspiration, or by a flat epithelial lining that is less active. The accuracy of ultrasound in distinguishing cystic from solid masses can be as high as 98% to 100% as reported by Hilton et al. Strict ultrasound criteria for a simple cyst include well-circumscribed mass margins, sharp anterior and posterior walls, a round or oval contour, absence of internal echoes, and posterior acoustic enhancement of

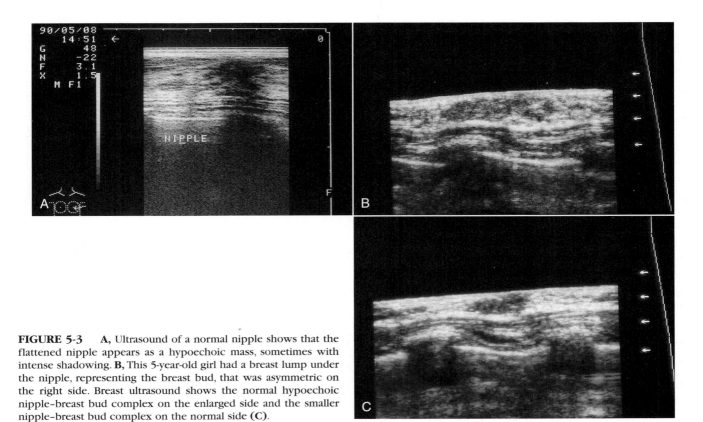

FIGURE 5-3   **A,** Ultrasound of a normal nipple shows that the flattened nipple appears as a hypoechoic mass, sometimes with intense shadowing. **B,** This 5-year-old girl had a breast lump under the nipple, representing the breast bud, that was asymmetric on the right side. Breast ultrasound shows the normal hypoechoic nipple–breast bud complex on the enlarged side and the smaller nipple–breast bud complex on the normal side **(C)**.

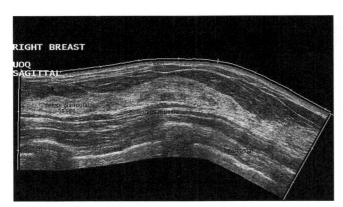

FIGURE 5-4   A landscape view shows normal dense tissue, the regular occurrence of ribs at the chest wall, and the pectoralis and intercostal muscles.

sound (Box 5-3, Fig. 5-5A). Cysts may be single or multiple, gathered into small clusters, or contain thin septations (Fig. 5-5B). Cysts are not premalignant, but they are important because they may cause lumps that mimic round cancer on physical examination or mammography. Depending on its location in the breast, a cyst is smooth, mobile, and tense on physical examination; it occasionally appears as a visible mass if the patient is supine and the

Box 5-3   Simple Cyst Criteria
Oval or round shape with circumscribed margins Anechoic Imperceptible back wall Enhanced transmission of sound

cyst is large. Cysts may be painful and may wax and wane with the patient's menstrual cycle. Once diagnosed, a patient with a simple cyst can be monitored by screening mammography because cysts are not cancer. Symptomatic cysts that are painful or cause a lump that is disturbing to the patient can be treated by aspiration alone.

Scanning breast cysts requires careful analysis of their internal characteristics to exclude mural masses or irregular thick walls, which can indicate intracystic tumors or necrotic neoplasms mimicking cysts. Attention to technical detail is especially important because increasing the TCG curve may produce artifactual echoes in benign cysts and suggest a solid mass (Fig. 5-5C and D). An improperly set DCG curve may inaccurately evaluate the internal matrix of the mass and make a cyst look solid and vice versa. At real-time imaging, cyst

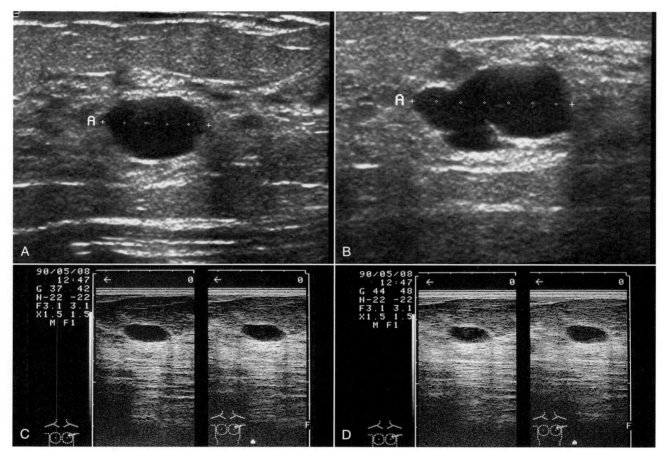

FIGURE 5-5   A, This simple cyst has an anechoic interior, an imperceptible wall, sharply marginated smooth borders, and enhanced transmission of sound. **B,** This simple cyst is lobulated and contains thin septations and imperceptible walls. **C** and **D,** Sequential images of the same cyst show that echoes can be produced in the middle of a simple cyst by increasing the time-compensated gain, in this case increased in each image from left to right.

contours may be flattened with compression, whereas solid masses are less compressible. Alternatively, small or deeply located cysts may be at the technical limits of ultrasound to distinguish the usually anechoic cyst from a solid mass.

Deeply located cysts may not show enhanced through-transmission of sound because of their location close to the chest wall, and lateral cyst walls may be obscured by refractive shadows. These problems may be resolved by repositioning the patient or the transducer to scan from a different angle to permit visualization of distal acoustic enhancement or eliminate the refractive shadows obscuring the sharp cyst walls.

At real-time imaging, speckle artifact from debris in cyst fluid may simulate a solid mass. Watching the debris in the cyst over time may show slow movement of the particulate matter, or placing the patient in the decubitus position and noting a difference in the sedimentation pattern may be diagnostic of a complex cyst, but not always (Fig. 5-6A). Doppler imaging may detect movement of particulate matter within complex breast cysts; on real-time imaging, such movement is shown as speckle artifact swirling in the cyst like fake snow swirls in paperweights containing water-filled artificial winter scenes (Fig. 5-6B and C). If it is still uncertain whether a mass is cystic or solid, color Doppler or power Doppler may be helpful by identifying a vessel in a solid mass (Fig. 5-6D and E). Doppler imaging will show no blood vessels in breast cysts. Unfortunately, the absence of blood flow in a mass is not diagnostic of a cyst because Doppler does not always detect blood flow in solid masses.

In everyday clinical practice, cysts do not fulfill all the strict sonographic criteria because of a variety of technical factors, or they may contain echoes from debris within the fluid (Fig. 5-7A). Posterior enhanced through-transmission of sound was not seen on all images in 25% of 80 cysts reported by Hilton et al. Internal cyst

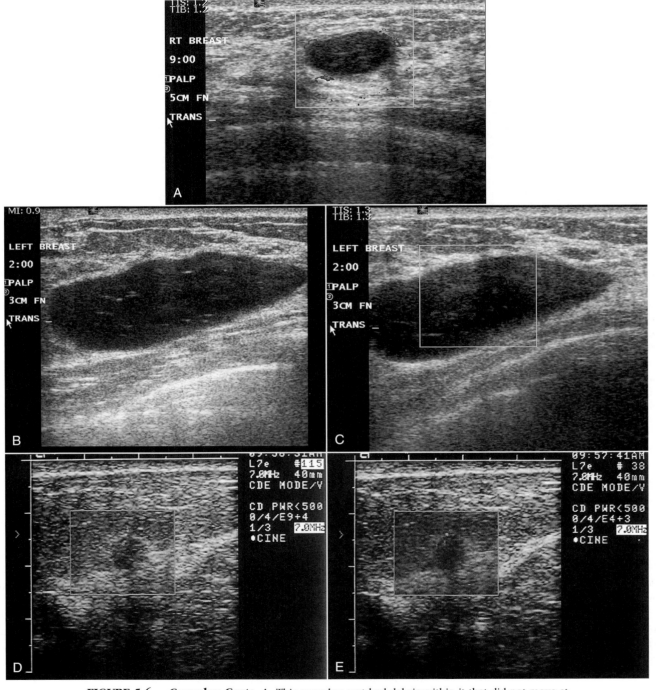

FIGURE 5-6   Complex Cysts. A, This complex cyst had debris within it that did not move at real-time imaging. Color Doppler ultrasound shows pulsating blood vessels around the cyst, but not within it. Aspiration yielded cloudy fluid. **B,** Ultrasound of a palpable mass showed speckle artifact within a complex cyst that moved at real-time imaging. **C,** Color Doppler detected movement of the debris in real time. In contradistinction, color Doppler **(D)** and power Doppler **(E)** show a pulsating vessel flowing into a round cancer, thus differentiating it from complex cysts.

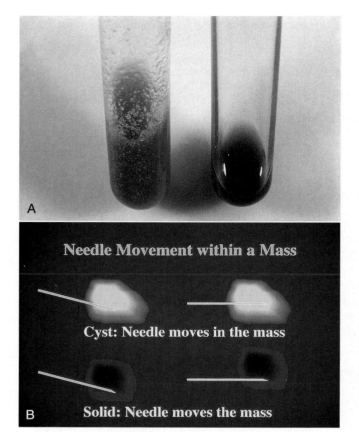

FIGURE 5-7   Simple Cyst Fluid Compared with Cyst Fluid Containing Debris. A, The complex cyst fluid in the left test tube, which contains debris consisting of particulate matter, is causing speckles within the cyst on ultrasound. The simple cyst fluid in the right test tube is clear and contains no debris. Both fluids are normal and may be discarded after aspiration. **B,** A simple way to tell whether a mass is cystic at needle biopsy is to move the needle tip within the mass. In a complex cyst, the needle will move within the mass. In a solid mass, the needle will move the mass up and down.

echoes may be produced by reverberation artifacts, although the near-field reverberations seen with linear transducers may be reduced by scanning through an offset. Fine-needle aspiration under x-ray or ultrasonographic guidance can be used to confirm or exclude the presence of a simple cyst. Berg et al. and others have shown that complex cystic masses with low-level internal echoes, no mural masses, thin walls, and septations rarely represent cancer and can either be monitored or aspirated with little or no morbidity.

Differentiation of complex cysts from benign or malignant cystic masses can be difficult (Box 5-4). Some cysts contain true internal echoes as a result of thick tenacious fluid or hemorrhage from previous aspirations. Some cysts have thick walls as a result of inflammation from cyst fluid leaking into the surrounding tissues. In

Box 5-4	Cystic or Fluid-Containing Masses

Simple cyst
Complex cyst
Intracystic papilloma
Intracystic carcinoma
Necrotic cancer
Hematoma
Abscess
Galactocele
Seroma/post-surgical scar (early)

cases in which all the sonographic criteria of a simple cyst are not met, needle aspiration may obviate the need for core or surgical biopsy. Once the needle is within the mass, the presence of cyst fluid rather than solid tissue can be confirmed by moving the needle in the mass, as suggested by Stavros et al. (Fig. 5-7B). Cyst fluid should be sent for cytologic analysis if it is bloody, if an intracystic mass is visualized on ultrasound or pneumocystography, or if the patient has an unusual clinical history of cancer in a cyst previously. Clear cyst fluid can be discarded if no clinical factors are present that require cytologic examination.

On the other hand, fluid-filled masses with thick walls or mural projections require biopsy to exclude the rare intracystic papilloma, intracystic carcinoma, or solid cancers with central necrosis (Fig. 5-8). Intracystic carcinomas are a rare subgroup of tumors that arise from the walls of a cyst; they represent 0.5% to 1.3% of all breast cancers. These tumors have a better prognosis than other malignant breast neoplasms do. On ultrasound, intracystic carcinomas often appear as solid mural excrescences projecting into the cyst fluid. Differentiation of intracystic carcinoma from benign intracystic papilloma is not possible, and surgical biopsy is thus necessary. This appearance may also occasionally be simulated by debris within complicated cysts or by reverberations in simple cysts produced by high gain settings, and aspiration or biopsy is necessary (Fig. 5-8C). Color or power Doppler imaging may be helpful if a blood vessel can be identified in the intracystic mass; such a finding confirms the presence of a tumor rather than debris or sludge.

Benign Solid Masses—Fibroadenoma and Fatty Pseudolesions

Fibroadenomas arise from breast lobules and are the most common solid benign masses in women younger

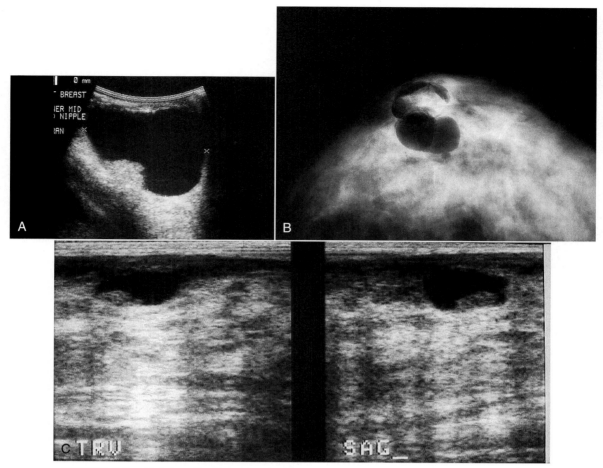

FIGURE 5-8   Intracystic Tumors. A, An intracystic carcinoma is shown as a mural mass projecting into the fluid-filled center of a cyst on ultrasound. **B,** In another patient, an intracystic papilloma is shown as a mass surrounded by air after fluid aspiration and pneumocystography. **C,** In a third patient, an apparent intracystic mass was shown to represent debris stuck to the side wall of a complex cyst at aspiration.

than 30 years. Once diagnosed, fibroadenomas may remain stable in 80% of cases, regress in about 15%, and grow in 5% to 10%. Fibroadenomas are benign, although cancer can occur within a fibroadenoma. Women with a specific histologic diagnosis of "complex fibroadenomas" have a small increased risk of future breast cancer, as described by DuPont et al. Fibroadenomas may be single or multiple and are called "giant" fibroadenomas if larger than 8 cm.

On ultrasound, fibroadenomas have been described by Cole-Beuglet et al. as having well-circumscribed, round or oval borders and containing weak low-level homogeneous internal echoes with enhanced, decreased, or unchanged sound transmission. Stavros et al. and Fornage et al. have described fibroadenomas as smooth, wider-than-tall structures. Stavros et al. further characterize fibroadenomas as having at most four gentle lobulations and homogeneous internal echo texture (Box 5-5) (Fig. 5-9A). Their appearance, however, can be highly

Box 5-5	Benign Mass Characteristics

Ellipsoid shape (wider than tall)
Four or fewer gentle lobulations
Intense homogeneous hyperechogenicity (in comparison to fat)
Thin, echogenic capsule
No malignant sonographic criteria

From Stavros AT, Thickman D, Rapp CL, et al: Solid breast nodules: Use of sonography to distinguish between benign and malignant lesions. Radiology 196:123-134, 1995.

variable (Fig. 5-9B and C). Fibroadenomas may occasionally display irregular margins, inhomogeneous echo texture, lobulated borders, or posterior acoustic shadowing and should prompt biopsy because they simulate cancer.

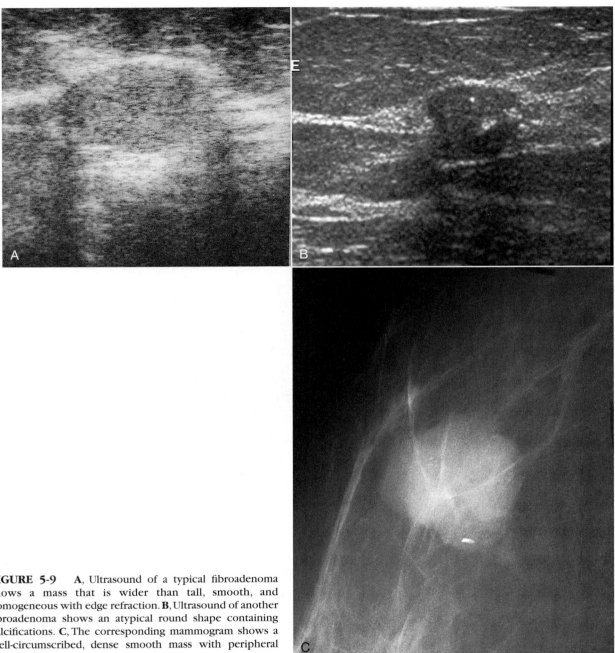

FIGURE 5-9   **A**, Ultrasound of a typical fibroadenoma shows a mass that is wider than tall, smooth, and homogeneous with edge refraction. **B**, Ultrasound of another fibroadenoma shows an atypical round shape containing calcifications. **C**, The corresponding mammogram shows a well-circumscribed, dense smooth mass with peripheral coarse calcifications. Biopsy revealed fibroadenoma.

Stavros et al. have described specific criteria for benign solid lesions (see Box 5-5): smooth margins with fewer than four gentle lobulations, intense homogeneous hyperechogenicity, thin echogenic pseudocapsule, wider-than-tall elongated appearance, and no malignant sonographic signs. Suspicious findings include acoustic shadowing, microlobulation, microcalcifications, ductal extension, angulated margins, or a very hypoechoic pattern (Box 5-6). In their 1995 study, large-core needle or surgical biopsy was performed on all masses, and findings were compared with prospective diagnoses by ultrasound. When the sonographic findings were benign by their criteria, the results yielded 424 true negatives and 2 false negatives. The negative predictive value was 99.5% and the sensitivity was 98.4% with strict adherence to the benign characteristics detailed earlier. Conversely, some well-circumscribed carcinomas may simulate fibroadenomas and should undergo biopsy (Fig. 5-9D-F) because not all round or oval solid masses are benign (Box 5-7).

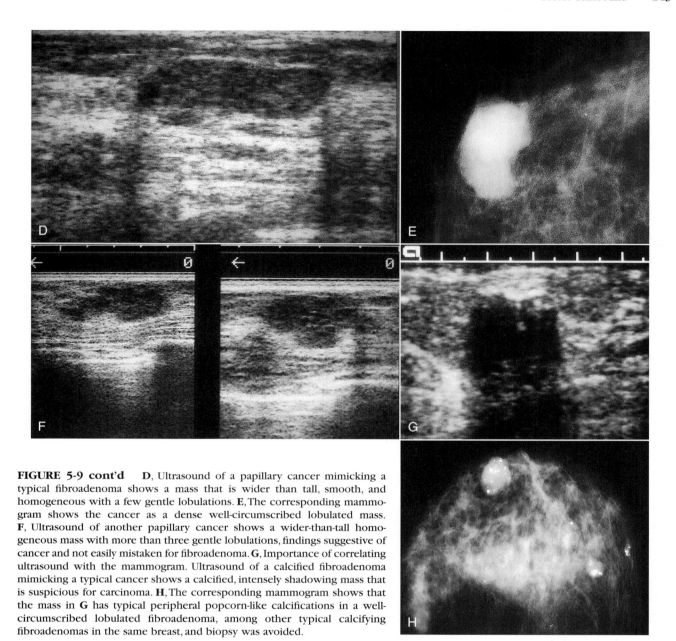

FIGURE 5-9 cont'd   **D,** Ultrasound of a papillary cancer mimicking a typical fibroadenoma shows a mass that is wider than tall, smooth, and homogeneous with a few gentle lobulations. **E,** The corresponding mammogram shows the cancer as a dense well-circumscribed lobulated mass. **F,** Ultrasound of another papillary cancer shows a wider-than-tall homogeneous mass with more than three gentle lobulations, findings suggestive of cancer and not easily mistaken for fibroadenoma. **G,** Importance of correlating ultrasound with the mammogram. Ultrasound of a calcified fibroadenoma mimicking a typical cancer shows a calcified, intensely shadowing mass that is suspicious for carcinoma. **H,** The corresponding mammogram shows that the mass in **G** has typical peripheral popcorn-like calcifications in a well-circumscribed lobulated fibroadenoma, among other typical calcifying fibroadenomas in the same breast, and biopsy was avoided.

After evaluation of a mass by ultrasound, it is important to re-evaluate the mammogram and correlate findings on the film with the ultrasound, not simply relying on only the ultrasound findings alone. The mammogram may provide important clues to the correct diagnosis, such as calcifications in a typical fibroadenoma, calcifications in benign fat necrosis, or suspicious pleomorphic calcifications suggestive of cancer that were lost in the normal speckled ultrasound background (Fig. 5-9G and H).

Pseudolesions produced by fatty deposits in the breast may simulate a solid hypoechoic mass. When a fatty pseudomass is scanned from various projections, the mass-like appearance of the fatty lobule should blend into the surrounding tissue and lack three-dimensional features.

Other benign solid breast masses in the breast include papillomas, lipomas, hamartomas, lymph nodes, and healed post-surgical scars. In these various benign conditions, the clinical setting and mammographic appearance usually help identify the true nature of the lesion because the sonographic features are rarely diagnostic. Examples of these masses are shown in Chapter 4.

Malignant Solid Masses

Cancers are generally hypoechoic relative to the brightly echogenic normal fibroglandular tissue; often have irregular, angulated, or spiculated margins; can show invasion by extension through normal breast planes ("taller than wide"); and may have an echogenic halo (Fig. 5-10A and B). Distal acoustic shadowing has been reported to occur in 60% to 97% of spiculated carcinomas and is thought to relate to fibrosis or collagen associated with the tumor (Fig. 5-10C). Acoustic shadowing should be differentiated from edge shadowing, an artifact caused by the edge of the mass against breast tissue, which has a different speed of sound. Scanning from different planes should distinguish edge shadowing from true acoustic shadowing because edge shadowing will not persist in all planes but true acoustic shadowing will (Fig. 5-11A and B).

By combining terms from the ACR BI-RADS lexicon and terms developed by Stavros et al., malignant solid masses often display angulated, indistinct, microlobulated, or spiculated margins; acoustic shadowing; microcalcifi-

Box 5-6	Suspicious Ultrasound Characteristics of Solid Breast Masses

Taller than wide
Acoustic shadowing
Spiculation
Microlobulation
Microcalcifications
Duct extension
Branch pattern
Angular margins
Markedly hypoechoic (in comparison to fat)

From Stavros AT, Thickman D, Rapp CL, et al: Solid breast nodules: Use of sonography to distinguish between benign and malignant lesions. Radiology 196:123-134, 1995.

Box 5-7	Round or Oval Solid Breast Masses

Fibroadenoma
Invasive ductal cancer—not otherwise specified
Medullary cancer
Mucinous (colloid) carcinoma
Papillary carcinoma
Metastasis
Phyllodes tumor
Papilloma

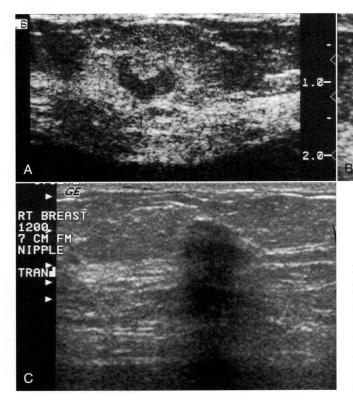

FIGURE 5-10   Transverse **(A)** and longitudinal **(B)** scans show a typical invasive ductal cancer: very hypoechoic relative to normal breast tissue and surrounded by a fuzzy echogenic halo. The irregular shape, angulated margins, invasive growth through normal tissue planes, and taller-than-wide configuration are all suspicious for cancer. Note that acoustic shadowing is absent in this cancer and that shadowing is not necessary to make the diagnosis. **C,** Ultrasound of a grade II invasive ductal carcinoma shows a very hypoechoic indistinct irregular mass with marked acoustic shadowing.

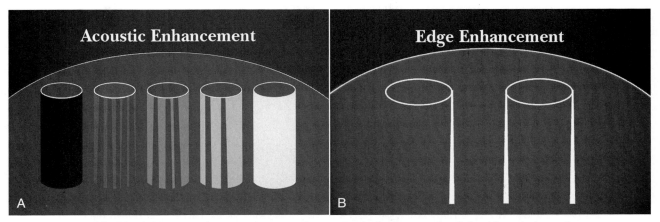

FIGURE 5-11 **A**, Schematic drawing of acoustic shadowing on the *left* with variations of shadowing and acoustic enhancement on the *right*. **B**, In comparison, the artifact of edge enhancement will be seen only at the edge of a mass, where it meets the surrounding breast tissue, and not in the middle of the mass.

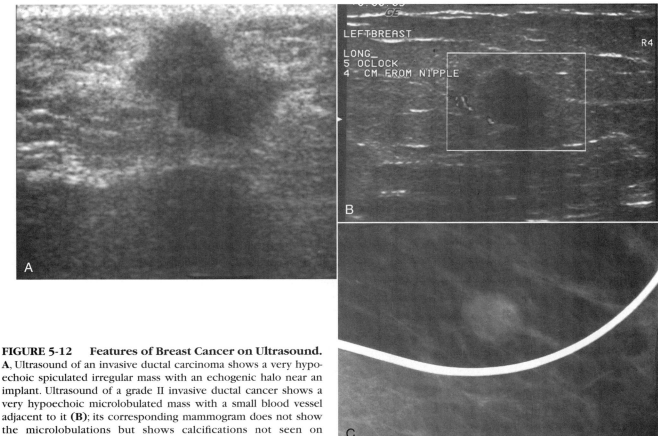

FIGURE 5-12   Features of Breast Cancer on Ultrasound. **A**, Ultrasound of an invasive ductal carcinoma shows a very hypoechoic spiculated irregular mass with an echogenic halo near an implant. Ultrasound of a grade II invasive ductal cancer shows a very hypoechoic microlobulated mass with a small blood vessel adjacent to it **(B)**; its corresponding mammogram does not show the microlobulations but shows calcifications not seen on ultrasound **(C)**.

cations; ductal extension; an echogenic halo; and a "taller-than-wide" configuration on ultrasound (see Box 5-6 and Table 5-1) (Fig. 5-12). Unfortunately, round circumscribed solid cancers can simulate benign breast masses on ultrasound, and the clinical history and mammographic findings must be taken into consideration in each case. The most common round breast malignancy is invasive ductal cancer (Box 5-8). Although the round circumscribed form is uncommon for invasive ductal cancer, this histology is so common that a round cancer is statistically

much more likely to be invasive ductal cancer than the
more rare medullary or mucinous cancer (Fig. 5-13A)
Circumscribed malignancies such as round invasive
ductal cancer and medullary, solid papillary, and colloid
(mucinous) carcinoma may simulate benign fibroadenomas
on ultrasound by appearing round or oval in shape with
enhanced transmission of sound (Fig. 5-13B and C).

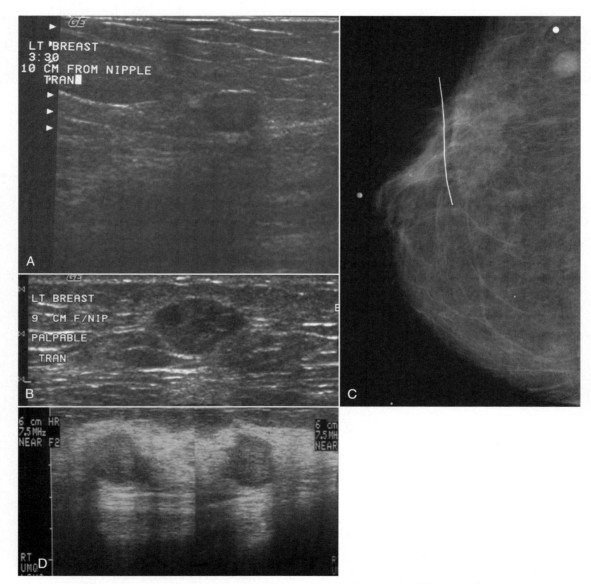

FIGURE 5-13   Breast Cancer Mimicking Benign Masses on Ultrasound. A, A well-
circumscribed, oval hypoechoic mass on ultrasound is an invasive ductal cancer that was new on the
mammogram from the previous year. Although medullary and mucinous cancers are often round,
invasive ductal cancer is more common (accounting for about 90% of all breast cancers) and is the
most common round cancer. **B,** Mucinous cancer mimicking a complex cyst on ultrasound. Ultrasound of a palpable mass shows an oval, circumscribed, complex cystic mass with rather thick septa.
Correlation with the mammogram shows a dense, slightly irregular mass that would be unusual for
a multilobulated cyst **(C)**. Biopsy revealed mucinous cancer. **D,** Medullary cancer. Ultrasound of a
palpable mass in a young woman shows a round mass with acoustic enhancement. Note that some
of the borders are circumscribed on one scan plane but one side of the mass has three spiculations,
thus demonstrating the importance of scanning all the margins of the mass in more than one plane.

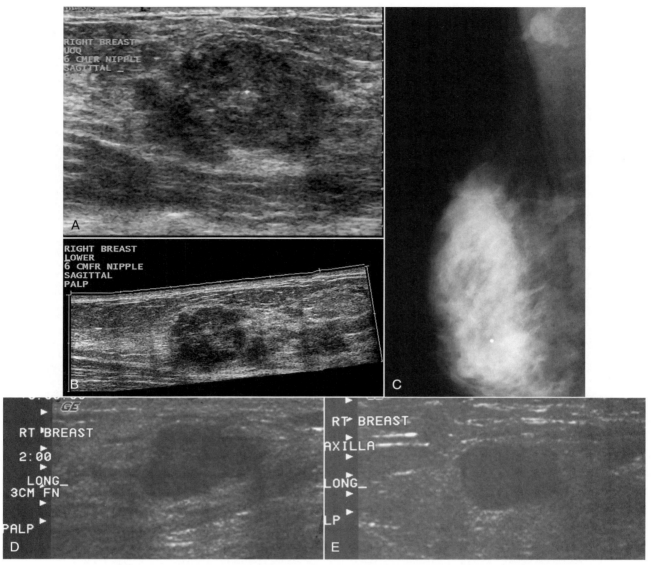

FIGURE 5-14   Features of Malignancy on Ultrasound. A, This invasive ductal cancer has microlobulated borders and bright internal echoes representing calcifications within the tumor. **B,** A landscape overview shows the invasive ductal cancer of **A** with its internal calcifications and a smaller second tumor slightly inferior and lateral to it. **C-G,** Axillary metastasis. **C,** A mediolateral oblique mammogram shows a dense breast with an abnormal dense lymph node in the axilla. Ultrasound of a palpable mass in the breast tissue on the ipsilateral side, not seen on the mammogram, shows a circumscribed lobulated mass with enhanced transmission of sound **(D)** that represents an invasive ductal cancer. **E,** Ultrasound of the abnormal lymph node in the axilla shows a hypoechoic mass without a fatty hilum that represents lymphadenopathy from the metastasis. Contrast the abnormal lymph node with a normal lymph node shown in Figure 5-1D.   *Continued*

Careful attention to the mass margins may prompt biopsy. The borders of some tumors may appear circumscribed in one scan plane, so it is important to scan in multiple planes to evaluate all mass borders for margin irregularity (Fig. 5-13D). Necrosis or mucin within cancers may produce anechoic regions resulting in posterior acoustic enhancement of sound, thereby mimicking the enhanced transmission of sound seen in cysts. Thus, some benign sonographic features of fibroadenomas and benign complex cystic lesions can also be seen in round malignancies.

Some of the larger calcifications in breast cancer may be seen by ultrasonography, but this important diagnostic sign is not generally visualized with regularity by ultrasound (Fig. 5-14A and B).

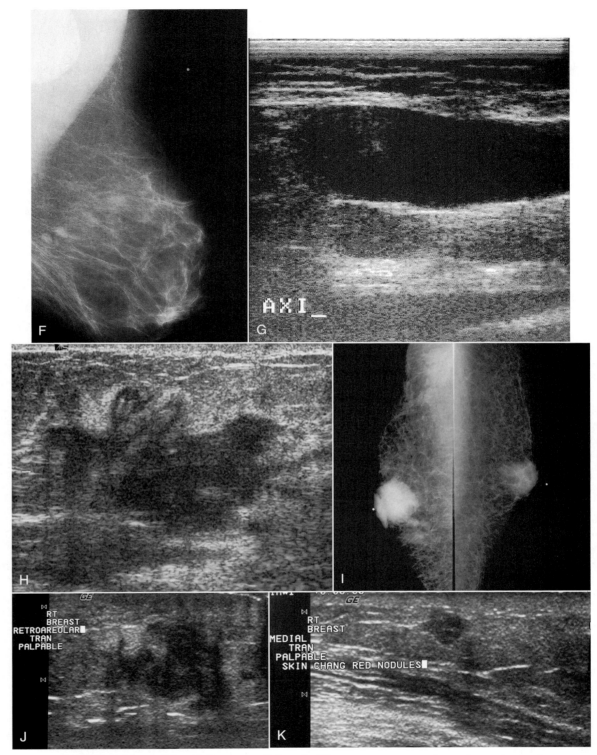

FIGURE 5-14 cont'd   F, On the mediolateral oblique mammogram, a huge dense abnormal lymph node is evident in the axilla. **G**, Ultrasound shows a hypoechoic mass that is so homogeneous that it almost looks like a cyst. Biopsy findings were consistent with lymphoma. **H**, A hypoechoic invasive ductal cancer with angulated margins and an echogenic halo has produced architectural distortion of the surrounding breast tissue. **I-K**, Inflammatory cancer in a male with red skin nodules. **I**, Mediolateral oblique mammograms show bilateral gynecomastia with an irregular right retroareolar mass, skin and nipple thickening, and a second mass in the axilla. **J**, Ultrasound shows a hypoechoic spiculated and angulated retroareolar mass with acoustic shadowing and thickening of the areola-nipple complex. **K**, Ultrasound of the skin changes and red nodules shows marked skin thickening and a hypoechoic mass in the skin from inflammatory cancer.

Box 5-9	Secondary Signs of Breast Cancer on Ultrasound

Calcifications
Lymphadenopathy
Skin thickening
Architectural distortion
Breast edema
Retraction of Cooper's ligaments

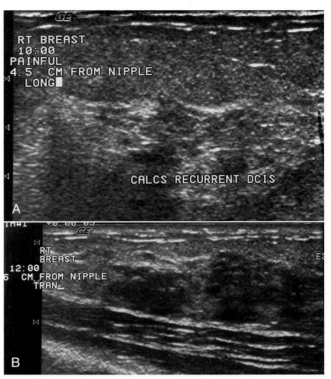

FIGURE 5-15   **A**, Ultrasound of recurrent ductal carcinoma in situ (DCIS) shows a few calcifications as bright echoes near hypoechoic dilated ducts, but they might easily be lost in the normal speckled background of normal breast tissue. **B**, Ultrasound of DCIS in another patient shows clumped hypoechoic nodular ducts on the chest wall and a few bright echoes within it, possibly representing the microcalcifications easily seen on mammography.

Unlike benign lymph nodes that contain a fatty hilum, lymphadenopathy in the axilla appears as hypoechoic oval masses without a fatty hilum (Fig. 5-14C-E). Benign reactive lymph nodes cannot be reliably differentiated from lymph nodes containing metastases or lymphoma (Fig. 5-14F and G). On the other hand, normal-appearing lymph nodes with fatty hila may contain occult metastases that are not detected by ultrasound.

Secondary signs of breast cancer include skin thickening, architectural distortion, breast edema, and retraction of Cooper's ligaments (Box 5-9) (Fig. 5-14H). Inflammatory carcinomas may have all of these signs, as well as marked attenuation of the sound beam (Fig. 5-14I-K).

Breast Calcifications

Breast calcifications are important because they may be the only indication of breast cancer on mammography and are often seen in ductal carcinoma in situ (DCIS). Calcifications may also be the only indication of invasive ductal cancer for which an associated mass has been obscured or hidden by dense breast tissue on the mammogram. Although mammography and micro–focal spot magnification views are the mainstay of calcification analysis, ultrasound performed in locations where suspicious microcalcifications are seen on mammography may detect an unsuspected hidden suspicious mass associated with the calcifications. The purpose of detecting these associated masses is to further analyze the finding and direct subsequent ultrasound-guided biopsy. If no suspicious mass or calcifications are discovered on targeted ultrasound, the decision to biopsy the calcifications is based solely on analysis of the calcification on mammography.

Although mammography effectively detects calcifications in DCIS, ultrasound is limited in finding calcifications in DCIS (Fig. 5-15A) because the calcifications may be lost in speckle artifact on ultrasound. Ultrasound is much better at depicting invasive breast cancer detected as breast masses than in detecting breast calcifications, unless the calcifications are associated with a mass. In a 2000 study of 40 women with breast cancer by Berg and Gilbreath in which mammography was compared with ultrasound for detection of invasive and noninvasive breast cancer, ultrasound showed 94% (45/48) of invasive breast cancers and 44% (7/16) of DCIS, whereas mammography depicted 81% (39/48) of invasive cancers and 88% (14/16) of DCIS. Thus, mammography is better at depicting calcifications than ultrasound is and should be used to screen the breast for DCIS.

On occasion, highly aggressive DCIS may be detected by ultrasound as hypoechoic masses, as reported by Soo et al., Huang et al., and Moon et al. (Fig.15-5B), but non-detection of DCIS calcifications was reported by others when ultrasound was used as a primary and stand-alone method of breast cancer screening. The non-detection of calcifications alone may limit ultrasound's use as a stand-alone screening modality, which will be discussed later in this chapter under "Breast Cancer Screening with Ultrasound."

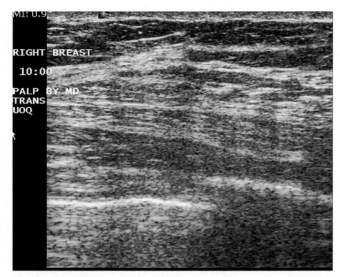

FIGURE 5-16 Ultrasound of a palpable mass felt by the patient's physician shows normal breast tissue and no discrete mass. This image was taken after the patient pointed out the mass prompting this examination; the mass was palpated by the operator who scanned over the mass. With a negative mammogram and ultrasound, management of the palpable finding is based on clinical grounds alone, and the patient is encouraged to follow up with her referring physician for the palpable finding. In this case, an image of the normal breast tissue was obtained; however, some facilities take no images of normal breast tissue and only take an image of areas specified by the words breast side, clock or quadrant position of the finding, number of centimeters from the nipple, and "palpable finding."

PALPABLE OR MAMMOGRAPHICALLY DETECTED FINDINGS UNDETECTED BY ULTRASOUND

Benign fibrofatty nodules, areas of dense glandular tissue, benign breast tissue, or breast cancer felt as a mass or lump by the patient or her physician may be shown as normal breast tissue on ultrasound when scanning directly over the palpable finding (Fig. 5-16). If the mammogram is normal, the patient is referred back to her referring physician for management of the palpable mass. In these cases, management of the palpable mass is based on clinical grounds alone.

For patients with suspicious physical findings and a normal mammogram and ultrasound, the decision to perform biopsy is based on the physical findings and the clinical situation alone. Invasive lobular cancer is especially notorious for producing extremely subtle or no mammographic findings, and although it may be seen as a mass on ultrasound, on occasion, invasive lobular cancer may be missed by breast ultrasound as well.

Some solid benign breast masses and breast cancers detected on mammography are ultrasonographically "invisible." In the setting of a mammographically suspicious lesion and a "normal" ultrasound examination, further investigation or biopsy should be based on analysis of the suspicious mammographic finding. If the suspicious mammographically detected finding is not found by targeted ultrasound, the mass is presumed to be composed of solid tissue and could be benign or malignant. In these cases, the decision to perform biopsy is based on the mammographic impression and clinical and physical findings.

YOUNG PATIENTS AND PALPABLE FINDINGS IN DENSE BREASTS

Ultrasound is commonly used as the first modality to evaluate palpable findings in young patients, particularly women younger than 30 years when the breasts are composed of mostly glandular tissue, which may hide a cancer. Similarly, ultrasound may be used to evaluate palpable masses in women with radiographically dense breasts on mammography.

If no mass is seen on breast ultrasound, the decision for biopsy of the palpable finding is based on clinical grounds alone because some cancers may not be seen with ultrasound.

CORRELATING MAMMOGRAPHIC FINDINGS WITH ULTRASOUND FINDINGS

Ultrasound is commonly used to characterize findings detected by mammography. Once a lesion is identified, it must be determined whether the ultrasound finding and the mammographic finding are the same thing. To accomplish this with nonpalpable findings, the operator places a metallic skin marker over the ultrasound finding and repeats the mammogram. To begin, the operator scans directly over the finding and slides a finger, a jumbo paper clip, or a cotton swab under the transducer so that it overlies the ultrasound finding (Fig. 5-17) and produces a ring-down shadow (Fig. 5-18). Once the ring-down shadow overlies the finding, the operator removes the transducer; leaves the fingertip, paper clip, or cotton swab on top of the skin over the mass; and marks this location with a permanent ink marker. The operator places a radiopaque skin marker on the ink spot for subsequent craniocaudal and mediolateral mammograms. The skin marker should correlate with the mammographic finding if the lesions are one and the same. Because the lesion may be deep in the breast, the skin marker may be compressed a few centimeters away from the lesion on the follow-up mammogram.

Alternatively, a radiopaque marker can be placed in the finding through a needle under ultrasound guidance.

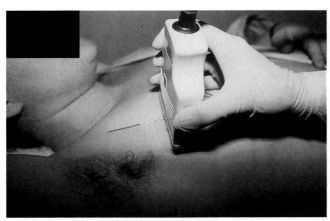

FIGURE 5-17   Correlating the Ultrasound Finding with the Mammogram. A large open paper clip is placed under the transducer over a finding.

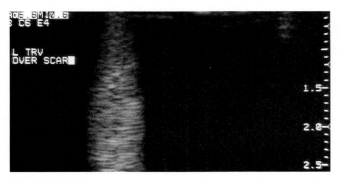

FIGURE 5-18 The ring-down shadow from the paper clip produces a bright shadow of the image. Superimposing this ring-down shadow over the lesion triangulates its location directly under the skin.

Follow-up orthogonal mammograms will determine whether the marker lies in the mammographic finding and thus shows that the mammographic finding and the ultrasound findings are one and the same.

On occasion, findings are seen on only one mammographic projection because of the finding's location in the breast or obscuration of it by adjacent breast tissue. Ultrasound of a one-view finding should be applied only in cases in which a full mammographic work-up has failed to visualize the finding in a second view. Once the lesion is seen on ultrasonography, confirmation that the mammographic abnormality corresponds to the ultrasonographic lesion should be accomplished by taking mammograms with skin markers or by placing a metallic marker in the finding and repeating the mammogram.

Box 5-10	Differential Diagnosis of Breast Edema

UNILATERAL	BILATERAL (SYSTEMIC PROBLEMS)
Mastitis	Anasarca
Inflammatory cancer	Congestive heart failure
Radiation therapy	Bilateral lymphadenopathy
Unilateral lymphadenopathy	Renal failure
Trauma (focal)	

BREAST EDEMA

Breast edema occurs in women with mastitis, inflammatory cancer, radiation therapy, post-biopsy trauma, or blockage of lymphatic drainage by various etiologies (Box 5-10). On breast physical examination an edematous breast is heavy and boggy. "Peau d'orange," or orange-peel skin, may be present as a result of skin pitting at locations where hair follicles hold the skin down and the surrounding tissues rise up with edema. On ultrasound, breast edema occasionally shows skin thickening greater than 2 to 3 mm. When compared with the contralateral breast, the edematous subcutaneous fat is gray as a result of leakage of fluid, the normally sharp Cooper ligaments are less well defined, and breast tissue loses the sharp clarity of individual structures because of breast edema blurring normal breast landmarks. On occasion, dermal and subdermal lymphatics may become engorged and filled with fluid and produce fluid-filled branching tubules simulating blood vessels or ducts (Fig. 5-19A). Fluid-filled lymphatics can be distinguished from blood vessels by Doppler ultrasound; blood vessels will show pulsation but fluid-filled lymphatics will not show flow (Fig. 5-19B). Normal fluid-filled breast ducts are larger than lymphatics and should branch and converge on the nipple. Fluid-filled lymphatics will parallel the skin surface and branch quickly along the superficial layers of the breast.

The key to identifying breast edema is to look for gray fat and thicker breast tissue and to compare the structures of the abnormal breast with the normal contralateral breast (Fig. 5-19C and D). In a normal breast the fat is dark, and Cooper's ligaments and breast structures will be sharply demarcated. In an edematous breast the fat is gray, and normal breast structures will be less well defined.

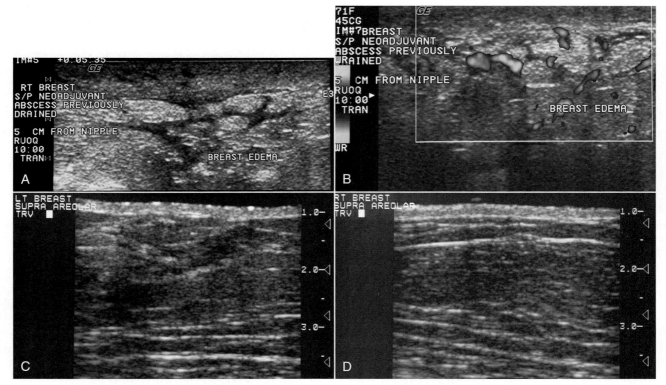

FIGURE 5-19   Breast Edema. A, Ultrasound shows marked skin thickening and a gray tinge to the normally markedly hypoechoic subcutaneous fat in this patient with marked breast edema. Just below the skin surface are numerous tubular fluid-filled structures representing blood vessels and fluid-filled lymphatics. Cooper's ligaments are not seen distinctly. **B,** Power Doppler shows that some of the structures represent blood vessels from hyperemia whereas others show no flow and represent fluid-filled dilated lymphatics. **C,** Breast edema in another patient shows gray-appearing fat, a marked hypoechoic streak through the normal breast tissue, and loss of the usual speckled appearance of Cooper's ligaments. In this case, there is no skin thickening or dermal lymphatic engorgement. **D,** For comparison, the normal opposite side shows normal dark hypoechoic fat, the normal thin lines of Cooper's ligaments, and a thinner breast.

BREAST ABSCESS

On occasion, mastitis progresses to a focal abscess, which is collection of pus within breast tissues. Mastitis can be focal or diffuse and causes inflammation. Early, the infection may percolate within breast tissue and, if untreated, give rise to a pus collection that forms a thick wall. The patient's breast will be painful to touch and may become hot, erythematous, or edematous, and the patient may have a fever and elevated white blood cell count. An abscess is commonly caused by *Staphylococcus aureus* or *Streptococcus* and is frequently subareolar because the infection is often introduced through a cracked duct during nursing. Antibiotics, though indicated for treatment, cannot reach the inside of the abscess to treat the infection because of the thick walls forming around the pus collection, and in many cases the abscess must be drained either percutaneously or surgically.

On ultrasound, an abscess is an irregular fluid collection that is ill defined along its edges in the early phases and may be either irregular or well encapsulated in later phases (Fig. 5-20A) with surrounding breast edema obscuring normal breast structures. An abscess can contain only one pocket of pus that can be drained by a needle (Fig. 5-20B), or it may have debris, thick pus, or septa that render percutaneous drainage difficult without using a larger needle or leaving a catheter in place (Fig. 5-20C and D). In larger abscesses, percutaneous drainage may help palliate the patient until surgery can be arranged. Air can be seen in abscesses that are drained percutaneously. Large abscesses are drained surgically,

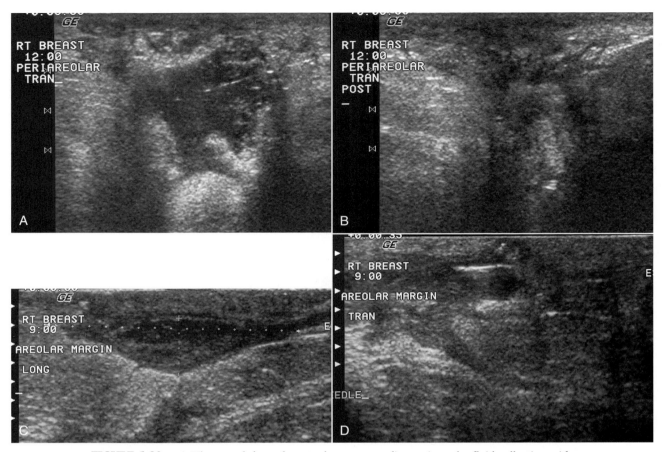

FIGURE 5-20   **A,** Ultrasound shows breast edema surrounding an irregular fluid collection with enhanced transmission of sound characteristic of a retroareolar abscess. Note the needle used to drain the abscess. **B,** After drainage of the pus, a post-aspiration ultrasound scan shows skin thickening and persistent edema, with less fluid in the abscess cavity. **C,** In another patient with an abscess, the fluid collection is just below the skin at the areolar margin, with marked skin thickening and surrounding edema. **D,** Unlike the patient in **A** and **B,** even though the fluid collection was in only one pocket, a 19-gauge needle could not drain the collection shown in **C** because of its thick tenacious nature, and the ultrasound image with the needle tip in the superior lateral portion of the collection shows no change in its size. This collection was drained surgically, although in some facilities a catheter might be placed percutaneously into the collection.

with irrigation of the abscess cavity and manual description of the septa, and the abscess is left to heal by granulation.

BREAST BIOPSY SCARS

In patients who have undergone lumpectomy for cancer, the lumpectomy cavity fills with fluid and the subcutaneous breast tissue and the skin are closed above it. On ultrasound, the biopsy cavity is predominantly filled with fluid, is hypoechoic, and may have a sharp or ill-defined edematous rim with or without shadowing in the immediate postoperative period. Careful scanning over the skin biopsy scar may show the thickened skin

at the incision and distortion of breast tissue along the incision from the skin surface to the biopsy scar (Fig. 5-21A). Later, serous fluid in the biopsy cavity may contain fibrous septa that move during real-time scanning, or the fluid may contain debris (Fig. 5-21B). Subsequently, the biopsy scar fills in with granulation tissue and becomes fibrotic, and the ultrasound appearance mimics a spiculated breast cancer by showing a hypoechoic breast mass with acoustic shadowing (Fig. 5-21C-F).

Breast cancers occurring near the biopsy site will have the same malignant characteristics and appearance of breast cancers on ultrasound, but they may be separated from the scar by normal breast parenchyma. Such separation can help distinguish breast cancer from the biopsy scar.

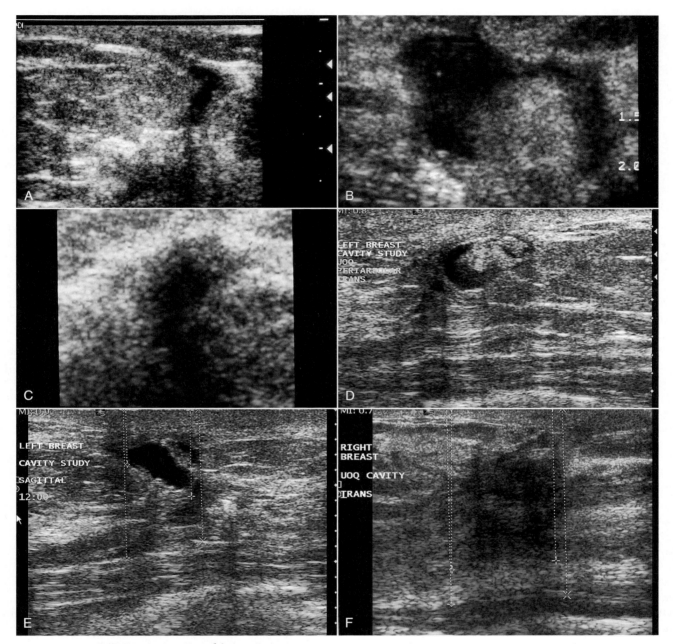

FIGURE 5-21   Post-biopsy Scars. A, Ultrasound of a post-biopsy scar after lumpectomy and radiation therapy shows a crescent-like fluid collection representing fluid in the biopsy cavity, with an edge trailing toward the skin representing the incision site. **B**, A post-biopsy scar in another patient is associated with an irregular fluid-filled mass and an echogenic ball within it representing fibrin and debris after biopsy. **C**, Ultrasound of the post-biopsy scar months later shows a hypoechoic irregular spiculated mass corresponding to the biopsy site. Without the correct history, the scar could easily be mistaken for breast cancer. **D**, Post-biopsy cavities before radiation therapy. Ultrasound for electron beam boost planning shows a fluid-filled biopsy cavity with echogenic solid debris within it. **E**, Imaging of a biopsy cavity in another patient shows the fluid-filled cavity with a thick septation and hypoechoic breast edema around the biopsy site. The measurements show the distance from the skin surface to the bottom of the cavity and the skin surface to the chest wall for electron beam boost planning. **F**, In a third patient, ultrasound shows the cavity as a hypoechoic spiculated mass with very little fluid within it.

CANCERS UNDERGOING NEOADJUVANT CHEMOTHERAPY

Locally advanced breast cancer, including inflammatory breast cancer and tumors larger than 5 cm that occasionally involve the chest wall or skin, accounts for a small fraction of all breast cancer in the United States. Such cancer may have bulky or matted lymph nodes containing metastatic disease. In past times, these women usually underwent mastectomy, with poor local control and poor survival 5 years after mastectomy.

Investigators have reported that preoperative neo-adjuvant chemotherapy combined with systemic therapy after local treatment by surgery and radiation improves disease-free and overall survival. Preoperative neoadjuvant chemotherapy is defined as combined chemotherapy given for local control before definitive surgical treatment to breast cancer patients who have large tumor masses (stage T3 or T4) and/or regional lymph node involvement. Neoadjuvant chemotherapy provides tumor shrinkage, decreases tumor burden, and improves local control and overall survival. However, poor outcomes in these patients are usually due to distant micrometastatic disease at the time of diagnosis.

In the setting of neoadjuvant chemotherapy, ultrasound is used to guide percutaneous biopsy to establish a histologic diagnosis as needed, determine initial tumor size and extent, document treatment response, and evaluate for residual tumor after neoadjuvant chemotherapy (Fig. 5-22). After neoadjuvant chemotherapy, the residual tumor site is often resected to establish the type and extent of residual tumor on pathologic analysis. This information is important for predicting prognosis and determining whether breast-conserving therapy is an option.

On occasion, neoadjuvant chemotherapy may produce a complete clinical response and the tumor may become undetectable by physical examination. However, the original tumor site may still require resection to determine whether there has been a complete pathologic response to neoadjuvant chemotherapy. The finding of no residual invasive or in situ tumor on pathologic evaluation has important positive prognostic implications.

Because some tumors become undetectable by both clinical examination and imaging after neoadjuvant chemotherapy, the radiologist may be asked to place a marker in the tumor under imaging guidance (Fig. 5-23). If all traces of the tumor fade with chemotherapy, the marker will show the location of the original tumor site and can be used for subsequent preoperative needle localization.

POST-BIOPSY BREAST MARKERS AND CORE BIOPSY SITES

Vacuum-assisted biopsy methods may remove an entire lesion. Usually, air or fluid may be seen in the biopsy track, in the biopsy site, or in a hematoma immediately after vacuum-assisted core biopsy. This air and fluid are absorbed relatively quickly after biopsy. After resorption, the only ultrasound findings are residua of the original mass, if any remains (Fig. 5-24A-C). Otherwise, very little, if any residua remain in the biopsy site. This is a problem if the entire lesion is removed and histologic evaluation shows cancer for which surgical excisional biopsy is needed. Fluid, air, or blood accumulating in the biopsy cavity may be resorbed before the surgery date and cannot be relied on to guide the surgeon. To solve this problem, tiny permanent metallic markers were developed to place in the biopsy site during percutaneous needle biopsy. The metallic marker in the biopsy cavity provides a landmark to guide subsequent mammographic or ultrasonographic preoperative needle localization.

On ultrasound, the metallic markers are seen as tiny bright echogenic lines, but the metallic marker echo can be lost in the speckle artifact of normal breast tissue (Fig. 5-24D). To overcome problems in imaging the metallic markers by ultrasound, some manufacturers have encased the metallic markers in echogenic pledgets composed of various materials. The pledgets and their encased metallic markers are placed in the biopsy site through a vacuum-assisted biopsy probe or directly through a separate needle deployment device under ultrasound guidance. The pledgets are radiolucent and invisible to mammography, but they are detectable as echogenic lines or plugs on ultrasound (Fig. 5-24E). These pledgets are absorbed by the body at a slower rate than blood or seromas and were developed as targets for subsequent ultrasound-guided preoperative needle localization. The facility should be familiar with the resorption rate of the pledget in any particular case if follow-up ultrasound-guided preoperative localization is anticipated.

COLOR DOPPLER, POWER DOPPLER, ULTRASOUND CONTRAST AGENTS, AND THREE-DIMENSIONAL IMAGING

Color Doppler and power Doppler ultrasound depict the location of blood vessels when planning percutaneous breast biopsy needle trajectories (Fig. 5-25). As a diagnostic tool, the finding of a blood vessel in an intracystic mass or within a cystic versus a solid mass is a helpful diagnostic sign.

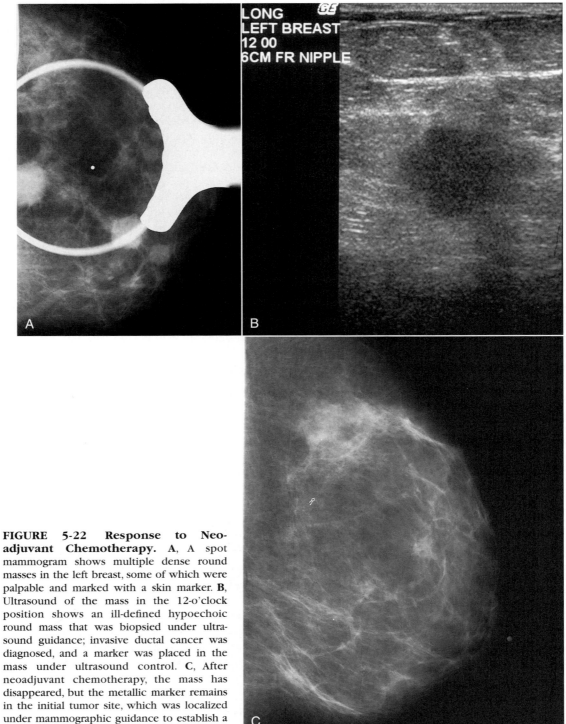

FIGURE 5-22 Response to Neo-adjuvant Chemotherapy. A, A spot mammogram shows multiple dense round masses in the left breast, some of which were palpable and marked with a skin marker. **B,** Ultrasound of the mass in the 12-o'clock position shows an ill-defined hypoechoic round mass that was biopsied under ultrasound guidance; invasive ductal cancer was diagnosed, and a marker was placed in the mass under ultrasound control. **C,** After neoadjuvant chemotherapy, the mass has disappeared, but the metallic marker remains in the initial tumor site, which was localized under mammographic guidance to establish a pathologic response.

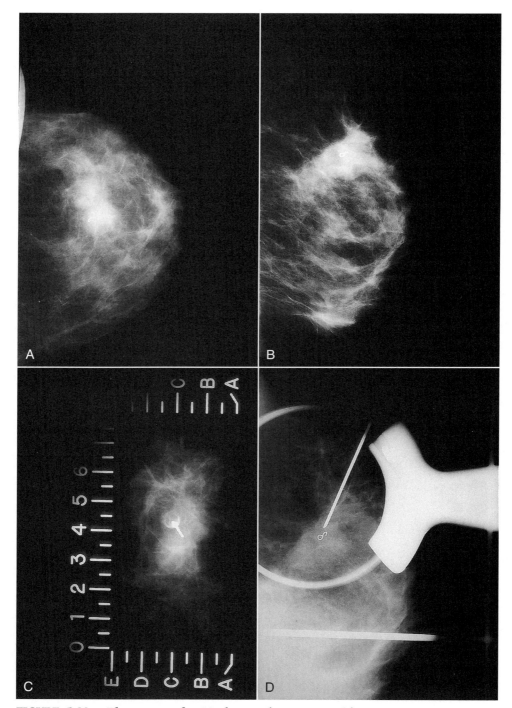

FIGURE 5-23   Placement of a Marker under X-ray Guidance. Craniocaudal (**A**) and mediolateral (**B**) mammograms show a 3-cm invasive ductal cancer in the 12-o'clock position of the breast. Because the patient was to undergo neoadjuvant chemotherapy, a marker was placed in the mass under x-ray guidance. An alphanumeric grid is placed over the tumor and a needle inserted into the tumor (**C**). An orthogonal view shows the tip of the needle in the middle of the tumor, the marker is deployed through the needle (**D**), and the needle is removed.   *Continued*

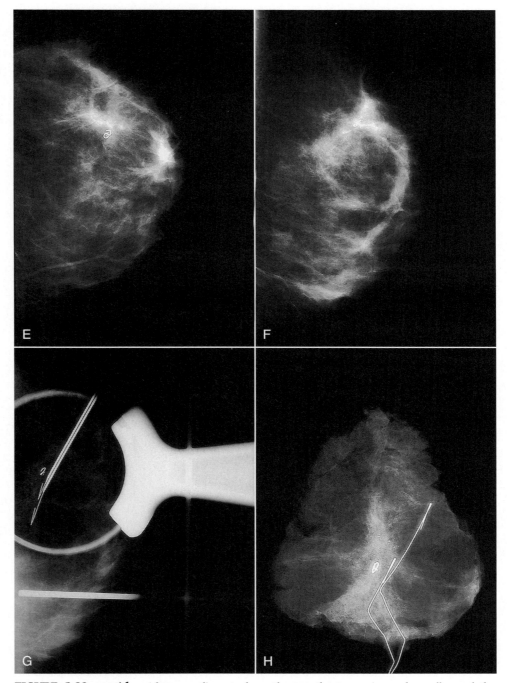

FIGURE 5-23 cont'd   After neoadjuvant chemotherapy, the tumor is much smaller and the marker is still in place on craniocaudal (**E**) and mediolateral (**F**) mammograms. Preoperative needle localization bracket wires are placed around the marker and residual tumor (**G**), which is resected in toto as shown on the specimen (**H**).

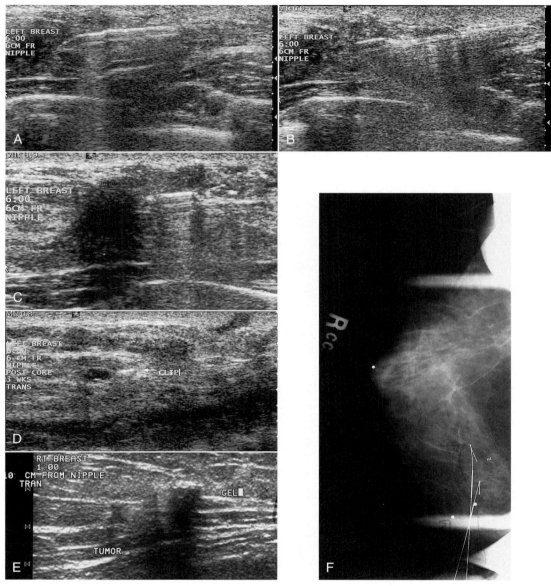

FIGURE 5-24   **A**, Ultrasound shows a core biopsy needle in the post-fire position in an irregular hypoechoic invasive ductal cancer. **B**, After biopsy, a second needle was placed in the mass and a marker deployed to a position near the biopsied mass. The marker is the thin, bright echogenic line just beyond the needle tip. **C**, Ultrasound after marker placement shows the mass and the bright echogenic linear clip, easily seen adjacent to the hypoechoic irregular mass, which is the residua after biopsy. In this case, either the clip or the mass would be used as a target for preoperative needle localization for subsequent excisional biopsy. **D**, Another portion of the same breast in **A** to **C** had undergone stereotactic vacuum-assisted biopsy 3 weeks before. Ultrasound shows a small oval fluid-filled cavity, and the marker was placed adjacent to the fluid collection by stereotaxis. The clip is a thin, bright echogenic line that might subsequently be lost in the speckle artifact of normal breast tissue once the fluid collection is resorbed. In another patient, an echogenic pledget with a metallic marker is placed near a tumor close to the chest wall **(E)**. The marker is the thick echogenic line to the left of the word "gel." In this case, the tumor was difficult to see on the craniocaudal mammogram because of its position in the high inner aspect of the breast, and the residual tumor and the clip were used for bracket localization, as shown in the craniocaudal post-localization mammogram **(F)**.

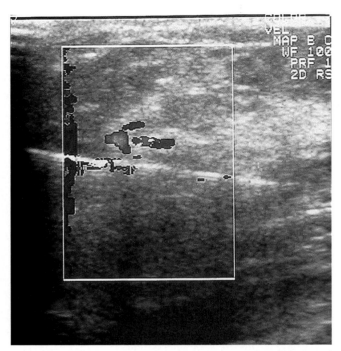

FIGURE 5-25 Color Doppler ultrasound shows a blood vessel that was avoided during biopsy of a mass deep in the breast tissue. Because the vessel's location was known, the needle was guided below it to approach the mass, which proved to be a cyst.

It was hoped that color Doppler and power Doppler imaging would distinguish cancer from benign breast lesions by showing increased blood flow in breast malignancies. The increased flow was thought to arise from tumor angiogenesis because increased vasculature was produced by carcinomas in pathologic specimens. However, color Doppler did not always detect increased flow in breast cancer, and there was overlap between benign and malignant blood flow patterns. Attempts to increase the sensitivity of ultra-sound for detecting blood flow with power Doppler improved these results, but not enough to advocate its use as a screening mechanism for breast cancer or to influence the decision to monitor a mass in lieu of biopsy. The use of contrast agents has been proposed as a means of increasing the ability of ultrasound vascular imaging techniques to detect small increases in vascular density, but such techniques are still experimental. Three-dimensional gray-scale and color Doppler imaging to depict gray-scale characteristics and vascular flow patterns, though promising, is also still being developed.

BREAST CANCER SCREENING WITH ULTRASOUND

X-ray mammography is the gold standard for breast cancer screening and diagnosis. It depicts calcifications in DCIS and effectively displays invasive breast cancer masses in fatty breasts, but its limitations are well known in dense breast tissue. Because breast ultrasound is not limited by dense breast tissue, requires only moderate breast compression, does not use ionizing radiation, is widely available, and is relatively easy to use, there was great hope that screening for breast cancer with ultrasound would be promising.

The initial clinical investigations of screening breast ultrasonography from the early 1980s were disappointing. An automated whole-breast ultrasound screening study by Kopans et al. depicted only 64% of 127 breast cancers in a study of 1140 women; in contrast, mammography detected 94% of the cancers. Another study with a similar number of patients by Sickles et al. resulted in sonographic detection of 58% (37 of 64) of cancers and mammographic detection of 97% (62 of 64). Only 8% of the ultrasound-detected tumors were smaller than 1 cm, but mammography detected all tumors less than 1 cm in size. Breast ultrasound produced very poor visualization of microcalcifications, and the limitations of ultrasound in studying fatty breasts resulted in an early recommendation that breast sonography not be used for breast cancer screening.

Later, subsequent improvements in transducer and ultrasound technology resulted in more optimistic results. Hand-held whole-breast ultrasound screening studies found small invasive cancers undetected by mammography in asymptomatic women. A 2002 study of 11,130 asymptomatic dense-breasted women undergoing screening mammography and whole-breast ultrasound screening by Kolb et al. showed 246 cancers in 221 women (1.98% of 11,130 women). Mammography had a sensitivity and specificity of 77.6% and 98.8% versus 75.3% and 96.8% for ultrasound. A 1995 study by Gordon et al. showed 1575 solid nonpalpable masses invisible by mammography but visualized by ultrasound in 12,706 women. Of these, 279 ultrasound-detected masses underwent biopsy, with 44 cancers found (16% of 279, 2.8% of the 1575 solid masses, 0.35% of 12,706 women).

However, the early promise and enthusiasm for whole-breast ultrasound screening to increase breast cancer detection have been dampened by limited operator resources, inherent issues of reproducibility, possible non-detection of calcifications in DCIS, and potential unnecessary biopsies of incidentally detected benign breast lesions. A follow-up large-scale trial of breast cancer screening with ultrasound is in progress under the American College of Radiology Imaging Network (ACRIN) to determine whether the sensitivity and specificity of screening breast ultrasound shown in the smaller pilot studies can be reproduced across multiple facilities.

KEY ELEMENTS

Breast ultrasound is a useful adjunct to mammography and clinical examination, particularly for the diagnosis of cysts and in certain other limited settings.

Ultrasound results should be considered in conjunction with mammographic and clinical findings to avoid misdiagnosis.

Cysts are anechoic, round or oval well-circumscribed masses with imperceptible walls and enhanced transmission of sound.

Fibroadenomas are classically described as ellipsoid, well-circumscribed masses with fewer than four gentle lobulations, and they are wider than tall.

There is overlap in the ultrasound appearance of benign fibroadenomas and well-circumscribed breast cancers.

Suspicious ultrasound findings in solid masses include acoustic spiculation; shadowing; taller-than-wide configuration; angulated, indistinct, microlobulated, or spiculated margins; irregular shape; and an echogenic halo.

Secondary signs of breast cancer on ultrasound are changes in Cooper's ligaments, breast edema, architectural distortion, skin thickening, skin retraction or irregularity, and suspicious microcalcifications.

Cystic breast masses include breast cysts, complex breast cysts, intracystic carcinoma or papilloma, mucinous cancer, necrotic cancer, abscess, seroma, hematoma, and galactocele.

Solid round or oval masses include fibroadenoma, papilloma, cancer (invasive ductal, medullary, mucinous, papillary), metastasis, and phyllodes tumor.

The most common round cancer is invasive ductal cancer, an uncommon form of a very common tumor.

Multiple solid masses include fibroadenomas, papillomas, multiple breast cancers, or metastases.

Breast edema is characterized by skin thickening, gray fat, loss of crisply defined breast structures, increased breast thickness when compared with the contralateral side, and occasionally, fluid-filled lymphatics.

Breast abscesses are usually caused by *Staphylococcus aureus* or *Streptococcus,* are generally subareolar, and cause a hot, painful hypoechoic pus-filled mass with surrounding breast edema.

Breast biopsy scars look just like cancer on ultrasound after the seroma is resorbed, and correlation with the skin scar and surgical history is necessary.

Metallic markers may be placed in breast biopsy cavities or in tumors before neoadjuvant chemotherapy to guide subsequent preoperative needle localization.

Current studies are under way to evaluate ultrasound for breast cancer screening.

SUGGESTED READINGS

American College of Radiology: American College of Radiology Standards. Reston, VA, American College of Radiology, 2002, pp 593-595.

American College of Radiology: Illustrated Breast Imaging Reporting and Data System (BI-RADS), 4th ed. Reston, VA, American College of Radiology (in press).

Baker JA, Soo MS: Breast US: Assessment of technical quality and image interpretation. Radiology 223:229-238, 2002.

Berg WA: Rationale for a trial of screening breast ultrasound: American College of Radiology Imaging Network (ACRIN) 6666. AJR Am J Roentgenol 180:1225-1228, 2003.

Berg WA, Campassi CI, Ioffe OB: Cystic lesions of the breast: Sonographic-pathologic correlation. Radiology 227:183-191, 2003.

Berg WA, Gilbreath PL: Multicentric and multifocal cancer: Whole-breast US in preoperative evaluation. Radiology 214:59-66, 2000.

Birdwell RL, Ikeda DM, Jeffrey SS, et al: Preliminary experience with power Doppler imaging of solid breast masses. AJR Am J Roentgenol 169:703-707, 1997.

Bruneton JN, Caramella E, Héry M, et al: Axillary lymph node metastases in breast cancer: Preoperative detection with ultrasound. Radiology 158:325-326, 1986.

Buchberger W, DeKoekkoek-Doll P, Springer P, et al: Incidental findings on sonography of the breast: Clinical significance and diagnostic workup. AJR Am J Roentgenol 173: 921-927, 1999.

Chopra S, Evans AJ, Pinder SE, et al: Pure mucinous breast cancer—mammographic and ultrasound findings. Clin Radiol 51:421-424, 1996.

Cole-Beuglet C, Soriano RZ, Kurtz AB, Goldberg BB: Ultrasound analysis of 104 primary breast carcinomas classified according to histologic type. Radiology 147:191-196, 1983.

Cole-Beuglet C, Soriano RZ, Kurtz AB, Goldberg BB: Fibroadenoma of the breast: Sonomammography correlated with pathology in 122 patients. AJR Am J Roentgenol 140:369-375, 1983.

Dennis MA, Parker SH, Klaus AJ, et al: Breast biopsy avoidance: The value of normal mammograms and normal sonograms in the setting of a palpable lump. Radiology 219:186-191, 2001.

Downey DB, Fenster A, Williams JC: Clinical utility of three-dimensional US. Radiographics 20:559-571, 2000.

DuPont WD, Page DL, Pari FF, et al: Long-term risk of breast cancer in women with fibroadenoma. N Eng J Med 351(1): 10-15, 1994.

Fornage BD, Lorigan JG, Andry E: Fibroadenoma of the breast: Sonographic appearance. Radiology 172:671-675, 1989.

Gordon PB: Ultrasound for breast cancer screening and staging. Radiol Clin North Am 40:431-441, 2002.

Gordon PB, Goldenberg SL: Malignant breast masses detected only by ultrasound. A retrospective review. Cancer 76:626-630, 1995.

Hashimoto BE, Kramer DJ, Picozzi VJ: High detection rate of breast ductal carcinoma in situ calcifications on mammographically directed high-resolution sonography. J Ultrasound Med 20:501-508, 2001.

Hilton SW, Leopold GR, Olson LK, Wilson SA: Real time breast sonography: Application in 300 consecutive patients. AJR Am J Roentgenol 147:479-486, 1986.

Huang CS, Wu CY, Chu JS, et al: Microcalcifications of non-palpable breast lesions detected by ultrasonography: Correlation with mammography and histopathology. Ultrasound Obstet Gynecol 13:431-436, 1999.

Kaplan SS: Clinical utility of bilateral whole-breast US in the evaluation of women with dense breast tissue. Radiology 221:641-649, 2001.

Kolb TM, Lichy J, Newhouse JH: Occult cancer in women with dense breasts: Detection with screening US—diagnostic yield and tumor characteristics. Radiology 207:191-199, 1998.

Kolb TM, Lichy J, Newhouse JH: Comparison of the performance of screening mammography, physical examination, and breast US and evaluation of factors that influence them: An analysis of 27,825 patient evaluations. Radiology 225:165-175, 2002.

Kopans DB, Meyer JE, Lindfors KK, et al: Breast sonography to guide cyst aspiration and wire localization of occult solid lesions. AJR Am J Roentgenol 143:489-492, 1984.

Kopans DB, Meyer JE, Lindfors KK: Whole-breast US imaging: Four year follow-up. Radiology 157:505-507, 1985.

Liberman L, Feng TL, Dershaw DD, et al: US-guided core breast biopsy: Use and cost-effectiveness. Radiology 208:717-723, 1998.

Mendelson EB, Berg WA, Merritt CR: Toward a standardized breast ultrasound lexicon, BI-RADS: Ultrasound. Semin Roentgenol 36:17-25, 2001.

Meyer JE, Amin E, Lindfors KK: Medullary carcinoma of the breast: Mammographic and US appearance. Radiology 170:79-82, 1989.

Moon WK, Im JG, Koh YH, et al: US of mammographically detected clustered microcalcifications. Radiology 217:849-854, 2000.

Moon WK, Myung JS, Lee YJ, et al: US of ductal carcinoma in situ. Radiographics 22:269-280, 2002.

Moon WK, Noh DY, Im JG: Multifocal, multicentric, and contra-lateral breast cancers: Bilateral whole-breast US in the pre-operative evaluation of patients. Radiology 224:569-576, 2002.

Parker SH, Jobe WE, Dennis MA, et al: US-guided automated large-core breast biopsy. Radiology 187:507-511, 1993.

Reuter K, D'Orsi CJH, Reale F: Intracystic carcinoma of the breast: The role of ultrasonography. Radiology 153:233-234, 1984.

Schneck CD, Lehman DA: Sonographic anatomy of the breast. Semin Ultrasound 3:13-33, 1982.

Sickles EA: Sonographic detectability of breast calcifications. SPIE 419:51-52, 1983.

Sickles EA, Filly RA, Callen RW: Breast cancer detection with sonography and mammography: Comparison using state-of-the-art equipment. AJR Am J Roentgenol 140:843-845, 1983.

Sickles EA, Filly RA, Callen PW: Benign breast lesions: Ultra-sound detection and diagnosis. Radiology 151:467-470, 1984.

Skaane P, Sauer T: Ultrasonography of malignant breast neoplasms. Analysis of carcinomas missed as tumor. Acta Radiol 40:376-382, 1999.

Soo MS, Baker JA, Rosen EL, et al: Sonographically guided biopsy of suspicious microcalcifications of the breast: A pilot study. AJR Am J Roentgenol 178:1007-1015, 2002.

Stavros AT, Thickman D, Rapp CL, et al: Solid breast nodules: Use of sonography to distinguish between benign and malignant lesions. Radiology 196:123-134, 1995.

Tabár L, Péntek Z, Dena PB: The diagnostic and therapeutic value of breast cyst puncture and pneumocystography. Radiology 141:659-663, 1981.

The WL, Wilson AR, Evan AJ, et al: Ultrasound guided core biopsy of suspicious mammographic calcifications using high frequency and power Doppler ultrasound. Clin Radiol 55:390-394, 2000.

Weind KL, Maier CF, Rutt BK, Moussa M: Invasive carcinomas and fibroadenomas of the breast: Comparison of microvessel distributions—implications for imaging modalities. Radiology 208:477-483, 1998.

CHAPTER 6

Image-Guided Breast Procedures

Introduction
Pre-biopsy Patient Work-up
Informed Consent
Local Anesthesia
Preoperative Needle Localization under Radiographic
Guidance Using a Fenestrated Alphanumeric Compression
Plate with Specimen Radiography
    Specimen Radiography after Preoperative Needle Localization and
        Pathology Correlation
    Stereotactic Preoperative Needle Localization
    Ultrasound Guidance for Preoperative Needle Localization
Biopsy of Palpable Breast Masses
    Cyst Aspiration
    Freehand Fine-Needle Aspiration of Palpable Breast Masses
    Fine-Needle Aspiration under Radiographic Guidance Using a
        Fenestrated Alphanumeric Compression Plate
    Ultrasound Guidance for Fine-Needle Aspiration or Core Needle
        Biopsy of Solid Masses
Core Biopsy
    Stereotactic Localization for Core Needle Biopsy
    Core Specimen Radiography
    Carbon Marking after Stereotactic Biopsy
    Patient Comfort after Biopsy
    Complete Lesion Removal
    Marker Placement, Marker Movement, and Ultrasound and MRI
        Marker Compatibility
    Calcification and Epithelial Displacement
    Review of Radiography and Pathology in Core Biopsy
        Specimens
    Controversy regarding Management of Specific Core
        Histologic Findings
    Follow-up of Breast Lesions Diagnosed as Benign
    Complications
Follow-up, Audits, and Patient Non-compliance
Key Elements

INTRODUCTION

Biopsy of nonpalpable imaging-detected breast lesions with correlation of imaging and pathologic findings is an important part of the breast-imaging service. The advantage of percutaneous biopsy is that it can provide a diagnosis with a minimum of patient trauma. A diagnosis of cancer by percutaneous needle biopsy allows the patient to decide on lumpectomy versus mastectomy. Furthermore, biopsy specimens showing invasive cancer allow both tumor excision and axillary node dissection at the first surgery. This chapter will describe percutaneous breast biopsy techniques, preoperative needle localization, and imaging-pathology correlation.

PRE-BIOPSY PATIENT WORK-UP

Nonpalpable, imaging-detected breast lesions are amenable to preoperative localization or percutaneous biopsy. Accurate and safe targeting and sampling require communication between the surgeon, patient, radiologist, and technologist to ensure successful results.

Nothing substitutes for a complete imaging work-up of nonpalpable breast lesions. Physicians must have the lesion's location firmly entrenched in three dimensions in their mind to plan an approach that will be successful in removing the lesion. Pre-biopsy mammographic work-up requires visualization of the lesion in craniocaudal and mediolateral orthogonal views (Box 6-1). When the finding is not seen definitively, additional work-up with fine-detail mammographic views, views with skin markers, ultrasound, and physical examination is necessary to ensure proper triangulation of the lesion. *Do not attempt to biopsy a breast lesion if you do not know whether it is real or if you do not know its location in the breast!*

A full work-up is essential to triangulate and analyze the lesion to prevent cancellation of the procedure. Philpotts et al. reported various reasons for cancellation of stereotactic biopsy in 89 cases, including 26 (29%) lesions that were not recognized; 17 (19%) lesions reassessed as benign; 12 (13%) and 11 (12%) cysts diagnosed by ultrasound or aspiration, respectively; 12 (13%) suboptimal lesion locations for targeting; and 7 (8%) patients intolerant of the procedure or 4 (4%) for other reasons. Canceled procedures and lost time would have been avoided by a full work-up or history in most of these cases.

On occasion, a lesion is seen in only one view and difficult to triangulate on mammography. In such cases, the location of the lesion can be approximated by using stereotactic targeting and estimating the predicted needle tip depth in the breast. Recording the depth and location (e.g., upper outer quadrant) of the lesion by stereotactic biopsy may help direct further imaging studies in the quadrant of interest.

Some calcifications prompting biopsy may be within the skin and not require biopsy at all. Calcifications in a peripheral location or radiolucent calcification centers may be a clue to the true origin of the calcifications. Tangential views can identify dermal calcifications, and the procedure can be canceled.

INFORMED CONSENT

Informed consent is an important part of any procedure (Box 6-2). For percutaneous breast biopsy, the patient is advised of the risks, benefits, and alternatives to biopsy, including surgery. Possible untoward outcomes include an inability to sample the lesion because of technical limitations (not seeing calcifications or the lesion being too deep, shallow, or dangerous to biopsy), insufficient samples requiring re-biopsy or surgery, pathology results requiring surgery, the probability of leaving a marker in the biopsy site, and follow-up scenarios for benign results *because it might be cancer.* Other risks include hematoma, uncontrollable bleeding requiring an emergency room visit or surgical intervention, pneumo-

thorax in cases of ultrasound-guided biopsy, and breast infection. The patient is also informed about wound management and when and how to obtain biopsy results.

LOCAL ANESTHESIA

Some facilities use local anesthesia routinely for breast biopsy and preoperative needle localization. A common local anesthetic for the skin in breast biopsies is 1% lidocaine buffered with 8% sodium bicarbonate in a 20:1 ratio. Because skin necrosis can occur with the injection of 1% lidocaine with 1:100,000 epinephrine, plain buffered lidocaine or topical anesthetics are used for skin anesthesia. For deep anesthesia, a common local anesthetic is 1% lidocaine with 1:100,000 epinephrine buffered with 8% sodium bicarbonate in a 20:1 ratio. To avoid a mix-up of plain and epinephrine-added lidocaine, the two solutions may be drawn up in different-sized syringes, with a 25-gauge skin injection needle placed only on the syringe containing plain lidocaine. The maximum dose of 1% lidocaine with epinephrine is 7 mg/kg (3.5 mg/lb) body weight, not to exceed 500 mg. The maximum dose of 1% lidocaine without epinephrine is 4.5 mg/kg (2 mg/lb), not to exceed 300 mg.

PREOPERATIVE NEEDLE LOCALIZATION UNDER RADIOGRAPHIC GUIDANCE USING A FENESTRATED ALPHANUMERIC COMPRESSION PLATE WITH SPECIMEN RADIOGRAPHY

This method involves the use of a compression plate containing an aperture that is lined by letters and numbers or a series of holes (Fig. 6-1A-D), and it is simple

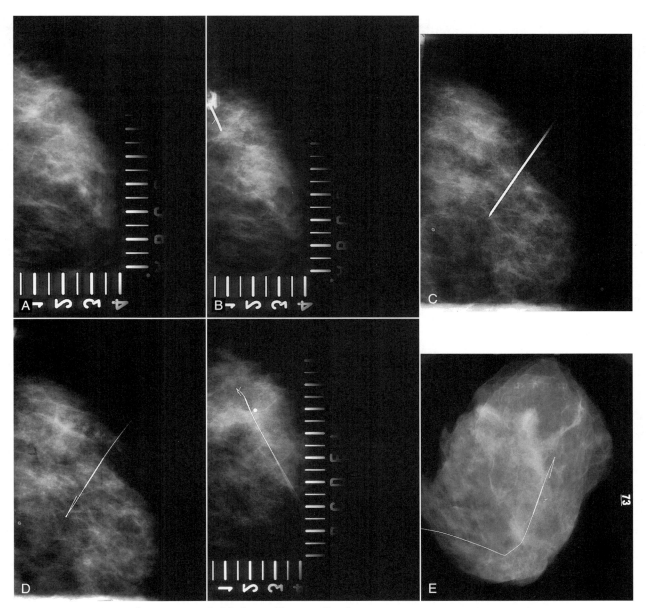

FIGURE 6-1   X-ray–Guided Needle Localization. Mammograms had shown a clip in a suspicious cluster of microcalcifications in the upper outer quadrant where core biopsy showed ductal carcinoma in situ (DCIS) and invasive ductal cancer. **A,** A lateral view shows an alphanumeric plate placed over the skin closest to the calcifications and the clip. **B,** After needle placement, a mammogram shows the hub over the coordinates specifying the calcifications. Note that the hub of the needle overlies the needle shaft to ensure that the needle is traveling straight through the finding. **C,** A craniocaudal view with the needle in place shows that the needle has traversed the calcifications. **D,** A hookwire is placed in the needle and the needle removed; a craniocaudal view shows that the hookwire tip is 1 cm medial to the clip. Correct hookwire placement is confirmed on the lateral view. **E,** A specimen radiograph shows inclusion of the hookwire, the hookwire tip, the clip, and the calcifications; these findings were reported to the surgeon in the operating room. Pathologic examination demonstrated invasive ductal cancer and high-grade DCIS with comedo necrosis and four of five positive lymph nodes.

and easy to implement with a minimum of equipment. The original mammograms are reviewed to identify the shortest distance to the lesion from the skin surface (Box 6-3). The aperture is placed over the skin closest to the lesion, and the patient is left in compression until the image is viewed. Permanent ink marks are placed at the edges of the aperture at its contact with skin to show whether the patient has moved between the time that the image was taken and the time that the image is interpreted. The image should show the lesion within the

Box 6-3 X-ray–Guided Needle Localization and Specimen Radiography Procedur

MATERIALS

1. Images showing the lesion
2. Informed consent
3. Povidone-iodine (Betadine) or alcohol
4. 1% Lidocaine without epinephrine
5. 21- and 25-gauge needles
6. Localizing needle/hookwire
7. Tuberculin and 5-mL syringes
8. Sterile vital blue dye
9. Skin markers
10. Sterile gauze pads and tape
11. 8% Sterile sodium bicarbonate

PROCEDURE

Put the grid on the skin closest to the lesion and mark with ink along the grid edge.
Take a mammogram. Find the coordinates of the lesion on the grid.
Mark the patient's skin at the coordinates and cleanse the skin.
Anesthetize the needle entry site and the deep portion of the breast with a 21-gauge needle.
Insert the localizing needle so the hub shadow projects directly over the needle shaft to verify straight insertion.
Take a mammogram showing the needle hub over the lesion.
Release compression with the needle still in place.
Take a 90-degree orthogonal mammogram to verify needle depth.
Adjust the depth so the needle tip is in or through the lesion.
Inject the vital dye/lidocaine through the needle.
Deploy the hookwire through the needle and remove the needle.
Place a skin marker at the entry site of the wire and on the nipple.
Take orthogonal mammograms.
Annotate the films and send them with the patient to surgery.
Wait for a breast specimen.
Radiograph the breast specimen.
Report whether the specimen contains the targeted lesion, hookwire, and hookwire tip.
If the specimen contains no lesion, direct the surgeon to the correct area.

open aperture; if not, the compression plate is repositioned appropriately. The coordinates of the lesion are taken from the image and marked on the patient's skin. A local anesthetic is applied or injected into the skin.

The depth of the lesion is estimated from the orthogonal view. The skin is cleansed, and a needle is passed into and through the lesion by sterile technique. To ensure that the needle path is straight, the shadow from the needle hub should lie directly over the needle shaft during insertion. After the needle is passed into the breast and lesion, an image is taken to ensure that the needle shaft projects over the lesion.

With the physician holding the needle deep in the breast, the technologist releases compression and takes an orthogonal view. The radiologist adjusts the needle depth according to the mammogram, and in some facilities, the radiologist injects a small amount of blue dye. The radiologist places a hookwire through the needle and removes the needle, with the hookwire left near or in the lesion. Orthogonal mammograms show the relationship of the lesion and the hookwire tip, the films are marked for the surgeon, and the patient is sent to the operating room with the films. The radiologist waits for the breast specimen for radiography (Fig. 6-1E).

Specimen Radiography after Preoperative Needle Localization and Pathology Correlation

The needle localization procedure is not over until the specimen is radiographed to ensure that the lesion has been removed (Box 6-4). On viewing the specimen radiograph, the radiologist reports whether the specimen contains the lesion; whether the lesion is at, is away

Box 6-4	**Breast Specimen Reporting**

Specimen includes lesion
Hookwire included
Hookwire tip included
Lesion is at or away from the specimen edge or is
    transected

from, or is transecting the specimen edge; and whether the hookwire and hookwire tip are included. The findings are reported to the surgeon in the operating room. If the lesion is not in the specimen, the radiologist directs the surgeon to the expected location by using landmarks in the excised tissue and on the mammogram (Fig. 6-2). If subsequent specimen radiographs still do not contain the lesion, the surgeon may close the breast and

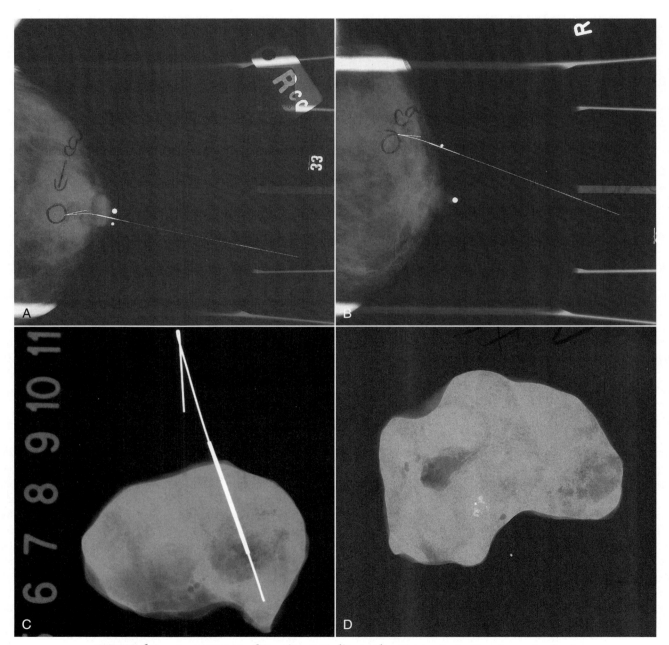

FIGURE 6-2   Importance of Specimen Radiography. The hookwire films from a freehand localization show the tip of the hookwire in microcalcifications on the craniocaudal (**A**) and mediolateral (**B**) views. **C,** The first specimen shows the hookwire but no calcifications. These findings were reported to the surgeon in the operating room. **D,** Calcifications are seen in the second specimen.

Table 6-1   Reasons Why Calcifications May Not Be Seen in the Pathology Report

Reason	Solution
Calcifications not removed	Check specimen radiograph
Calcifications in vacuum tubing	Radiograph fluid and debris in the tubing
Calcifications are calcium oxalate	Use polarized light on slides
Calcifications still in paraffin blocks	Paraffin block radiograph
Calcifications are milk of calcium	Check preoperative mammogram
Chatter from the slicing device removes large calcifications	Check postoperative mammogram

obtain a mammogram to determine whether the targeted lesion is still in the breast. This procedure is usually done a few weeks after the biopsy, although there is one report in the literature of immediate postoperative mammograms.

Radiologic-pathologic correlation ensures that the targeted lesion analyzed at pathologic evaluation is concordant with the imaging finding and, specifically, that the pathology report describes a histologic pattern that is known to correlate with the findings. For example, pathology reports for biopsies prompted by calcifications should contain a description of calcifications in the specimen.

Pathologic-radiologic correlation of targeted calcifications is a special subset of breast biopsy correlation. Calcifications may not be seen on pathology slides for several reasons (Table 6-1). First, the calcifications may not have been removed by biopsy. In such cases, the specimen radiograph should be checked to ensure that the calcifications are in the specimen and were indeed removed (see Fig. 6-2).

Second, the calcifications may be calcium oxalate. In these cases, the calcifications are seen in the specimen but are not described on the pathology report. Unlike calcium phosphate calcifications, which are easily seen on hematoxylin and eosin (H&E) staining, calcium oxalate is not visualized with H&E staining and requires a special polarized light to show the calcifications.

Third, the calcifications may be in the paraffin blocks. During specimen processing, thin breast tissue samples are embedded in paraffin blocks, which are then sliced and placed on slides for staining. Each block is several millimeters thick, but each slide contains only micromillimeters of paraffin and tissue. The calcifications may be left in the block and never placed on a slide for review. Radiographing the blocks may show the calcifications, and re-sectioning of that particular block will show the calcifications (Fig. 6-3).

Other calcifications may be removed from the specimen if the microtome cutting device that slices the tissue/paraffin block for slides pushes large calcifications out of the specimen at the time of sectioning. Finally, milk of calcium may fall out of the tiny benign cysts containing the calcifications and not be seen on the specimen slides. In such cases, the mammograms should be re-reviewed to determine whether the calcifications prompting biopsy might be milk of calcium.

If there are still no calcifications in the pathology report, in the specimen, or in the paraffin blocks, a repeat mammogram can determine whether the calcifications are still in the breast and were not removed at surgery.

A special scenario occurs when surgeons use "brackets" to remove a large area of the breast containing calcifications (Fig. 6-4). In this situation, the calcifications are localized with two wires or "brackets" so that the surgeon can remove all the calcifications between the two wires in toto. These specimens should include the two wires and the calcifications between them.

Stereotactic Preoperative Needle Localization

With this technique, a lesion is visualized under stereotactic guidance, as described for stereotactic core biopsy later in this chapter. Once the needle is placed in the lesion, blue dye is instilled, a hookwire is placed, and the patient is removed from the stereotactic device for standard orthogonal mammograms. The usual problem with stereotactic wire placements is adjusting the depth of the needle in the z-axis.

Ultrasound Guidance for Preoperative Needle Localization

Real-time hand-held ultrasound units with a small transducer provide an easy method to place a needle for preoperative needle localization into an ultrasonographically detected breast lesion (Fig. 6-5). With the patient in the supine position, the radiologist rolls the patient until the needle path is directed safely away from the chest wall to prevent pneumothorax. Using sterile technique and under direct ultrasound visualization, the radiologist plans the needle path to the lesion. The skin is anesthetized, and then a longer needle for deep anesthesia is inserted under direct ultrasound visualization so that the entire shaft of the needle and the target are seen in the same plane. The anesthesia needle can be used as a "trial run" to judge the safety of the needle path

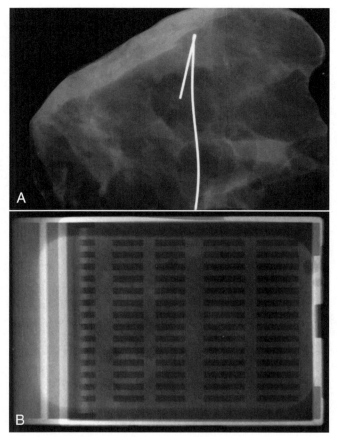

FIGURE 6-3   Importance of Correlation of Pathology and the Specimen Radiograph.
A, The specimen radiograph shows a hookwire and calcifications, but pathologic examination showed no calcifications. **B,** Radiography of the paraffin block containing breast tissue from the biopsy shows that the calcifications are still in the paraffin block. Further sectioning of this block showed the calcifications. Pathologic examination revealed benign fibrocystic change and microcalcifications.

and the difficulty of needle insertion. The needle tip for preoperative localization is then inserted into the lesion under real-time ultrasound guidance, with both the shaft and the needle tip visualized at all times to prevent pneumothorax. Once the needle is within the lesion, some facilities inject blue dye through the needle. Then, under direct ultrasound visualization, the radiologist places the hookwire through the needle, makes sure that the hookwire tip is in the correct place, and gently removes the needle while leaving the hookwire tip in place. Some facilities place an "x" over the skin where the lesion lies and mark the skin with two BBs that are displayed on the mammogram.

Some facilities place a skin marker at the skin entry site and take a mammogram to show the surgeon the location of the lesion, the hookwire, and the hookwire tip. Post-wire placement mammograms direct the surgeon to the correct location. The radiologist waits for the specimen; performs specimen radiography to ensure that the lesion, hookwire, and hookwire tip are removed; and reports the results to the surgeon in the operating room.

On occasion, the specimen radiograph may show the hookwire and hookwire tip but not show the lesion prompting biopsy. Specimen ultrasound to show the lesion in the biopsy tissue is performed by scanning directly over the breast specimen with a covered transducer.

In some facilities, radiologists or surgeons perform intraoperative ultrasound to direct the breast biopsy.

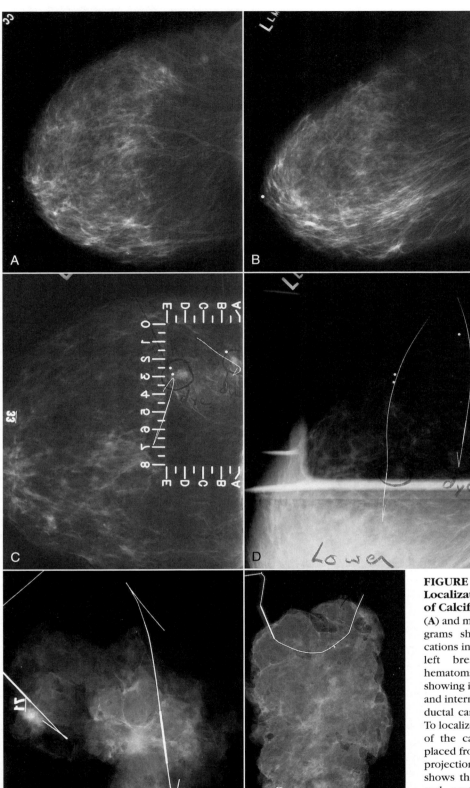

FIGURE 6-4 Bracket Localization for a Large Area of Calcifications. Craniocaudal (**A**) and mediolateral (**B**) mammograms show suspicious calcifications in the outer aspect of the left breast and two small hematomas from core biopsies showing infiltrating ductal cancer and intermediate-grade solid-type ductal carcinoma in situ (DCIS). To localize the outermost aspects of the cancer, two wires were placed from the craniocaudal (**C**) projection. The lateral view (**D**) shows the wires at the anterior and posterior aspects of the calcifications. The specimen radiograph (**E**) shows the hookwires/ hookwire tips, the two hematomas, and the calcifications in their entirety. Another bracket specimen radiograph shows the inclusion of other calcifications in a different patient (**F**) with intermediate-grade DCIS and calcifications.

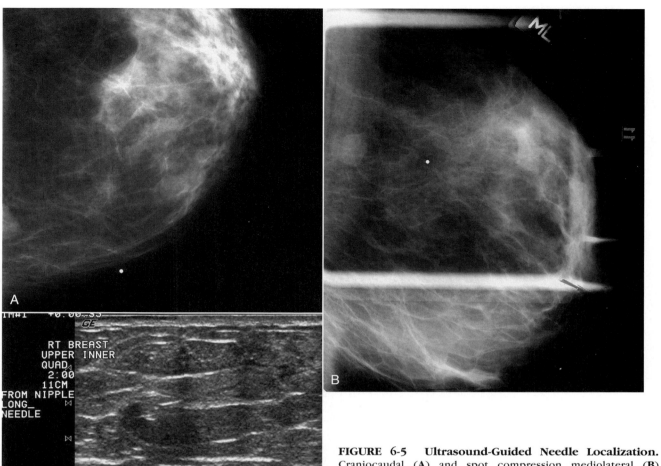

FIGURE 6-5   Ultrasound-Guided Needle Localization. Craniocaudal (**A**) and spot compression mediolateral (**B**) mammograms show a mass in the medial portion of the breast that was solid on ultrasound, and excisional biopsy was requested by the patient. Ultrasound was used to guide a needle into the mass for preoperative localization, and the image shows the needle tip in the middle of the mass (**C**).   *Continued*

BIOPSY OF PALPABLE BREAST MASSES

Cyst Aspiration

Cyst aspiration can be performed by any of the aforementioned methods with a fine needle. The physician advances the fine needle into a mass, and fluid wells up into the needle hub. The physician attaches a syringe to the needle, and fluid is drawn into the syringe until no more fluid is obtained (Fig. 6-6). The physician should be able to watch the cyst disappear in real time with ultrasound.

Some facilities perform pneumocystograms, or injection of air into the cyst cavity to help identify the cyst cavity. Air is thought to be therapeutic in preventing cyst recurrence (Fig. 6-7). Once the fluid has been aspirated completely, the radiologist disengages the

syringe and holds the needle carefully so that its tip is not displaced out of the decompressed, flattened cyst cavity. After attaching an air-filled syringe to the needle, the radiologist injects a small amount of air into the cavity, and the needle is withdrawn. A normal pneumocystogram shows an air-filled, thin-walled, round or oval cavity. In certain cases, two orthogonal mammograms are obtained to determine whether an intracystic mass is present and to ensure that the aspirated cyst corresponds to the mammographic finding prompting biopsy. The fluid is sent for cytologic evaluation only if an intracystic mass is present or the fluid is bloody. A large series of cyst aspirations by Tabar et al. showed that cyst fluid cytology is often falsely negative, even in the presence of an intracystic mass. In these cases the pneumocystogram was enough to diagnose an intracystic mass and prompt biopsy of the rare intracystic cancer.

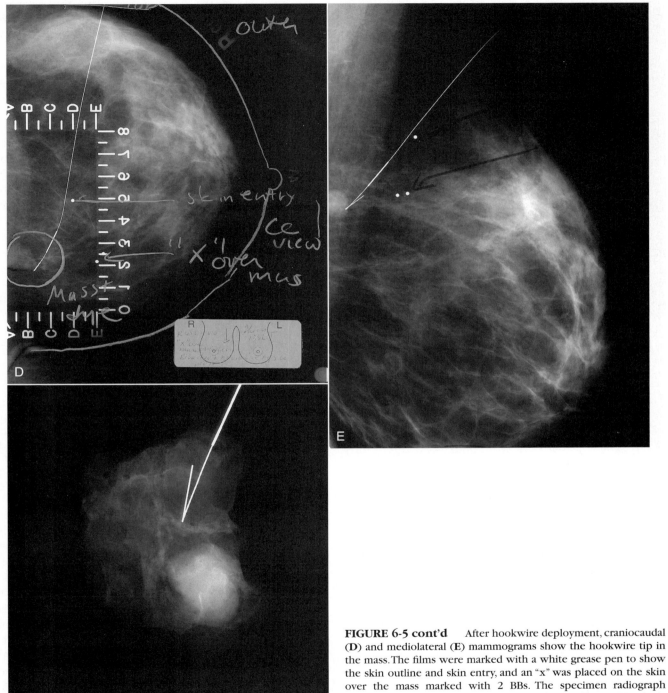

FIGURE 6-5 cont'd   After hookwire deployment, craniocaudal (**D**) and mediolateral (**E**) mammograms show the hookwire tip in the mass. The films were marked with a white grease pen to show the skin outline and skin entry, and an "x" was placed on the skin over the mass marked with 2 BBs. The specimen radiograph (**F**) shows inclusion of the mass and the hookwire. Histologic examination revealed a fibroadenoma.

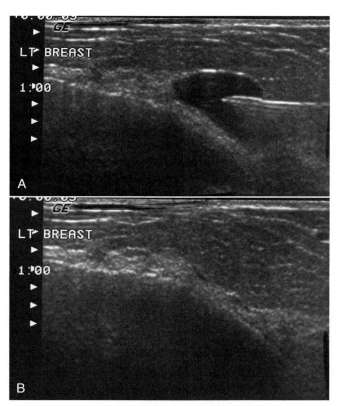

FIGURE 6-6   Cyst Aspiration. A, Ultrasound shows a needle in a cyst near an implant. **B,** The following ultrasound shows that the cyst is gone.

Freehand Fine-Needle Aspiration of Palpable Breast Masses

Fine-needle aspiration or core biopsy can be performed on palpable masses. With this method, craniocaudal and mediolateral mammograms and other imaging studies are reviewed, but the biopsy is guided by physical findings.

For aspiration of a palpable mass, the patient is placed in the supine position and the radiologist determines whether the mass is far enough away from the chest wall to prevent pneumothorax. After injection of a local anesthetic, the physician holds the breast mass firmly away from the chest wall. The needle is inserted into the lesion while ensuring that its trajectory is well away from the chest wall. Fine-needle aspiration is performed by making several short excursions through the mass. The radiologist prepares slides and washings and achieves hemostasis by direct pressure.

Fine-Needle Aspiration under Radiologic Guidance Using a Fenestrated Alphanumeric Compression Plate

This method was initially used as a diagnostic breast biopsy procedure in the 1980s. The technique is similar to preoperative needle localization, but instead of placing a hookwire through the needle, the radiologist aspirates the lesion for fluid or cells for cytologic examination. Once the needle has been placed through the aperture of the compression plate, the physician estimates the depth of the lesion (z-axis) from the orthogonal view and measures the thickness of the compressed breast. The depth of the lesion is estimated by determining how deep the lesion should reside from the skin in the compressed breast. For example, if the lesion is in the upper third of the breast and the breast is 9 cm thick, the needle is passed 3 cm into the breast.

The needle is connected to a syringe or to tubing connected to a syringe. Suction is applied to the needle, and the needle is passed vigorously through the lesion 15 times with at least a 5- to 10-mm excursion. The needle is rotated during the up-and-down motion of the aspiration procedure to increase the amount of material aspirated. Suction is terminated before the needle is withdrawn, and the material is smeared on slides for analysis or rinsed in a cytology solution for cell blocks.

At least four passes should be performed, and optimally, the material should be analyzed immediately to ensure that adequate cellular material has been obtained for diagnosis. After aspiration, the patient is released from compression and direct pressure is applied to the site.

Ultrasound Guidance for Fine-Needle Aspiration or Core Needle Biopsy of Solid Masses

When compared with stereotactic biopsy, ultrasound-guided biopsy has the advantage of using readily available equipment and is fast and cost-effective. With high-frequency transducers, some investigators use ultrasound to guide biopsy of microcalcifications or their associated masses.

For fine-needle aspiration, the radiologist introduces a needle in the plane of the transducer under direct visualization and with sterile technique to show the entire shaft of the needle and the lesion (Fig. 6-8) to prevent pneumothorax. The needle is introduced into the lesion perpendicular to the skin along the transducer axis. Once the needle is within the lesion, the radiologist aspirates the mass with a vigorous to-and-fro movement to obtain material for cytologic evaluation and then withdraws the needle.

To perform a core biopsy under ultrasound guidance, the radiologist determines whether the lesion is in a safe location for biopsy. Specifically, the lesion must be away from the chest wall and in a location so that the throw of the needle does not produce a pneumothorax or extend through the skin on the opposite side of the breast. The needle throw should be calculated to ensure that the core trough is in the middle of the lesion. The lesion

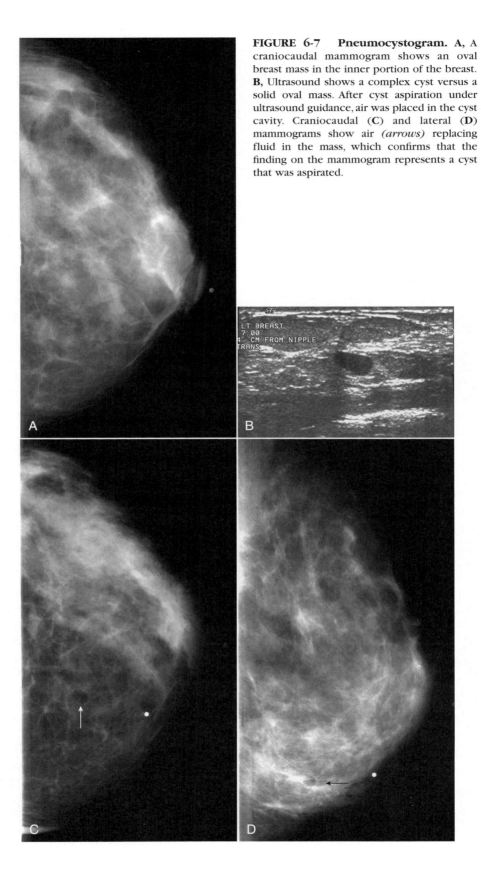

FIGURE 6-7   Pneumocystogram. A, A craniocaudal mammogram shows an oval breast mass in the inner portion of the breast. **B,** Ultrasound shows a complex cyst versus a solid oval mass. After cyst aspiration under ultrasound guidance, air was placed in the cyst cavity. Craniocaudal (**C**) and lateral (**D**) mammograms show air *(arrows)* replacing fluid in the mass, which confirms that the finding on the mammogram represents a cyst that was aspirated.

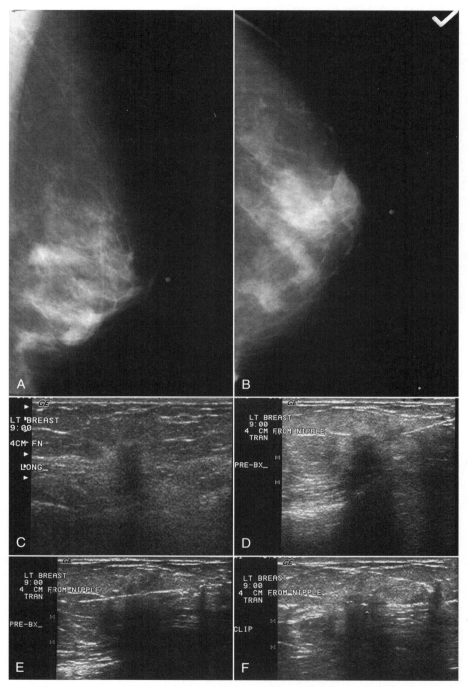

FIGURE 6-8   Ultrasound-Guided Core Biopsy with Clip Placement and Subsequent Needle Localization. Lateral medial (**A**) and craniocaudal (**B**) mammograms show a spiculated mass in the midportion of the left breast at the 9-o'clock position. **C,** Ultrasound shows a hypoechoic, spiculated shadowing mass. **D,** Ultrasound-guided needle placement shows the tip of the core biopsy needle before biopsy just proximal to the mass. Note that the trajectory of the needle is well away from the chest wall and will not produce a pneumothorax. **E,** A post-fire ultrasound scan shows the needle traversing the mass and the expected location of the sampling trough inside the mass. All post-fire films are imaged. **F,** A clip is placed in the mass and is displayed as a bright echo in the middle of the mass.   *Continued*

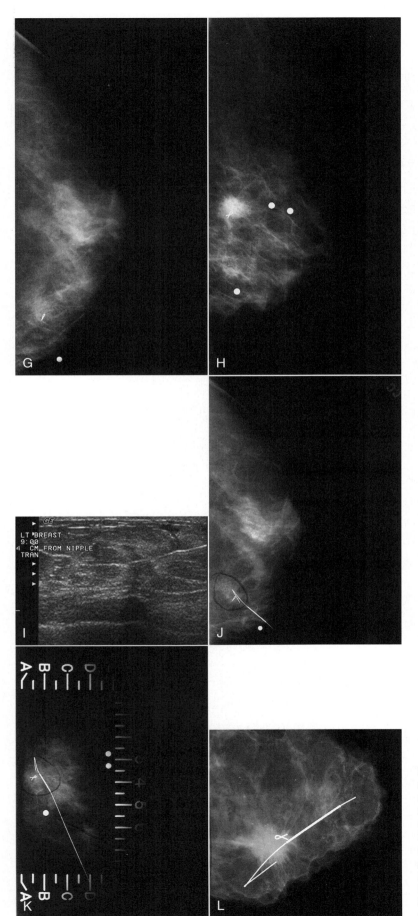

FIGURE 6-8 cont'd   Follow-up craniocaudal (**G**) and mediolateral (**H**) views show the clip in the mass. A single marker shows the skin entry site for the core needle, and two BBs show the location of the mass on the skin. **I,** Subsequent ultrasound-guided needle localization shows a wire in the mass. Craniocaudal (**J**) and lateral (**K**) mammograms taken after ultrasound-guided needle localization show the wire tip in the mass. **L,** The specimen radiograph shows the mass, hookwire tip, and the clip. Pathologic examination revealed invasive ductal cancer, lobular carcinoma in situ, and one of three sentinel lymph nodes was positive.

cannot be so close to the skin that the core biopsy will obtain epidermis. For vacuum-assisted biopsies, the trough is aimed at the lesion, and the breast must be thick enough to accommodate the probe.

To perform an ultrasound-guided core biopsy, the lesion is localized by ultrasound, the skin is sterilized and anesthetized, and a scalpel is used to make a skin nick in the sterilized and anesthetized breast. The core biopsy needle track is anesthetized with local anesthesia under ultrasound guidance. During the anesthesia procedure, the entire shaft of the needle and the bevel of the needle tip are visualized to get an idea of the needle trajectory. Under direct ultrasound visualization, the large-core biopsy needle is introduced into the breast. If the lesion is large enough, the needle is introduced into the edge of the lesion to hold it in place. The biopsy core needle is deployed under direct visualization, the core is harvested, and direct pressure is held on the breast afterward.

Vacuum-assisted ultrasound-guided multidirectional core biopsies produce results similar to those of stereotactic core biopsy. In one study involving 71 lesions biopsied under ultrasound guidance, 52 cores were benign (51 benign and 1 cancer at surgery), 18 cores were cancerous (17 cancers and 1 benign at surgery), and 1 core was premalignant (benign at surgery). Complications included a bleeding rate of 7% (bleeding beyond 10 minutes in 5 of 71 biopsy samples) and one vasovagal reaction. These findings show that ultrasound-guided vacuum-assisted core biopsy is accurate but has a higher bleeding rate than multifire large-core needle biopsy under ultrasound guidance does. Complete excision of benign lesions has been reported with this technique. After vacuum-assisted 11-gauge core biopsy, hematomas were seen in most patients by ultrasound 1 week after biopsy.

CORE BIOPSY

Stereotactic Localization for Core Needle Biopsy

This method uses a compression device with a small aperture and an x-ray tube that has the ability to take two stereotactic views about 10 to 15 degrees off perpendicular (Fig. 6-9). Stereotactic localization is performed with the patient in an upright or prone position and a fenestrated compression paddle. Pre-biopsy craniocaudal and mediolateral mammograms are reviewed to determine the location of the lesion on orthogonal views, evaluate the architecture of breast tissue around the lesion to ensure accurate targeting, and provide landmarks for subsequent needle localization if the entire lesion is removed and a marker cannot be placed (Table 6-2). The aperture is placed on the skin surface closest to the breast lesion. Two stereo views of

the lesion are obtained, the lesion is located on the stereo views, and a needle is passed into the center of the lesion. Two more stereo views are taken to ensure that the trough of the needle is within the breast lesion. Post-fire images show whether the lesion has been sampled. After the specimens are collected, specimen radiographs are obtained to make sure that the calcifications or mass has been sampled. These are labeled and sent to the pathology laboratory. At this point a clip may be deployed into the biopsy cavity with vacuum-assisted devices. Immediate post-biopsy craniocaudal and mediolateral mammograms show the biopsy cavity, confirm removal of all or a portion of the lesion, and show the location of the marker and its position relative to the targeted lesion.

Various techniques can be used to increase the amount of breast tissue to perform vacuum-assisted stereotactic biopsy in a thin breast, including the use of two paddles to increase the amount of tissue thickness, anesthesia to increase the thickness of the skin, and skin hooks to cover the vacuum-assisted trough. Accurate deployment of clips or markers can be tricky. Inaccurate clip placement or non-deployment can be due to the marker being blocked by tissue fragments retained in the probe, blood in the probe, or aspiration of the marker out of the tissue (Table 6-3).

Vacuum-assisted biopsy was developed as an alternative to multiple-fire large-core biopsies to increase the quantity of tissue extracted. Burbank has shown that 14-gauge tissue specimens were twice as large when assisted by vacuum-type aspiration biopsy devices, with even more tissue obtained when 11-gauge probes were used. The 0.14% complication rate (3 of 2093 biopsies, including 2 hematomas and 1 infection) with vacuum-assisted biopsy is similar to the 0.16% complication rate (6 of 3765, 3 hematomas and 3 infections) with multiple-fire large-core biopsy reported by Parker et al. in 1994. Even larger samples may be obtained with 8-gauge probes or 1- to 2-cm probes.

The larger amount of tissue obtained with vacuum-assisted biopsy aids in the diagnosis of atypical hyperplasia as shown by both Jackman and Liberman, and the number of ductal carcinoma in situ (DCIS) cases decreased at subsequent excisional biopsy. The 11-gauge vacuum-assisted biopsy system also allows placement of a small metallic marker in the biopsy site if the lesion is totally excised. Marker placement helps locate a cancer core biopsy site if the mass or calcifications are totally removed because very few mammographic findings remain after core biopsy. Immediate post–stereotactic core biopsy craniocaudal and mediolateral mammograms are required to determine the location of the marker relative to the biopsied lesion. It is well known that clips can move within the breast after initial placement, before subsequent preoperative needle localization or

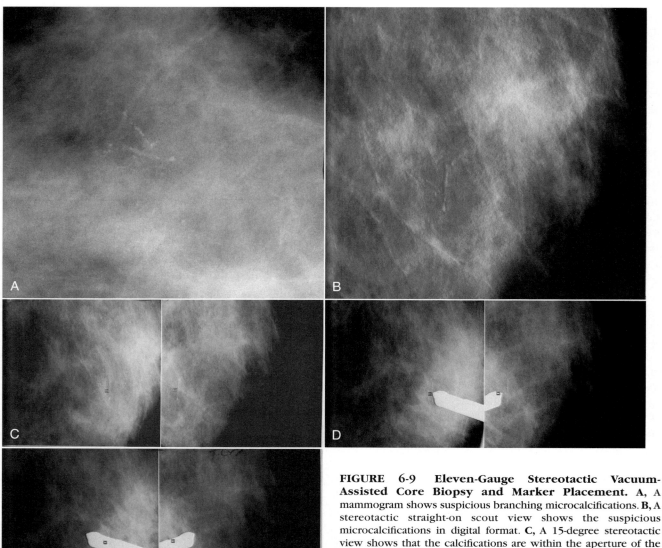

FIGURE 6-9 Eleven-Gauge Stereotactic Vacuum-Assisted Core Biopsy and Marker Placement. A, A mammogram shows suspicious branching microcalcifications. **B,** A stereotactic straight-on scout view shows the suspicious microcalcifications in digital format. **C,** A 15-degree stereotactic view shows that the calcifications are within the aperture of the compression plate. **D,** Pre-fire films demonstrate that the stereotactic needle is directed toward the calcifications. **E,** Post-fire stereotactic views show that the needle is traversing the suspicious microcalcifications.

re-biopsy. Thus, after marker placement and before preoperative needle localization, the radiologist reviews the pre-biopsy mammograms, the post–marker placement mammograms, and the pre–needle localization/post–marker placement mammograms to ensure that the cancer site is removed if the marker moves in the breast.

Core Specimen Radiography

After core biopsy for calcifications, core specimen radiography is mandatory to ensure that the lesion that prompted biopsy has been removed. Magnification specimen radiography may help identify small microcalcifications difficult to see on conventional imaging.

The specimen radiograph is reviewed by the radiologist to ensure that the lesion has been removed or sampled. If the targeted lesion is not present in the specimen, repeat cores can be obtained.

Friedman et al. reported finding calcifications in the tubing and debris from vacuum-assisted biopsies when the calcifications are not in the specimen radiograph but appear to have been removed by biopsy. They suggest straining the contents of the tubing and debris and performing specimen radiography on the retrieved material in this circumstance.

At times, interpretation of the results of specimen radiography may be equivocal. In such cases, the findings on breast specimen pathology should be compared with

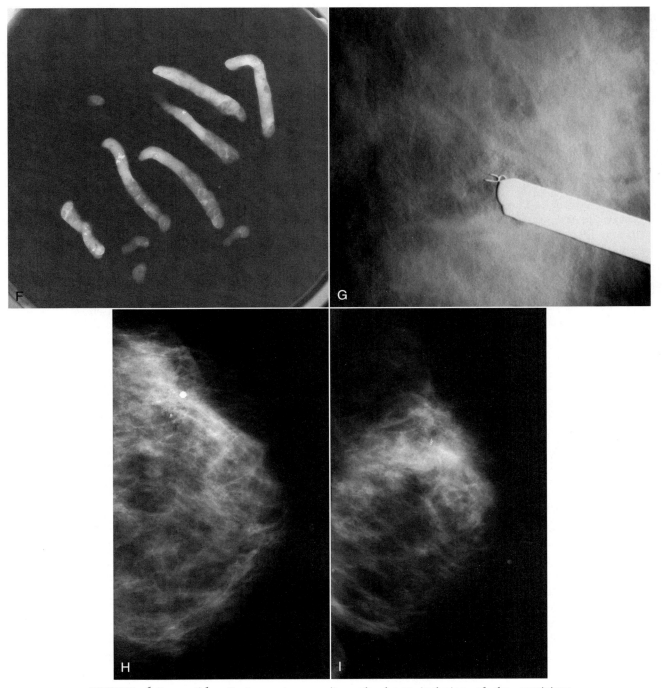

FIGURE 6-9 cont'd   **F,** A specimen radiograph shows inclusion of the suspicious microcalcifications corresponding to the mammographic finding. **G,** A stereotactic view at clip placement demonstrates that the clip is near the biopsy cavity on the stereo view. Immediate post-biopsy craniocaudal (**H**) and lateral (**I**) mammograms show that the clip is near the biopsy site and that air is present in the biopsy site.

Table 6-2 Reasons for Mammograms in Women Undergoing Stereotactic Biopsy	
Reason	**Solution**
Lesion location on orthogonal views	CC and ML pre-biopsy mammograms
Marker relationship to biopsy site	Immediate post-biopsy CC and ML mammograms
Marker migration before preoperative needle localization	CC and ML pre-localization mammograms

CC, craniocaudal; ML, mediolateral.

Table 6-3 Methods to Obtain Accurate Stereotactic Marker Deployment in Vacuum-Assisted Biopsies	
Reason for Inaccurate Deployment	**Solution**
Did not pull back probe for deployment	Pull back probe when suggested
Aspirated marker back into probe	Turn aspiration off
Marker stuck on fragment retained in probe	Dry tap probe
Too much blood, puffed-up gel plug	Dry tap probe

those of the specimen radiograph. If there is a discrepancy between the appearance of the mammographic finding and the pathology report, the patient's immediate post-biopsy mammograms should be reviewed to see whether the lesion that prompted biopsy has been sampled or removed.

Carbon Marking after Stereotactic Biopsy

This method uses activated charcoal USP (Mallinckrodt, Phillipsburg, NJ) sterilized and suspended as a 4% weight/weight aqueous suspension. It is mixed with 0.3 mL sterile saline or water and injected in a to-and-fro motion after core biopsy along the stereotactic needle track to yield a dark line of carbon particles in the breast. This line of carbon particles can be used as a guide for excisional biopsy days to weeks after the percutaneous biopsy.

Patient Comfort after Biopsy

After biopsy, adequate hemostasis is achieved by direct pressure. In some institutions, after hemostasis is confirmed, the patient is instructed to "hold pressure" on the biopsy site so that she knows what to do if subsequent untoward bleeding occurs. After adequate hemostasis is achieved, some institutions close the wound with Steri-Strips and cover the Steri-Strips with Opsite, a self-adhesive saran wrap–like sterile material used to cover operative wounds. Opsite prevents the Steri-Strips from getting wet and keeps the wound clean and dry. The patient can take a shower with the Opsite on but is instructed to not "scrub" the Opsite, take a bath, swim, or engage in other activities that might immerse the wound site. Patients are told to expect a quarter-sized spot of blood on the Steri-Strips, expect a bruise at the biopsy site that may travel to dependent sites, and put direct pressure on the biopsy site if oozing or unexpected bleeding occurs. The patient is instructed to remove the Opsite and Steri-Strips after 4 days. Some facilities also bind the breast with wraparound bandages or the commercially available binders used after mastectomy to hold the breasts tight to the chest wall, restrict breast motion while the patient is awake, and limit breast motion during the night.

Part of recovery is pain control. If the patient is not allergic to acetaminophen, and has no liver problems, she may take acetaminophen initially and then every 6 hours as needed, up to 4 g per day. Rarely, as needed on the follow-up call, stronger medication such as Tylenol No. 3 or Vicodin may be prescribed for pain. The patient is given an ice pack to put on the biopsy site for 60 minutes initially and then for 10 minutes every hour on the hour as needed. She is *not* to keep it on longer because of the possibility of frostbite. Facilities that use a breast binder consisting of a stretchy cloth with Velcro keep the ice pack in place when in use. Patients are given verbal and written post-biopsy wound care instructions and a phone number to call for problems. They are instructed on where and how to obtain their biopsy result. Most patients do well with these instructions. Some facilities call the patient later in the afternoon, early evening, or the next day as a courtesy call to see how the patient is doing and answer any questions.

Complete Lesion Removal

If the entire lesion has been removed by core biopsy and shows cancer on pathology, the region where the stereotactic core biopsy was taken should be excised to completely remove any residual tumor. In a study of 15 cancers in which the radiographic finding was completely removed by stereotactic core biopsy, follow-up pathology showed residual invasive ductal cancer (3 cases) or DCIS (8 cases) for a total of 11 (73%) of the 15 lesions. Thus, even when the entire radiographic finding suggestive of cancer has been removed by core biopsy, surgical excision is essential to ensure clean margins.

How is the core biopsy site localized when the entire lesion has been removed and no marker was placed in the biopsy site? In many cases there are no findings on the follow-up mammogram to indicate the location of the biopsy after stereotactic needle biopsy has been performed, although a small hematoma or air may sometimes be seen in the immediate post-biopsy period. In 226 benign 11-gauge directional vacuum-assisted biopsies, 5 (2%) had a density in a projection parallel to the biopsy needle track, and in 422 specimens harvested by 14-gauge automated large-core biopsy, no findings were detected. Because air can move along the biopsy track, air alone is not enough to exactly identify the biopsy site. With complete removal of the lesion, Dr. Brenner suggests using landmarks within the breast to localize the approximate regions of the stereotactic biopsy site. Others have suggested localizing the fluid collection in the biopsy site by ultrasound.

Marker Placement, Marker Movement, and Ultrasound and MRI Marker Compatibility

Immediate post-biopsy craniocaudal and lateral views will identify the location of the biopsy cavity, which usually shows air and fluid and absence of all or part of the targeted lesion. If the finding is benign, a mammogram 6 months later will show little change from the pre-biopsy mammograms except for resorption of air and fluid, removal of or a decrease in calcifications, or a hole in the biopsied mass. In general, at 6 months almost no mammographic changes remain except for the removed portions of the lesion and the marker, if placed.

Immediate post–stereotactic biopsy mammograms show the location of the marker in relation to the biopsy site. Usually, the marker is located in the biopsy site; however, it may be deployed near the site instead of in it. If the marker stays in the same location on the subsequent mammogram for preoperative needle localization, the marker can be used for targeting to excise the biopsy site. If biopsy is performed on two sites in the same breast, markers with two unique shapes can be used to differentiate the two sites. Some patients request removal of a biopsy marker, which can be performed percutaneously with a vacuum-assisted large-core device.

Various types of clips or markers are available, including stainless steel or metallic clips alone and markers embedded in plugs of various types. The plugs are composed of Gelfoam/metallic markers, bovine or porcine collagen, or other materials. If markers containing bovine or porcine collagen are used, the patient should be asked about allergies to either beef or pork before deployment of the markers. It has been noted anecdotally that some plugs may get stuck during deployment and make it impossible to push the plunger in or difficult to withdraw or close the needle. This problem is possibly due to the plugs filling with fluid, expanding in the deployment device, and getting stuck in the trough, or the deployment device can get stuck on a retained fragment in the vacuum needle and be extruded out of the trough.

Some markers placed by stereotaxis are embedded in plugs visible by ultrasound. Some facilities use ultrasound to localize these plugs for subsequent needle localization after stereotactic biopsy.

Magnetic resonance imaging (MRI) is increasingly being used to stage the breast for cancer and to plan surgical management. Because biopsy site markers placed by stereotaxis, ultrasound, or MRI may be imaged by subsequent MRI studies, marker MRI compatibility, safety, and artifact are becoming increasingly important. Accordingly, facilities considering subsequent MRI studies may place MRI-compatible metallic markers in biopsy sites, with the understanding that subsequent breast MRI will be performed to stage the patient if the biopsy proves to be cancer. There is a difference between MRI marker "compatibility," meaning that the marker can be used in the MRI magnet and will cause little artifact, and marker "safety," meaning that the marker will produce no harm to the patient in the magnet. Some markers are "MRI compatible" but still cause large artifacts of up to 2 cm, thus rendering the MRI less readable than when using other markers. MRI testing of markers for artifact by using phantoms on the facility's pulse sequences before inserting metallic clips for marking tumors or biopsy sites is an easy way to determine the feasibility of using a particular marker after percutaneous biopsy.

Markers can move considerably within the breast after the completion of stereotactic biopsy. On follow-up mammograms taken days, weeks, or months after initial marker placement, markers occasionally move far from the original biopsy site, even to another breast quadrant. If the clip has moved away from an original biopsy site in which cancer has been demonstrated, the location of the original targeted lesion is determined by the use of breast architecture and landmarks (Fig. 6-10) because the goal of subsequent localization is to remove any residual cancer. Whether it is necessary to also localize the migrated clip is controversial. In an article in the surgical literature, Kass et al. found that the clip moved more than 20 mm from the targeted site in 93 cases that could be evaluated, thus leading to the use of intraoperative ultrasound to determine the location of the biopsy site when feasible. However, this group did not state the average time after biopsy or the ease of visualization of the biopsy site by ultrasound.

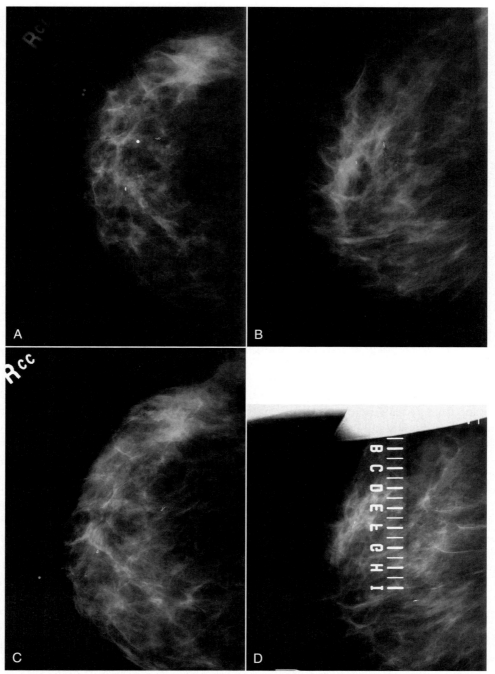

FIGURE 6-10   Value of Two Different Types of Clips for Two Stereotactic Biopsy Sites and Clip Migration. Because this patient had two suspicious microcalcification clusters, two different clips were placed at stereotactic biopsy. Craniocaudal (**A**) and mediolateral (**B**) mammograms show the difference in clip configuration, which clearly identifies the biopsy site. If the same type of clip had been placed in both sites, it would be difficult to determine the location of each biopsy site on subsequent mammograms. Cancer was found in the upper biopsy site, and the lower biopsy site was benign. Two months later, preoperative craniocaudal (**C**) and lateral (**D**) views show that the upper clip has migrated to the inferior portion of the breast. Because cancer was taken from the upper biopsy site, breast architecture was used to target the original upper biopsy site for excision since the clip is now in a different quadrant. This case shows the importance of correlation of the pre–stereotactic biopsy scout mammogram, the immediate post–clip placement mammogram, which documents orientation of the clip to the biopsy site, and scout mammograms before preoperative needle localization.

Box 6-5   Specimen Pathology Requiring Surgical Excision or Re-biopsy after Core Biopsy

Noncongruent results of pathology and imaging
Insufficient samples
Cancer, even if an entire lesion appears to be removed
Ductal carcinoma in situ
Atypical ductal hyperplasia
Papillary lesions with atypia
Phyllodes tumor

Calcification and Epithelial Displacement

Calcifications may be displaced by percutaneous biopsy needles to locations distant from the original biopsy site. One case report describes displacement of a few of the targeted calcifications 3 cm medial to the target site during stereotactic biopsy. Two clips were also displaced medially in this case. The biopsy specimen was benign, and 6 months later the calcifications and clips were unchanged. Follow-up mammography immediately after a core procedure can identify such displacements. It is controversial whether displaced clips or displaced calcifications far from the biopsy site require surgical excision when the percutaneous biopsy specimen shows cancer.

With 11-gauge vacuum-assisted probes, epithelial displacement of breast cancer cells into benign tissue along the needle track may occur and simulate breast cancer invasion or a second focus of tumor. Pathologists should be informed that a stereotactic core biopsy has been performed so that they do not mistakenly diagnose displaced epithelium as invasive cancer in a DCIS lesion or erroneously stage a tumor as multifocal when only one cancerous site is present.

Review of Radiography and Pathology in Core Biopsy Specimens

Routine correlation between the mammographic appearance of the breast lesion and the pathology report is an essential part of quality assurance to reduce the number of false-negative results and to excise cancers. In reviewing 1003 stereotactic core biopsies, Brenner et al. showed a working sensitivity of 95%, a specificity of 98%, and an accuracy of 96%. In their report they stressed the importance of correlating the clinical and imaging findings. Such correlation ensures that the suspicious lesion that prompted biopsy was actually sampled. Specific histologic findings require surgical excision after core biopsy (Box 6-5).

Biopsy samples showing cancer routinely undergo subsequent excisional biopsy to remove residual cancer at the core biopsy location, including both invasive cancers and DCIS. Invasive cancer of any sort should be re-excised even if the entire radiographic finding has been removed by percutaneous biopsy because occult invasive cancer has been demonstrated in the core biopsy site in 73% of cases at subsequent surgery. In addition, tumor size may be underestimated by stereotactic core biopsy and the true size determined only at excision.

Surgical excision is advised for all DCIS lesions, the same as for invasive cancer, but women with DCIS may not undergo axillary node dissection at surgery. Stereotactic biopsy specimens with DCIS will be shown to have invasive carcinoma in 15% to 36% of cases at subsequent excisional biopsy. Thus, a small percentage of patients with DCIS may eventually need axillary node dissection because of the presence of invasive cancer on subsequent excisional biopsy.

Atypical ductal hyperplasia (ADH) diagnosed by core biopsy should undergo surgical excisional biopsy. ADH may be associated with DCIS or may represent a histologic underestimation of DCIS. ADH is diagnosed 2.7 times more reliably by vacuum-assisted biopsy than by multiple-fire core biopsy, with no increase in complications. Excisional biopsy of masses diagnosed as ADH may show fibrocystic change, ADH, DCIS, or invasive ductal carcinoma at surgical excision. Because cancer is found in up to 25% of specimens obtained with an 11-gauge vacuum-assisted needle, excisional biopsy is advised for ADH. There are no patient risk factors that might obviate excision after stereotactic core biopsy showing ADH; specifically, no favorable ages, previous history of cancer, family history of cancer, or other factors were significant in determining that the percutaneously biopsied site would be negative on surgical excision.

Phyllodes tumor, though generally benign, has a small percentage of malignant forms that may sometimes be diagnosed only by complete histologic examination. Phyllodes tumor also tends to recur in the biopsy site and should be completely excised by surgery.

Nonconcordant findings on core biopsy (incongruent imaging and pathologic findings) should be re-biopsied or excised if considered suspicious by imaging or clinical findings. For example, a spiculated mass found on mammography that shows fibrocystic change on a core biopsy specimen indicates a miss of the needle and should be re-biopsied by core or surgical excisional biopsy.

Papillary lesions with atypia are excised to exclude papillary carcinoma.

Fibroadenomas, or benign-appearing calcifications that correspond to the calcifications in benign fibrocystic change or benign lymph nodes, are usually managed by follow-up imaging.

Controversy regarding Management of Specific Core Histologic Findings

Certain histologic findings on core biopsy may require surgical excision, but these indications are controversial (Box 6-6). Radial scars or nonencapsulated sclerosing lesions are benign lesions that produce a spiculated mass on mammography, and they are sometimes associated with DCIS. Lee et al. found malignancy at excision in one of four radial scars found by core biopsy. Jackman et al. detected cancer in two of five radial scars found by core biopsy. Philpotts and colleagues found no cancers in eight of nine radial scars that were excised, but they detected atypical ductal hyperplasia in four (50%) cases at surgery. Brenner et al. found cancer at surgery in 28% (8/29) of women with radial scar core biopsies containing atypical hyperplasia and in 4% (5/128) of women with radial scars without atypia. Their study further showed that radial scars with noncongruent radiologic-pathologic correlation, less than 12 cores by 11-gauge vacuum-assisted biopsy, or with atypical ductal hyperplasia are most likely to show cancer at subsequent excisional biopsy. Though controversial, some pathologists believe that a radial scar is a precursor to tubular carcinoma and is often associated with DCIS, and they recommend that all radial scars be excised.

Pseudoangiomatous stromal hyperplasia (PASH) is a proliferative lesion seen in older women; it is visualized as a mass on mammography. Growing PASH should be excised because of overlap with low-grade angiosarcoma.

Papillary breast lesions are rare and account for less than 10% of biopsy cases and 1% to 2% of breast cancers. Liberman et al. reviewed 26 papillary lesions (7 benign papillomas, 2 cases of papillomatosis, 10 papillomas with ADH, 7 cases of papillary DCIS) found on core biopsy. At surgery, no cancers were detected in the 7 benign papillary lesions, 1 DCIS was found in the 2 papillomatosis cases, 3 cases of DCIS were detected in the 10 papilloma/ADH cases, and 3 invasive cancers were found in the 7 papillary DCIS cases. Phillpotts and associates found papillary carcinoma in three of four suspicious papillary breast lesions on stereotactic core biopsy and one focus of DCIS in a microscopic papillary lesion. Mercado et al. reviewed 26 papillary lesions and found 1 cancer at surgery in 6 benign papillary lesions detected at core biopsy, five of six atypical lesions at excision that were atypical at core biopsy, and eight cancers in eight malignant core biopsies. These data suggest that surgical excision should follow all malignant and atypical papillary lesions and that until further data are available, excision of benign papillomas should be considered because of the possibility of underestimating the papillary lesion on core histology and the paucity of cases and follow-up in the literature.

Lobular carcinomas in situ (LCIS) and atypical lobular hyperplasia (ALH) are both high-risk markers for breast cancer. If a mammographic finding prompted biopsy and either of these histologic findings result from the biopsy, consideration should be given to surgical excision because of their high association with carcinoma. Liberman et al. reviewed 13 women with 14 core biopsy diagnoses of LCIS and an additional 4 women with core biopsies showing ALH. In five women with LCIS *and* a radial scar (three) or ADH (two), surgery showed one patient with DCIS and four with no cancer. In 4 women, the LCIS found on core biopsy had histologic features overlapping with DCIS, and DCIS was detected in 2 of 4 surgical excisions for a total of 3 (21%) cases of DCIS in the 14 specimens determined to have LCIS on core biopsy. In the remaining five cases, LCIS was found incidentally in the core biopsy specimen, and after surgical excision, LCIS was detected in four of the five cases, but no invasive cancer. Of four women with ALH in the core biopsy specimen, LCIS was found in two after surgical excision and benign lesions in two. Irfan and Brem reviewed seven patients with ALH on core biopsy and showed four with ALH (one with a radial scar), one with fibrocystic change, one with DCIS, and one with LCIS. Phillpotts et al. found DCIS at surgery in one case in which LCIS was diagnosed at stereotactic core biopsy, and they therefore recommend excisional biopsy for LCIS cases. This matter remains controversial.

Follow-up of Breast Lesions Diagnosed as Benign

Large-core needle biopsies sample rather than wholly remove breast lesions, which leaves the potential for the lesion or the region around the sampled area to change during the follow-up period, at times leading to re-biopsy. Follow-up strategies can be based on the results of long-term studies that monitored lesions with benign core biopsy pathologic findings. One study by Lee et al. reviewed 540 such cases and showed change in 21 (7%) of 298 with follow-up after initial core biopsy. Repeat biopsy showed two cancers, one mass that changed at 6 months, and calcifications changing at 24 months, for a delayed false-negative rate of 2% of all patients. Another study by Jackman et al. reviewed 310 lesions diagnosed as benign at core biopsy and showed cancer in 14 (58%) of 24 ADH lesions and 2 of 5 radial scars. Repeat core biopsy showed two cancers (one invasive ductal carcinoma, one DCIS) in two benign lesions that had mammographic progression at 6 and 18 months, for a false-negative rate of 1.2% (2 of 161 total cancers in the study period). In another study by Adler et al., 152 lesions were monitored after stereotactic core biopsy, with benign results showing cancer in 6 women 1 to 30 months after biopsy; in 64 women no follow-up data were available, and other information was missing for another 7 women.

These studies show that core biopsy can occasionally be falsely negative and emphasize the importance of a good follow-up program to minimize the potential for missing cancer. These studies suggest a 6-month follow-up of lesions with nonspecific benign results and concordant mammographic findings and a 12- and 24-month follow-up of lesions with specific benign results and concordant mammographic findings.

Complications

Invasive procedures carry potential risks and complications that must be recognized and treated (Box 6-7). Many of the complications of core needle biopsy are the same as for any invasive procedure: excessive bleeding, infection, failure to excise the lesion, insufficient sampling, and vasovagal reactions. A prospective survey of 370 cases over a 1-year period showed that 7% of needle localization and fine-needle aspiration procedures resulted in one of these complications. Thus, all personnel in the room must be able to recognize and treat a vasovagal reaction and be able to release the breast from compression for mammographic procedures. A stretcher and resuscitation cart should be in close vicinity to the percutaneous biopsy procedure room, and the patient should never be unaccompanied in the room during the procedure. The patient must be able to respond, be alert, be able to remain motionless during the procedure, and be able to cooperate with the radiologist during the biopsy.

Box 6-7	Complications from Percutaneous Biopsy
Hematoma
Untoward bleeding
Infection
Pneumothorax
Pseudoaneurysm

Bleeding and hematoma are known possible complications of percutaneous stereotactic core biopsy. In one case report of a woman undergoing a 14-gauge multiple-fire stereotactic biopsy procedure for a 5-mm invasive ductal carcinoma, a large 15-cm hematoma subsequently developed that occupied almost half of her breast. The hematoma developed because of an unsuspected factor IX deficiency. Instead of proceeding to preoperative needle localization, the 15-cm hematoma limited immediate patient management to excision of a large portion of the breast because of the hematoma and waiting for the hematoma to resolve or for mastectomy to be performed. Because the initial cancer was so small and the patient desired breast-conserving therapy, she waited 3 months for the hematoma to resolve to a few centimeters. The small hematoma was subsequently excised, along with the residual cancer, thus showing that hematomas can resolve with time. In another report, Melotti and Berg described the development of three hematomas ranging in size from 13 to 40 mm after 11-gauge core biopsy in eight anticoagulated patients, which suggests that core biopsy can be performed in anticoagulated patients if the need for biopsy is urgent.

Methods to decrease untoward bleeding include familiarity with the patient's current medications, over-the-counter self-prescribed drugs, herbs, and vitamins and the recommended times for which the patient should refrain from taking them. The radiologist works with the referring physician to determine whether administration of these medications should and can be safely curtailed in patients receiving anticoagulants. Patients should be instructed to refrain from taking all pain medications except for Tylenol for 1 week before the biopsy because aspirin, nonsteroidal anti-inflammatory drugs, and other medications can inactivate platelets if medically indicated. Similarly, patients should be instructed to stop taking all herbal medications (particularly *Ginkgo biloba,* which potentiates anticoagulants) and vitamins (particularly vitamin E or fish oils) for 1 week before the biopsy.

Mastitis is an uncommon complication of percutaneous biopsy. Common antibiotics prescribed for breast infection include cephalexin (Keflex) or amoxicillin-clavulanate (Augmentin). Serious infections with abscess formation require surgical consultation, and treatment may involve percutaneous drainage or surgical incision and drainage.

For ultrasound-guided biopsies, pneumothorax is an unusual but reported complication and is especially important if the patient is unable to hold still or is coughing, if the angle needed to biopsy the lesion is very steep, if the lesion is on the chest wall, and particularly if the lesion lies between ribs. Pneumothorax has been reported as a complication of both fine-needle breast aspiration and large-core biopsy. It is imperative that the radiologist identify the chest wall and the expected location of the pleura before the biopsy to evaluate the trajectory of the needle throw. Taking the extra time to roll the patient to obtain the perfect position so that the needle trajectory is parallel to the chest wall is especially important. When there is a possibility of pneumothorax during the biopsy, the radiologist should obtain consent from the patient specifically for the possibility that the "needle could puncture the lung and result in the need for an emergency room visit and possible stay in the hospital, which is very unusual." Knowledge of this possibility and strict instructions to the patient to remain immobile during the biopsy are important for informed consent. If there are serious concerns about pneumothorax during a procedure, one should consider using a needle or probe with a coring or firing device that stops at the needle tip and has no "throw" beyond the tip. An alternative is needle localization and surgical excision.

Pseudoaneurysms can occur in the breast after core biopsy, and some authors have reported treating these lesions percutaneously with sonographically guided embolization, alcohol, or thrombin.

FOLLOW-UP, AUDITS, AND PATIENT NON-COMPLIANCE

The true sensitivity and specificity of large-core biopsy techniques for nonpalpable breast lesions should be audited in one's own practice. Though deemed useful in the radiology literature for patients who have indeterminate breast lesions, the efficacy, sensitivity, and specificity of the core biopsy service should be audited to establish and justify the core procedure in a particular practice. In addition, standard mammographic surveillance after the fine-needle or core biopsy is essential to diagnose missed cancers. Several facilities request either short-term mammographic follow-up at 6 months or follow-up at 12, 24, and 36 months after cytologic or histologic sampling. In addition, the initial informed consent indicates that imaging follow-up is expected and that the patient is to return for all three or four visits after the procedure.

The problem of follow-up and compliance with follow-up is a difficult one even in the best of hands because as many as 40% of women do not return for all their follow-up mammograms after benign results and 15% do not complete the recommended surgery after an abnormal core or fine-needle aspiration result. As a result of the Mammography Quality Standards Act of 1992, U.S. federal law mandates follow-up on all abnormal mammograms. However, tracking in clinical practice is complicated, time-consuming, and expensive, with multiple costs for personnel, computer updates, and mailing. This requirement is a cause of frustration for many radiologists because despite computerized follow-up programs, women's outcomes may be difficult to track as a result of relocation, changing of insurance, decisions by their referring physicians contrary to recommended follow-up, or other reasons. Accordingly, informed consent before biopsy assumes even more importance so that proper patient management can be ensured.

KEY ELEMENTS

Know the location of the target lesion in three dimensions—do not attempt biopsy of a lesion not known to be genuine or one whose location in the breast is not known.

Do not attempt biopsy of skin calcifications.

Specimen radiography should show the hookwire, the hookwire tip, and the lesion; if not present in the specimen, the surgeon should be informed in the operating room.

Reasons that calcifications may not be visualized on the specimen radiograph include non-removal, calcium oxalate, location in the paraffin block, not present because it is pushed out of the specimen by the microtome, or milk of calcium.

Untoward complications of core biopsy include hematoma, infection, re-bleeding, pneumothorax, and pseudoaneurysm.

Correlation between the pathology results and imaging studies establishes concordance.

Markers placed in the core biopsy site may move significantly after placement.

Surgical excisional biopsy is recommended for core biopsy specimens showing invasive ductal cancer, DCIS, ADH, phyllodes tumors, atypical papillary lesions, and noncongruent imaging/pathology findings.

It is controversial whether surgical excisional biopsy should always be performed after obtaining core biopsy samples showing radial scar, pseudoangiomatous stromal hyperplasia, non-atypical papillary lesions, LCIS, and ALH.

SUGGESTED READINGS

Adler DD, Ligut RJ, Granstrom P, et al: Follow-up of benign results of stereotactic core breast biopsy. Acad Radiol 7(4): 248-253, 2000.

Bates T, Davidson T, Mansel RE: Litigation for pneumothorax as a complication of fine-needle aspiration of the breast. Br J Surg 89:134-137, 2002.

Bazzocchi M, Francescutti GE, Zuiani C, et al: Breast pseudoaneurysm in a woman after core biopsy: Percutaneous treatment with alcohol. AJR Am J Roentgenol 179:696, 2002.

Berkowitz JE, Gatewood OM, Donovan GB, Gayler BW: Dermal breast calcifications: Localization with template-guided placement of skin marker. Radiology 163:282, 1987.

Birdwell RL, Ikeda DM, Brenner RJ: Methods of compliance with Mammography Quality Standards Act regulations for tracking positive mammograms: Survey results. AJR Am J Roentgenol 172:691-696, 1999.

Bober SE, Russell DG: Increasing breast tissue depth during stereotactic needle biopsy. AJR Am J Roentgenol 174:1085-1086, 2000.

Brem RF, Schoonjans JM: Local anesthesia in stereotactic, vacuum-assisted breast biopsy. Breast J 7:72-73, 2001.

Brenner RJ: Lesions entirely removed during stereotactic biopsy: Preoperative localization on the basis of mammographic landmarks and feasibility of freehand technique—initial experience. Radiology 214:585-590, 2000.

Brenner RJ: Percutaneous removal of postbiopsy marking clip in the breast using stereotactic technique. AJR Am J Roentgenol 176:417-419, 2001.

Brenner RJ, Bassett LW, Fajardo LL, et al: Stereotactic core-needle breast biopsy: A multi-institutional prospective trial. Radiology 218:866-872, 2001.

Brenner RJ, Jackman RJ, Parker SH, et al: Percutaneous core needle biopsy of radial scars of the breast: When is excision necessary? AJR Am J Roentgenol 179:1179-1184, 2002.

Burbank F: Stereotactic breast biopsy: Comparison of 14- and 11-gauge Mammotome probe performance and complication rates. Am Surg 63:988-995, 1997.

Burbank F, Forcier N: Tissue marking clip for stereotactic breast biopsy: Initial placement accuracy, long-term stability, and usefulness as a guide for wire localization. Radiology 205:407-415, 1997.

Burnside ES, Sohlich RE, Sickles EA: Movement of a biopsy-site marker clip after completion of stereotactic directional vacuum-assisted breast biopsy: Case report. Radiology 221:504-507, 2001.

Carr JJ, Hemler PF, Halford PW, et al: Stereotactic localization of breast lesions: How it works and methods to improve accuracy. Radiographics 21:463-473, 2001.

Dershaw DD, Morris EA, Liberman L, Abramson AF: Nondiagnostic stereotaxic core breast biopsy: Results of rebiopsy. Radiology 198:323-325, 1996.

Deutch BM, Schwartz MR, Fodera T, Ray DM: Stereotactic core breast biopsy of a minimal carcinoma complicated by a large hematoma: A management dilemma. Radiology 202:431-433, 1997.

Dondalski M, Bernstein JR: Disappearing breast calcifications: Mammographic-pathologic discrepancy due to calcium oxalate. South Med J 85:1252-1254, 1992.

Fine RE, Boyd BA, Whitworth PW, et al: Percutaneous removal of benign breast masses using a vacuum-assisted hand-held device with ultrasound guidance. Am J Surg 184:332-336, 2002.

Frenna TH, Meyer JE, Sonnenfeld MR: US of breast biopsy specimens. Radiology 190:573, 1994.

Friedman PD, Sanders LM, Menendez C, et al: Retrieval of lost microcalcifications during stereotactic vacuum-assisted core biopsy. AJR Am J Roentgenol 180:275-280, 2003.

Goodman KA, Birdwell RL, Ikeda DM: Compliance with recommended follow-up after percutaneous breast core biopsy. AJR Am J Roentgenol 170:89-92, 1998.

Harris AT: Clip migration within 8 days of 11-gauge vacuum-assisted stereotactic breast biopsy: Case report. Radiology 228:552-554, 2003.

Harvey JA, Moran RE, DeAngelis GA: Technique and pitfalls of ultrasound-guided core-needle biopsy of the breast. Semin Ultrasound CT MR 21:362-374, 2000.

Helvie MA, Ikeda DM, Adler DD: Localization and needle aspiration of breast lesions: Complications in 370 cases. AJR Am J Roentgenol 157:711-714, 1991.

Huber S, Wagner M, Medl M, Czembirek H: Benign breast lesions: Minimally invasive vacuum-assisted biopsy with 11-gauge needles—patient acceptance and effect on follow-up imaging findings. Radiology 226:783-790, 2003.

Husien AM: Stereotactic localization mammography: Interpreting the check film. Clin Radiol 45:387-389, 1992.

Ikeda DM, Helvie MA, Adler DD, et al: The role of fine-needle aspiration and pneumocystography in the treatment of impalpable breast cysts. AJR Am J Roentgenol 158:1239-1241, 1992.

Irfan K, Brem RF: Surgical and mammographic follow-up of papillary lesions and atypical lobular hyperplasia diagnosed with stereotactic vacuum-assisted biopsy. Breast J 8:230-233, 2002.

Jackman RJ, Birdwell RL, Ikeda DM: Atypical ductal hyperplasia: Can some lesions be defined as probably benign after stereotactic 11-gauge vacuum-assisted biopsy, eliminating the recommendation for surgical excision? Radiology 224:548-554, 2002.

Jackman RJ, Burbank F, Parker SH, et al: Stereotactic breast biopsy of nonpalpable lesions: Determinants of ductal carcinoma in situ underestimation rates. Radiology 218:497-502, 2001.

Jackman RJ, Marzoni FA Jr: Stereotactic histologic biopsy with patients prone: Technical feasibility in 98% of mammographically detected lesions. AJR Am J Roentgenol 180:785-794, 2003.

Jackman RJ, Nowels KW, Rodriguez-Soto J, et al: Stereotactic, automated, large-core needle biopsy of nonpalpable breast lesions: False-negative and histologic underestimation rates after long-term follow-up. Radiology 210:799-805, 1999.

Kass R, Kumar G, Klimberg S, et al: Clip migration in stereotactic biopsy. Am J Surg 184(4):325-331, 2002.

Lamm RL, Jackman RJ: Mammographic abnormalities caused by percutaneous stereotactic biopsy of histologically benign lesions evident on follow-up mammograms. AJR Am J Roentgenol 174:753-756, 2000.

Lee CH, Carter D, Philpotts LE, et al: Ductal carcinoma in situ diagnosed with stereotactic core needle biopsy: Can invasion be predicted? Radiology 217:466-470, 2000.

Lee CH, Egglin TK, Philpotts L, et al: Cost-effectiveness of stereotactic core needle biopsy: Analysis by means of mammographic findings. Radiology 202:849-854, 1997.

Lee CH, Philpotts LE, Horvath LG, Tocino I: Follow-up of breast lesions diagnosed as benign with stereotactic core-needle biopsy: Frequency of mammographic change and false-negative rate. Radiology 212:189-194, 1999.

Lee SG, Piccoli CW, Hughes JS: Displacement of microcalcifications during stereotactic 11-gauge directional vacuum-assisted biopsy with marking clip placement: Case report. Radiology 219:495-497, 2001.

Lehman CD, Shook JE: Position of clip placement after vacuum-assisted breast biopsy: Is a unilateral two-view postbiopsy mammogram necessary? Breast J 9:272-276, 2003.

Liberman L, Bracero N, Vuolo MA, et al: Percutaneous large-core biopsy of papillary breast lesions. AJR Am J Roentgenol 172:331-337, 1999.

Liberman L, Dershaw DD, Glassman JR: Analysis of cancers not diagnosed at stereotactic core breast biopsy. Radiology 203:151-157, 1997.

Liberman L, Dershaw DD, Rosen PP, et al: Percutaneous removal of malignant mammographic lesions at stereotactic vacuum-assisted biopsy. Radiology 206:711-715, 1998.

Liberman L, Drotman M, Morris EA, et al: Imaging-histologic discordance at percutaneous breast biopsy. Cancer 89:2538-2546, 2000.

Liberman L, Kaplan J, Van Zee KJ, et al: Bracketing wires for preoperative breast needle localization. AJR Am J Roentgenol 177:565-572, 2001.

Liberman L, Sama M, Susnik B, et al: Lobular carcinoma in situ at percutaneous breast biopsy: Surgical biopsy findings. AJR Am J Roentgenol 173:291-299, 1999.

Liberman L, Smolkin JH, Dershaw DD, et al: Calcification retrieval at stereotactic, 11-gauge, directional, vacuum-assisted breast biopsy. Radiology 208:251-260, 1998.

Liberman L, Vuolo M, Dershaw DD, et al: Epithelial displacement after stereotactic 11-gauge directional vacuum-assisted breast biopsy. AJR Am J Roentgenol 172:677-681, 1999.

March DE, Coughlin BF, Barham RB, et al: Breast masses: Removal of all US evidence during biopsy by using a handheld vacuum-assisted device—initial experience. Radiology 227:549-555, 2003.

McNamara MP Jr, Boden T: Pseudoaneurysm of the breast related to 18-gauge core biopsy: Successful repair using sonographically guided thrombin injection. AJR Am J Roentgenol 179:924-926, 2002.

Melotti MK, Berg WA: Core needle breast biopsy in patients undergoing anticoagulation therapy: Preliminary results. AJR Am J Roentgenol 174:245-249, 2000.

Mercado CL, Hamele-Bena D, Singer C, et al: Papillary lesions of the breast: Evaluation with stereotactic directional vacuum-assisted biopsy. Radiology 221:650-655, 2001.

Mullen DJ, Eisen RN, Newman RD, et al: The use of carbon marking after stereotactic large-core-needle breast biopsy. Radiology 218:255-260, 2001.

Pal S, Ikeda DM, Birdwell RL: Compliance with recommended follow-up after fine-needle aspiration biopsy of nonpalpable breast lesions: A retrospective study. Radiology 201:71-74, 1996.

Parker SH, Burbank F, Jackman RJ, et al: Percutaneous large-core breast biopsy: A multi-institutional study. Radiology 193:359-364, 1994.

Philpotts LE, Lee CH, Horvath LJ, Tocino I: Canceled stereotactic core-needle biopsy of the breast: Analysis of 89 cases. Radiology 205:423-428, 1997.

Philpotts LE, Shaheen NA, Jain KS, et al: Uncommon high-risk lesions of the breast diagnosed at stereotactic core-needle biopsy: Clinical importance. Radiology 216:831-837, 2000.

Rebner M, et al: Paraffin tissue block radiography: Adjunct to breast specimen radiography. Radiology 173:695-696, 1989.

Rosen EL, Vo TT: Metallic clip deployment during stereotactic breast biopsy: Retrospective analysis. Radiology 218:510-516, 2001.

Ross BA, Ikeda DM, Jackman RJ, Nowels KW: Milk of calcium in the breast: Appearance on prone stereotactic imaging. Breast J 7:53-55, 2001.

Smathers RL: Marking the cavity site after stereotactic core needle breast biopsy. AJR Am J Roentgenol 180:355-356, 2003.

Smith LF, Henry-Tilman R, Rubio T, et al: Intraoperative localization after stereotactic breast biopsy without a needle. Am J Surg 182:584-589, 2001.

Tabar L, Pentek Z, Dean PB: The diagnostic and therapeutic value of breast cyst puncture and pneumocystography. Radiology 141:659-663, 1981.

Teh WL, Wilson AR, Evans AJ, et al: Ultrasound guided core biopsy of suspicious mammographic calcifications using high frequency and power Doppler ultrasound. Clin Radiol 55:390-394, 2000.

Tornos C, Silva E, el-Naggar A, Pritzker KP: Calcium oxalate crystals in breast biopsies. The missing microcalcifications. Am J Surg Pathol 14:961-968, 1990.

Whaley DH, Adamczyk DL, Jensen EA: Sonographically guided needle localization after stereotactic breast biopsy. AJR Am J Roentgenol 180:352-354, 2003.

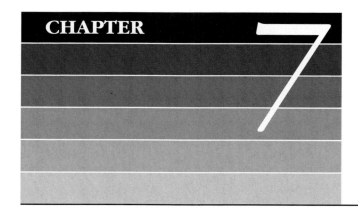

CHAPTER 7

Magnetic Resonance Imaging of Breast Cancer and MRI-Guided Breast Biopsy

BRUCE L. DANIEL

DEBRA M. IKEDA

Basic Principles
  Breast Cancer
Technique
  Patient Selection
  Equipment
  MRI Protocols
Interpretation of Breast MRI
  Normal Breast MRI Findings
  Common Breast MRI Artifacts
  Breast Lesions—Approach and Lexicon
    Morphology
    Dynamic Contrast Enhancement
    T2-Weighted Imaging
  Breast MRI Atlas
    Benign Breast Conditions
    Breast Cancers
  Diagnostic Limitations
Indications
  Screening
  Diagnosis
  Staging
  Management
MRI-Guided Biopsy
  Second-Look Ultrasound
  Preoperative Needle Localization
  Percutaneous Core Biopsy

BASIC PRINCIPLES

Magnetic resonance imaging (MRI) uses repeated radiofrequency pulses in concert with precise spatial modulation of a strong magnetic field to image the distribution and nuclear magnetic resonance characteristics of hydrogen atoms within human tissue. MRI provides either two-dimensional thin slices or three-dimensional volumetric tomographic images without ionizing radiation. Like mammography, MRI is comprehensive, reproducible, and operator independent. Like sonography, MRI is not limited by dense breast tissue.

Different MRI pulse sequences can be used to create images that reflect different tissue properties, such as T1, T2, or T2* relaxation times, proton density, apparent diffusion coefficient, and others. Pulse sequences can also be made specific for particular tissues, such as fat, water, or silicone, by a variety of techniques. MRI is exquisitely sensitive to paramagnetic substances such as intravenously injected gadolinium chelate contrast agents. Even minimal concentrations of these agents in tissues substantially shorten the T1 relaxation time and thereby result in high signal on T1-weighted images and improved tissue differentiation.

Breast Cancer

Invasive breast tumors are characterized by an ingrowth of neovascularity at their periphery. Tumor angiogenesis is associated with abnormal leaky endothelium leading to preferential enhancement of tumors versus normal breast tissue (Box 7-1). With bolus administration of an intravenous contrast agent, increased vascular flow and the rapid exchange rate of contrast between blood and the extracellular compartment cause invasive breast tumors to enhance more rapidly and more avidly than normal fibroglandular tissue, even in patients with dense breasts. This greater enhancement of tumors means that invasive breast cancers have high signal and show up whiter than the surrounding normal tissue. As a result, MRI exquisitely reveals invasive tumors that are occult on mammography (Fig. 7-1). The sensitivity of MRI for invasive breast cancer is extremely high, over 90%. However, as discussed in detail later, contrast enhancement on MRI is seen in many benign conditions as well; the specificity of MRI varies between 39% and 95%. As will be detailed later, both morphology and the time course of contrast enhancement help differentiate benign from malignant lesions (Box 7-1).

TECHNIQUE

Patient Selection

Benign hormone-related enhancement of normal breast tissue may occur before the onset of menses and

---

Box 7-1   Principles of Breast Cancer MRI

MRI is extremely sensitive to enhancement by contrast regardless of breast density or composition.

Tumor angiogenesis leads to preferential enhancement of cancers with intravenous contrast.

Lesion morphology helps distinguish cancer from benign conditions.

The time course of contrast enhancement helps distinguish cancer from benign conditions:

Cancers initially enhance rapidly ("rapid wash-in").

Cancers subsequently have a stable signal intensity ("plateau") or gradually declining signal intensity ("washout").

Benign and normal conditions enhance gradually and continuously.

---

can lead to false-positive studies. When possible, patients should be imaged 7 to 10 days after the onset of their menstrual cycle when spurious contrast enhancement of normal breast tissue is at its nadir (Box 7-2).

Before MRI scanning, the patient should be interviewed to exclude contraindications to entering the strong magnetic field, such as ferromagnetic vascular clips, metallic ocular fragments, pacemakers, implanted electromechanical devices, and others. A standardized MRI safety form (e.g., Fig. 7-2) should be completed by the patient and reviewed by a qualified person before scanning.

As with mammography, an MRI-specific breast history form is helpful. The patient places MRI-compatible markers on her breast to indicate lumps, complaints, or previous biopsies and annotates them on the history form. The patient also details the location, date, and results of previous breast biopsies because recent healing breast biopsies normally cause enhancement. The patient documents exogenous hormone therapy and the phase of the menstrual cycle or menopause and provides a brief family and risk factor history.

Equipment

An intravenous catheter is placed before scanning and continuously flushed by using the "keep vein open" setting of an MRI-compatible remote power injector. Placement of the catheter in the antecubital fossa contralateral to any known, previous, or suspected malignancy

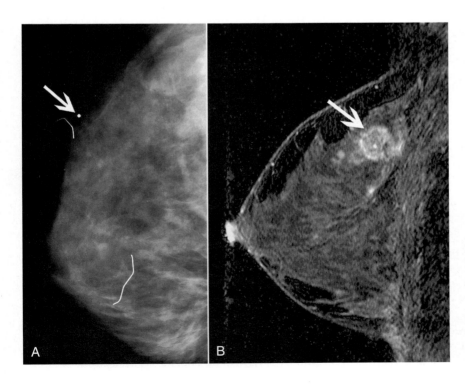

FIGURE 7-1   Mammographically Occult Breast Cancer. A mediolateral oblique x-ray mammogram (**A**) in a woman with a palpable mass in the upper portion of the breast indicated by a metallic skin marker *(arrow)* revealed only dense tissue. Contrast-enhanced water-specific three-dimensional MRI (**B**) demonstrated a 1-cm rim-enhancing lesion *(arrow).* Lumpectomy revealed a 1-cm invasive ductal carcinoma.

Box 7-2	**Patient Selection and Preparation**

Image on day 7 to 10 after the onset of menses to minimize false-positive enhancement.
Screen patients for MRI safety.
Use an MRI-specific breast history form.

MAGNETIC RESONANCE (MR) PROCEDURE SCREENING FORM FOR PATIENTS

Date _____/_____/_____   Patient Number _____

Name _____   Age _____   Height _____   Weight _____
      Last name   First name   Middle Initial

Date of Birth _____/_____/_____   Male ☐ Female ☐   Body Part to be Examined _____

     month day year
Address _____   Telephone (home) (_____) _____-_____

City _____   Telephone (work) (_____) _____-_____

State _____ Zip Code _____

Reason for MRI and/or Symptoms _____

Referring Physician _____   Telephone (_____) _____-_____

---

1. Have you had prior surgery or an operation (e.g., arthroscopy, endoscopy, etc.) of any kind?   ☐ No   ☐ Yes
   If yes, please indicate the date and type of surgery:
   Date _____/_____/_____   Type of surgery _____
   Date _____/_____/_____   Type of surgery _____
2. Have you had a prior diagnostic imaging study or examination (MRI, CT, Ultrasound, X-ray, etc.)?   ☐ No   ☐ Yes
   If yes, please list: Body part   Date   Facility

	Body part	Date	Facility
MRI	_____	___/___/___	_____
CT/CAT Scan	_____	___/___/___	_____
X-Ray	_____	___/___/___	_____
Ultrasound	_____	___/___/___	_____
Nuclear Medicine	_____	___/___/___	_____
Other_____	_____	___/___/___	_____

3. Have you experienced any problem related to a previous MRI examination or MR procedure?   ☐ No   ☐ Yes
   If yes, please describe: _____
4. Have you had an injury to the eye involving a metallic object or fragment (e.g., metallic slivers, shavings, foreign body, etc.)?   ☐ No   ☐ Yes
   If yes, please describe: _____
5. Have you ever been injured by a metallic object or foreign body (e.g., BB, bullet, shrapnel, etc.)?   ☐ No   ☐ Yes
   If yes, please describe: _____
6. Are you currently taking or have you recently taken any medication or drug?   ☐ No   ☐ Yes
   If yes, please list:_____
7. Are you allergic to any medication?   ☐ No   ☐ Yes
   If yes, please list:_____
8. Do you have a history of asthma, allergic reaction, respiratory disease, or reaction to a contrast medium or dye used for an MRI, CT, or X-ray examination?   ☐ No   ☐ Yes
9. Do you have anemia or any disease(s) that affects your blood, a history of renal (kidney) disease, or seizures?   ☐ No   ☐ Yes
   If yes, please describe: _____

For female patients:
10. Date of last menstrual period:_____/_____/_____   Post menopausal?   ☐ No   ☐ Yes
11. Are you pregnant or experiencing a late menstrual period?   ☐ No   ☐ Yes
12. Are you taking oral contraceptives or receiving hormonal treatment?   ☐ No   ☐ Yes
13. Are you taking any type of fertility medication or having fertility treatments?   ☐ No   ☐ Yes
    If yes, please describe: _____
14. Are you currently breastfeeding?   ☐ No   ☐ Yes

A

© F.G. Shellock, 2002   www.IMRSER.org

FIGURE 7-2   A and **B,** MRI safety form. As part of routine safety interview procedures before MRI, patients fill out a history form to screen for implanted devices or other conditions that might affect the safety of MRI. (Courtesy of Dr. Frank Shellock, MRI-Safety.com. Reprinted by permission.)
Continued

WARNING: Certain implants, devices, or objects may be hazardous to you and/or may interfere with the MR procedure (i.e., MRI, MR angiography, functional MRI, MR spectroscopy). **Do not enter** the MR system room or MR environment if you have any question or concern regarding an implant, device, or object. Consult the MRI Technologist or Radiologist BEFORE entering the MR system room. **The MR system magnet is ALWAYS on.**

Please indicate if you have any of the following:

☐ Yes ☐ No   Aneurysm clip(s)
☐ Yes ☐ No   Cardiac pacemaker
☐ Yes ☐ No   Implanted cardioverter defibrillator (ICD)
☐ Yes ☐ No   Electronic implant or device
☐ Yes ☐ No   Magnetically-activated implant or device
☐ Yes ☐ No   Neurostimulation system
☐ Yes ☐ No   Spinal cord stimulator
☐ Yes ☐ No   Internal electrodes or wires
☐ Yes ☐ No   Bone growth/bone fusion stimulator
☐ Yes ☐ No   Cochlear, otologic, or other ear implant
☐ Yes ☐ No   Insulin or other infusion pump
☐ Yes ☐ No   Implanted drug infusion device
☐ Yes ☐ No   Any type of prosthesis (eye, penile, etc.)
☐ Yes ☐ No   Heart valve prosthesis
☐ Yes ☐ No   Eyelid spring or wire
☐ Yes ☐ No   Artificial or prosthetic limb
☐ Yes ☐ No   Metallic stent, filter, or coil
☐ Yes ☐ No   Shunt (spinal or intraventricular)
☐ Yes ☐ No   Vascular access port and/or catheter
☐ Yes ☐ No   Radiation seeds or implants
☐ Yes ☐ No   Swan-Ganz or thermodilution catheter
☐ Yes ☐ No   Medication patch (Nicotine, Nitroglycerine)
☐ Yes ☐ No   Any metallic fragment or foreign body
☐ Yes ☐ No   Wire mesh implant
☐ Yes ☐ No   Tissue expander (e.g., breast)
☐ Yes ☐ No   Surgical staples, clips, or metallic sutures
☐ Yes ☐ No   Joint replacement (hip, knee, etc.)
☐ Yes ☐ No   Bone/joint pin, screw, nail, wire, plate, etc.
☐ Yes ☐ No   IUD, diaphragm, or pessary
☐ Yes ☐ No   Dentures or partial plates
☐ Yes ☐ No   Tattoo or permanent makeup
☐ Yes ☐ No   Body piercing jewelry
☐ Yes ☐ No   Hearing aid
              (Remove before entering MR system room)
☐ Yes ☐ No   Other implant _____
☐ Yes ☐ No   Breathing problem or motion disorder
☐ Yes ☐ No   Claustrophobia

Please mark on the figure(s) below the location of any implant or metal inside of or on your body.

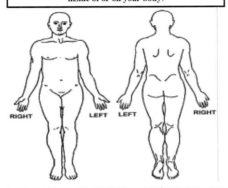

RIGHT   LEFT   LEFT   RIGHT

⚠ **IMPORTANT INSTRUCTIONS**

Before entering the MR environment or MR system room, you must remove <u>all</u> metallic objects including hearing aids, dentures, partial plates, keys, beeper, cell phone, eyeglasses, hair pins, barrettes, jewelry, body piercing jewelry, watch, safety pins, paperclips, money clip, credit cards, bank cards, magnetic strip cards, coins, pens, pocket knife, nail clipper, tools, clothing with metal fasteners, & clothing with metallic threads.

Please consult the MRI Technologist or Radiologist if you have any question or concern BEFORE you enter the MR system room.

NOTE: You may be advised or required to wear earplugs or other hearing protection during the MR procedure to prevent possible problems or hazards related to acoustic noise.

I attest that the above information is correct to the best of my knowledge. I read and understand the contents of this form and had the opportunity to ask questions regarding the information on this form and regarding the MR procedure that I am about to undergo.

Signature of Person Completing Form: _____   Date _____/_____/_____
                                          Signature

Form Completed By: ☐ Patient ☐ Relative ☐ Nurse _____   _____
                                                   Print name   Relationship to patient

Form Information Reviewed By: _____   _____
                                            Print name   Signature

☐ MRI Technologist   ☐ Nurse   ☐ Radiologist   ☐ Other_____

© F.G. Shellock, 2002   www.IMRSER.org

B

FIGURE 7-2 cont'd

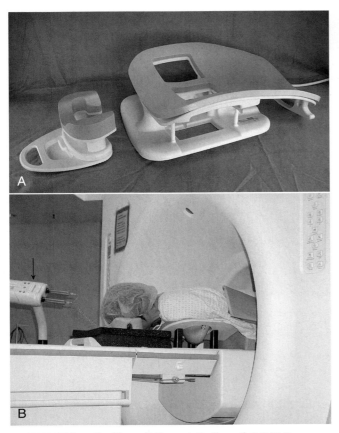

FIGURE 7-3   Dedicated Breast Coil and 1.5-T Scanner.
Prone positioning with the breasts in the apertures of a dedicated,
phased-array breast coil (**A**) improves image quality by maximizing
the image's signal-to-noise ratio and minimizing respiratory
motion. (Courtesy of Tom Tynes, MRI-Devices Inc, Waukesha, WI.
Used by permission.) Imaging at 1.5 T enables more robust fat
suppression and produces a higher signal-to-noise ratio than
imaging at lower field strengths does. Conventional closed-bore
scanners (**B**) have stronger, faster gradient systems than open MRI
systems do; these systems enable faster scans with more slices and
higher spatial resolution. Use of a remote power injector *(arrow)*
enables administration of contrast during the dynamic scan
protocol while the patient is within the magnet.

density of 1.5 T provide the best signal-to-noise ratio.
Magnets with "high-performance gradients" enable the
fastest, highest resolution scans (Box 7-3).

MRI Protocols

Conventional breast MRI begins with T1-weighted
images to define the position and anatomy of the breast.
T1-weighted images using the signal from the "body coil"
rather than the breast coil enable basic evaluation of the
axillae, anterior mediastinum, chest wall, and supraclavicular fossa for enlarged regional lymph nodes. The
dedicated breast coil signal should be used to perform all
subsequent sequences. T2-weighted fast spin echo (FSE)
images are then obtained to characterize the breast and
any lesions. T2-weighted scans with an FSE, turbo spin
echo (TSE), or rapid acquisition with relaxation inhibition
(RARE) technique enable high-quality images within
reasonable scan times of 5 to 6 minutes. High fat signal
on T2-weighted FSE images can be prevented with fat
suppression, and is most successful if unilateral scanning
is performed.

Considerable variation exists worldwide in methods
for the contrast-enhanced portion of the examination.
Most investigators agree that both the time course of
enhancement provided by dynamic scanning and the
morphology of lesions revealed by high–spatial resolution
scanning provide distinct and useful information about
the risk of malignancy in enhancing lesions. However,
commercially available MRI pulse sequences necessitate
a compromise between the dynamic and high–spatial
resolution approaches. In general, three basic approaches
have been developed: bilateral dynamic scanning, unilateral
high–spatial resolution scanning, and unilateral combined
dynamic and high-resolution scanning (Box 7-4).

In bilateral dynamic scanning, volumetric T1-weighted
three-dimensional spoiled gradient echo imaging is
repeated as rapidly as possible (preferably every minute
or faster if possible) before, during, and for approximately
5 to 7 minutes after a rapid intravenous bolus of
0.1 mmol/kg gadolinium contrast agent. Most investigators

is preferred. The patient is placed prone on a dedicated
breast coil (Fig. 7-3A). Prone positioning minimizes
respiratory motion in the breast. Phased-array breast
coils maximize the image's signal-to-noise ratio. Patient
discomfort is the primary cause of motion; the majority
of patients remain most comfortable for the entire scan
duration with both arms at their sides and wearing
hearing protection (Fig. 7-3B). Optional mild breast
stabilization or "compression" may be used to reduce
breast motion and decrease the volume of tissue to be
scanned so that the whole breast is included. However,
firm compression (as used routinely for mammography)
should be avoided because it may negatively affect
contrast enhancement. Scanners with a magnetic flux

Box 7-4   Breast Cancer MRI Protocols

Bilateral Rapid Dynamic	Unilateral High Spatial Resolution	Unilateral Combined Rapid Dynamic and High Spatial Resolution
Axial T1*	Axial T1*	Axial T1*
Axial T2[†]	Sagittal T2[†]	Sagittal T2[†]
Axial T1 3D Dynamic scans[‡];	Sagittal T1 3D Hi-Res[§]	Sagittal T1 3D Dynamic scans[‡]
Inject Gd contrast during scan[¶]	Inject Gd contrast[¶]	Inject Gd contrast during scan[¶]
Subtraction processing	Immediate sagittal T1 3D Hi-Res	Sagittal T1 3D Hi-Res[§]
	5-Minute delayed sagittal T1 3D Hi-Res	Sagittal T1 3D Dynamic scans[‡]

Note: Both fat suppression and high spatial resolution are essential to assess lesion morphology. Bilateral fat saturation suppression is unreliable.

  *Axial T1-weighted images: Use a body coil for this sequence only to interrogate for enlarged lymph nodes throughout the neck, chest, and axillae.

  [†]T2-weighted images: Use fast spin echo (FSE, RARE, TSE, etc.) with an effective echo time (TE) of 80 to 100 msec. Use 3- to 4-mm-thick slices, fat suppression, and a 256×192 matrix or higher for unilateral protocols with sagittal images. Use to evaluate cysts and cancer versus fibroadenoma. If fat suppression is poor, repeat after correcting the shim.

  [‡]T1-weighted three-dimensional images: Use "fast" spoiled three-dimensional gradient echo with a relaxation time (TR) of 6 msec or less. The flip angle (FA) is approximately 15 degrees for T1 weighting. Use a fractional k-space ("½ NEX," etc.) and a rectangular field of view (if used for bilateral imaging) to maximize speed. Adjust the number of slices and matrix to achieve a scan time of approximately 10 to 20 seconds. Some investigators sacrifice speed, especially on bilateral scans, to improve spatial resolution. Repeat rapidly for dynamic scans totaling at least 6 to 8 minutes. Subtraction processing is critical for detection of subtle enhancing lesions on non–fat-suppressed T1-weighted scans.

  [§]T1-weighted three-dimensional high-resolution images: Use "fast" spoiled three-dimensional gradient echo. Use a TR of 5 to 35 msec and an FA of approximately 15 to 45 degrees for T1 weighting. Fat suppression is critical to assess lesion morphology and is reliable only with a unilateral scan. High spatial resolution (≤2 mm) is also critical to assess lesion morphology and is most efficient in the sagittal plane. Elliptical-centric encoding increases sensitivity for early-enhancing lesions (e.g., cancers). Scan time is ideally 5 minutes or less.

  [¶]Use 2 to 3 mL/sec of intravenous gadolinium contrast agent, 0.1 mmol/kg, followed by a 20-mL saline flush.

---

use axial or coronal images with a rectangular field of view to maximize efficiency. Images are processed by subtracting the pre-contrast baseline images from subsequent dynamic images to reveal areas of enhancement. Region-of-interest analysis is used to assess the time course of contrast enhancement. Subtraction processing suppresses signal from bright fat because adipose tissue does not enhance significantly. Spatial resolution is limited by the need for rapid scan times and the large field of view required for bilateral scanning.

In unilateral high–spatial resolution scanning, volumetric T1-weighted three-dimensional spoiled gradient echo imaging is performed with voxel sizes of approximately 1 to 2 mm in greatest dimension before, immediately after, and approximately 5 minutes after bolus intravenous contrast injection. Sagittal volumes maximize unilateral breast imaging most efficiently, with a 20-cm field of view. Ideally, scan times are less than 5 minutes so that enhancement is captured during the initial period after injection when benign and malignant lesions are best discriminated. Intrinsic fat suppression is used to maximize the conspicuity of enhancing lesions and depiction of the margins of enhancing lesions where they abut fat, which would otherwise have high signal on non–fat-suppressed images. "Partial" or "intermittent" fat suppression can speed scan times significantly. Proper shimming and choice of center frequency are essential to ensure adequate fat suppression. Bilateral high–spatial resolution imaging is currently impractical because of the compromises required for bilateral shimming and because the added spatial coverage leads to impractically long scan times. Enhancing lesions are primarily characterized by their morphology; however, rudimentary time course information is available by comparing the initial post-contrast and 5-minute post-contrast images to look for early "washout" of contrast (see later).

In unilateral combined dynamic and high–spatial resolution imaging, sophisticated protocols and scanning techniques capture both rapid dynamic and high–spatial resolution images of one breast during and after intravenous contrast injection. Early approaches included "keyhole" imaging. Interleaved protocols, in which dynamic scanning is interrupted for high–spatial resolution imaging, provide very high-quality images and dynamic data but incomplete dynamic data and require rapid switching between different pulse sequences. Recent advances in true simultaneous combined imaging include variable-resolution projection reconstruction imaging and variable-density three-dimensional spiral imaging.

INTERPRETATION OF BREAST MRI

Normal Breast MRI Findings

Typical images from a patient who underwent both bilateral dynamic imaging and unilateral combined dynamic and high–spatial resolution imaging are provided in Figure 7-4. On T1-weighted non–contrast-enhanced images, aqueous tissues, including skin, fibroglandular

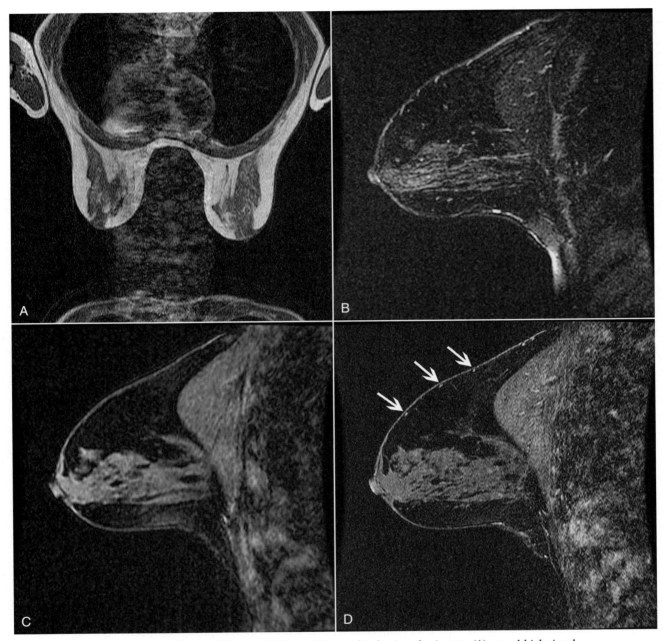

FIGURE 7-4   Normal Breast MRI. Axial T1-weighted spin echo images (**A**) reveal high-signal fat within the breast and axilla. Soft tissues, including skin, fibroglandular tissue, lymph nodes, and muscles, are dark. Sagittal, fat-saturated, T2-weighted fast spin echo images (**B**) reveal dark signal within fat and moderately low signal within the pectoralis muscle. Glandular tissue has mixed T2-weighted signal intensity. Pre-contrast water-specific three-dimensional gradient echo MRI with magnetization transfer contrast (3DSSMT, **C**) reveals dark fat and moderately low fibroglandular and muscle tissue signal. High–spatial resolution 3DSSMT after the intravenous administration of a 0.1-mmol/kg bolus of contrast (**D**) reveals enhancing peripheral vessels *(arrows)* and mild nipple enhancement.   *Continued*

tissue, muscle, and lymph nodes, have moderately low signal intensity when compared with the higher signal intensity of fat, which has a short T1 relaxation time. In the absence of previous surgery or pathology, a layer of subcutaneous and retromammary fat completely surrounds the mammary gland tissue except where it enters the nipple-areola complex. The mammary gland itself is composed of a mix of low-signal fibroglandular tissue and high-signal fat lobules. The mix and distribution of fat and fibroglandular tissue vary greatly

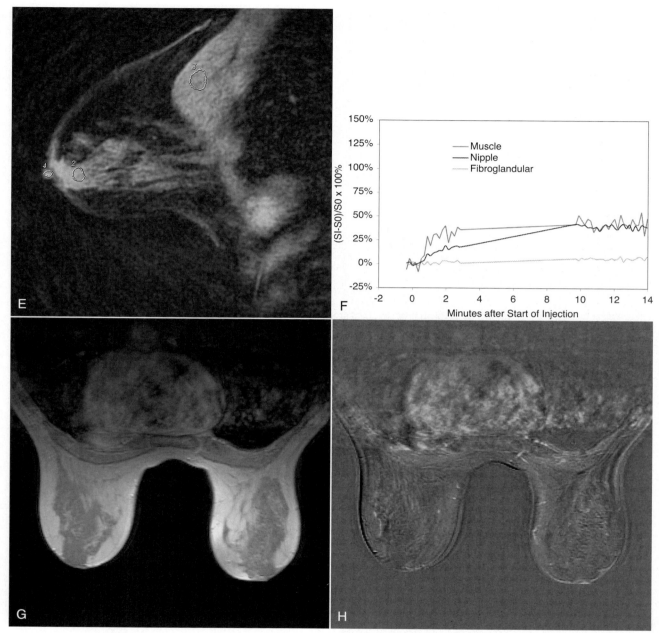

FIGURE 7-4 cont'd   Rapid dynamic three-dimensional spiral imaging (**E**) reveals mild (<50%) gradual enhancement in the nipple and fibroglandular tissue and mild (<50%) rapid enhancement in the pectoralis muscle (**F**). Subtraction processing of early post-contrast multiplanar two-dimensional spoiled gradient echo images (**G**) minus pre-contrast baseline images reveals diffuse low-level fibroglandular and muscle enhancement (**H**).

between patients—from dense, uniformly glandular tissue with almost no visible fat, to heterogenous, to predominantly fatty tissue separated by thin strands or septa of fibroglandular tissue.

T2-weighted non–contrast-enhanced images reveal heterogeneous fibroglandular tissue that is usually higher in signal intensity than adjacent muscle, but still not as bright as the small subcutaneous blood vessels commonly seen at the periphery of the breast or pure fluid (i.e., cysts, ducts—see later).

After injection of contrast, there is normal enhancement of peripheral small subcutaneous vessels and normal enhancement of the nipple and adjacent retroareolar tissue to a variable degree. Dynamic imaging reveals that fibroglandular tissue enhances mildly and slowly. Nipple enhancement is more avid, but still gradual. Muscle

Table 7-1	**Common Artifacts**
Artifact	**Cause**
Ghosting	Wrong phase-encoding direction
Blurring	Patient motion
Bright and dark edges on subtraction	Patient motion
Poor enhancement	Slow or missed injection
Poor fat suppression	Poor shimming or center frequency

enhances rapidly at first, but never enhances very avidly. Subtraction imaging of a normal breast should show mild glandular and muscle enhancement.

Common Breast MRI Artifacts

Ghosting from cardiac or respiratory motion occurs in the phase-encoding direction (Table 7-1). It can be prevented from obscuring breast tissue by careful selection of phase- and frequency-encoding directions. Poor fat suppression is usually due to poor shimming or incorrect choice of the excitation center frequency (Fig. 7-5).

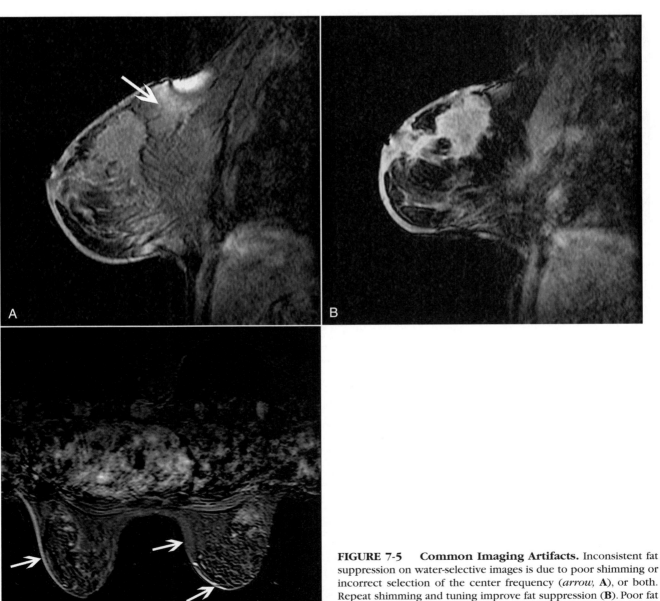

FIGURE 7-5   Common Imaging Artifacts. Inconsistent fat suppression on water-selective images is due to poor shimming or incorrect selection of the center frequency (*arrow,* **A**), or both. Repeat shimming and tuning improve fat suppression (**B**). Poor fat suppression on subtraction images is due to patient motion causing misregistration artifacts at fat-skin or fat-glandular interfaces (*arrows,* **C**).

Patient motion may cause blurring of the image, so it is especially important that the patient hold still and breathe quietly during scanning. On subtraction imaging, patient motion causes alternating bright and dark bands at fat-glandular tissue interfaces (Fig. 7-5). Poor breast tissue enhancement may be due to failed contrast injection and can be confirmed by abnormal dynamic enhancement curves from the heart, which normally show rapid, avid initial enhancement and rapid washout.

Breast Lesions—Approach and Lexicon

Initial studies of contrast-enhanced MRI reported a sensitivity of over 90% for invasive breast cancer. The sensitivity of contrast enhancement has remained high for invasive breast cancer. However, achieving high specificity remains difficult because some benign breast conditions enhance more avidly than normal breast tissue and may resemble breast cancer when enhancement alone is used for interpretation. Specifically, benign fibroadenomas, papillomas, and proliferative fibrocystic change also enhance to a greater degree than normal surrounding breast tissue.

Two strategies have evolved to improve the specificity of contrast-enhanced breast MRI: high–spatial resolution and dynamic imaging. In addition, T2-weighted imaging plays a secondary role in distinguishing some benign and malignant lesions. The American College of Radiology (ACR) Breast Imaging Reporting and Database System (BI-RADS) provides a valuable standard for the terminology used to analyze breast lesions on MRI (Table 7-2) and is recommended for all breast MRI reporting. Reporting should include a brief summary of the scan technique, including the scanner, field strength, and pulse sequences used; the specifics of contrast injection; and imaging findings and management recommendations.

Table 7-2   Breast MRI Lexicon and Reporting: Morphologic Categories and Terms for Each Lesion Type

Lesion Type	Internal Enhancement	Shape	Margin
Focus, foci			
Mass	Homogeneous	Round	Smooth
	Homogeneous	Oval	
	Rim enhancement	Lobulated	Irregular
	Enhancing internal septations	Irregular	Spiculated
	Dark internal septations		
	Central enhancement		
Linear	Smooth, clumped		
Ductal	Smooth, clumped		
Focal area	Homogeneous, heterogeneous, stippled, clumped		
Segmental	Homogeneous, heterogeneous, stippled, clumped		
Regional	Homogeneous, heterogeneous, stippled, clumped		
Multiple regions	Homogeneous, heterogeneous, stippled, clumped		
Diffuse	Homogeneous, heterogeneous, stippled, clumped, reticular/dendritic		

Note: stippled = sand-like or dot-like
Heterogeneous = nonuniform
Clumped = cobblestone-like
Homogeneous = confluent, uniform enhancement
Reticular/Dendritic = trabecular thickening
Symmetric or asymmetrical

Associated Findings

Nipple retraction	Nipple invasion	Pectoralis and/or chest wall invasion
Skin retraction	Skin thickening	Skin invasion
Edema	Lymphadenopathy	Hematoma/blood
Fluid-filled ducts	Abnormal signal void	Pre-contrast high duct signal
Cysts		Skin retraction

Reporting of Kinetic Data
Region-of-interest size: >3 pixels
Region-of-interest location: most intensely enhancing area, most suspicious curve
Initial enhancement: slow, medium, rapid
Enhancement pattern over time: persistent rise, plateau, washout

From American College of Radiology: ACR BI-RADS—MRI, 4th ed. *In* ACR Breast Imaging Reporting and Database System, Breast Imaging Atlas. Reston, VA, American College of Radiology, 2003.

Box 7-5   Lesion Morphology

Benign Features	Malignant Features
Minimal (mild) enhancement	Bright (strong) enhancement
Smooth border	Spiculated, very irregular border
Lobulated border	Rim enhancement (beware of fat necrosis, inflamed cyst)
Homogeneous	Heterogeneous
Nonenhancing (dark) internal septations	Enhancing (bright) septations
Parallels Cooper's ligaments	Grows through Cooper's ligaments
Microcysts	Ductal/linear-branching form

Morphology

In the high–spatial resolution approach, lesion morphology is evaluated on fat-nulled, three-dimensional images to look for characteristic shapes, borders, or internal enhancement patterns characteristic of cancer. With this approach, Nunes et al. reported a sensitivity of 96% and a specificity of 80% for cancer. Leong et al. reported similar results. The morphologic characteristics of benign and malignant lesions are summarized in Box 7-5 and shown in Figure 7-6. As with mammography, spiculated or very irregular borders are suspicious. Bright enhancement, particularly rim enhancement and enhancing septations, are usually specific for tumor angiogenesis. A ductal or linear-branching pattern of clumped or segmental enhancement is suspicious for ductal carcinoma in situ (DCIS), but it can also be seen in benign duct ectasia or fibrocystic change. As with mammography, entirely smooth, oval or lobulated masses suggest benign lesions. As with sonography, oval masses oriented parallel to Cooper's ligaments suggest benign lesions. Nonenhancing internal septations in smooth, oval, or lobulated masses are highly specific for a benign fibroadenoma (see later). Nonenhancing lesions are also benign. However, it is important to evaluate the dynamic curves of benign-appearing enhancing masses because round or oval homogeneous cancers do exist.

Dynamic Contrast Enhancement

In the dynamic MRI approach, the signal intensity of lesions is evaluated as a function of time during bolus intravenous administration of contrast material (Box 7-6). The dynamic curves are evaluated according to the initial enhancement in the first 2 minutes during the bolus or when the curve begins to change, as well as according to the late phase of enhancement, which is described as persistent, plateau, or washout in keeping with the ACR BI-RADS MRI lexicon. The entire spectrum of the time course of enhancement may be categorized from most benign to most suspicious according to the following scheme of Daniel et al. (Fig. 7-7): nonenhancing (type I); gradually enhancing (type II); or rapidly enhancing with a sustained gradual enhancement, plateau, or early

"washout" (types III, IV, and V, respectively). In reference to the curve shapes depicted in Figure 7-7, types I and II typically indicate benignancy and types IV and V indicate a high likelihood of malignancy. Type III curves are indeterminate. Using a similar approach, Kuhl et al. reported a sensitivity of 91% and a specificity of 83%. There are a few exceptions to these general principles. DCIS may exhibit any of the curve types, including nonenhancing or gradually enhancing curves shown as types I and II in Figure 7-7. Benign papillomas may exhibit the type I, II, III, or even type IV curves shown in Figure 7-7. The geographic distribution of dynamic enhancement also appears to be predictive, with tumors usually enhancing most rapidly at their periphery and benign lesions enhancing most rapidly at the center.

A variety of image-processing techniques have been developed to automate analysis of dynamic images throughout the breast on a pixel-by-pixel basis, including the saturation model, the two-compartment pharmaco-kinetic model, the "three time point method," and simpler enhancement ratios, wash-in slopes, and washout rates. Stand-alone workstations are available to perform these calculations and produce "functional images" that display abnormal areas of dynamic enhancement on corresponding anatomic images.

Not surprisingly, the highest sensitivity and specificity arise when both morphologic information and dynamic enhancement curves are taken into account, with a sensitivity of 95% and a specificity of 86% reported by Daniel et al. and a sensitivity of 91% and a specificity of 83% reported by Kinkel et al. Pharmacokinetic scans or physiologic scans are scans that superimpose physiologic information such as enhancement information on morphologic images, thereby combining both types of information into one format. This type of scan usually shows the morphologic appearance of a lesion with the physiologic image superimposed in color.

T2-Weighted Imaging

T2-weighted imaging also plays an important role in discriminating which enhancing lesions are likely to be benign or malignant (Table 7-3, Fig. 7-8). Lesions with

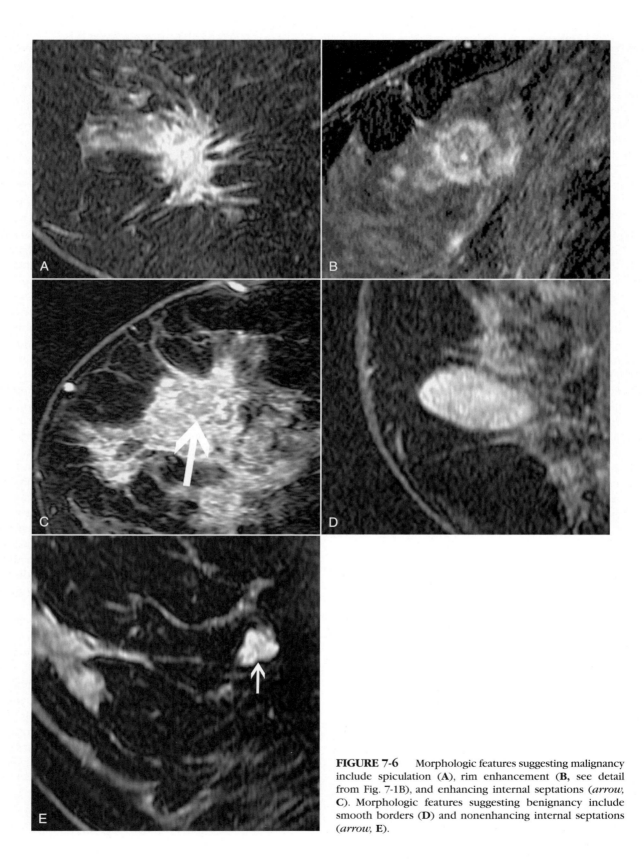

FIGURE 7-6 Morphologic features suggesting malignancy include spiculation (**A**), rim enhancement (**B**, see detail from Fig. 7-1B), and enhancing internal septations (*arrow,* **C**). Morphologic features suggesting benignancy include smooth borders (**D**) and nonenhancing internal septations (*arrow,* **E**).

very high signal in which the lesion is much brighter than glandular tissue and even higher than fat on non–fat-suppressed T2-weighted FSE images suggest benign lesions such as cysts, fluid-filled ducts, lymph nodes, or fibroadenomas. Invasive tumor, on the other hand, usually has a T2 signal similar to that of glandular tissue, that is, higher than muscle but not as high as fluid. Low-signal septations within very high-signal smooth oval or lobulated lesions on T2-weighted imaging also suggest benign fibroadenomas (see later).

Breast MRI Atlas

Benign Breast Conditions

Fluid-filled cysts and milk ducts are normal and occur frequently (Fig. 7-9). Simple cysts are round or oval with sharp margins. Adjacent cysts may be separated by thin, low-signal septations. Simple cysts have very high T2 signal and display no internal enhancement with

contrast, although a faint thin rim of gradual enhancement may be seen on high-resolution images. Occasionally, benign cysts may demonstrate high signal on unenhanced T1-weighted images, with corresponding lower signal on T2-weighted images, presumably because of their protein content. Dilated fluid-filled ducts are linear, radiate from the nipple, and may branch. Their signal and enhancement characteristics are the same as for cysts.

Hormone-related enhancement occurs in premenopausal women and women taking oral contraceptives (Fig. 7-10). Usually, diffuse gradual glandular enhancement is seen. Dynamic enhancement is generally gradual and progressive (Daniel type II, III); thus the appearance is rarely confused with invasive carcinoma on dynamic imaging. Less commonly, hormone-related enhancement may be focal (Fig. 7-10) and resemble lobular carcinoma or DCIS (see later). Hormone-related enhancement is minimized by scanning during the second week of a woman's menstrual cycle.

Fibrocystic change is commonly associated with focal (geographic) or regional nonspecific enhancement, especially in premenopausal women (Fig. 7-11), with

Box 7-6	Patterns of Dynamic Contrast Enhancement
Pattern suggests a benign lesion:	Pattern suggests malignancy:
No enhancement	Rapid initial enhancement
Gradual, sustained, early and late enhancement	Late plateau (stable enhancement)
Center enhances first	Washout (decreasing late signal intensity)
	Periphery enhances first

Table 7-3   Use of T2-Weighted Imaging

	T2 ≫ Glandular Tissue	T2 ≤ Glandular Tissue
Rapidly enhances with contrast	Probably benign, e.g., lymph node or fibroadenoma	Possible cancer
Nonenhancing with contrast	Benign, e.g., cyst or duct	Benign, e.g., sclerotic fibroadenoma

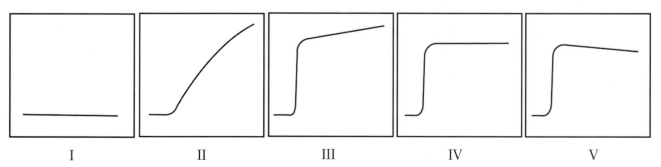

I   II   III   IV   V

FIGURE 7-7   Classification of the time course of dynamic contrast enhancement from the most likely benign (type I) through the most likely malignant (type V). No enhancement (type I) or gradual enhancement (type II) suggests a benign lesion. Rapid initial enhancement followed by gradual late enhancement (type III) is indeterminate. Rapid initial enhancement followed by a "plateau" signal intensity (type IV) or early "washout" of signal intensity (type V) is suspicious for invasive malignancy. (From Daniel BL, Yen YF, Glover GH, et al: Breast disease: Dynamic spiral MR imaging. Radiology 209:499-509, 1998.)

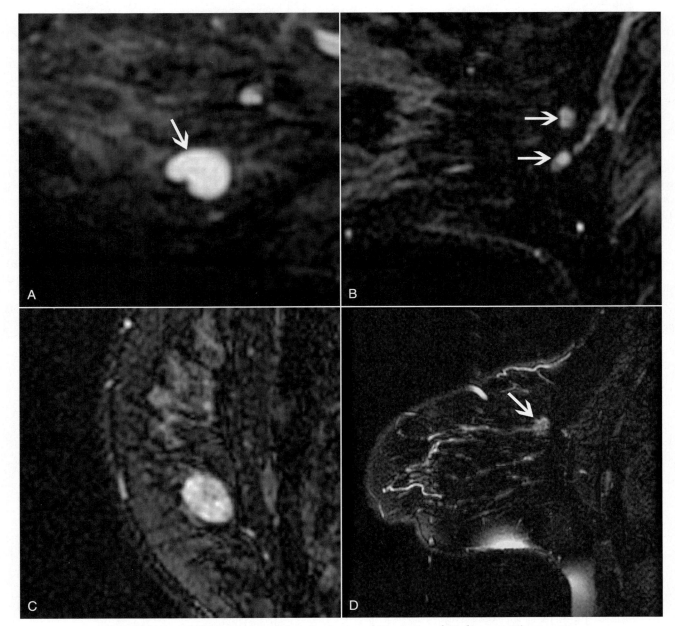

FIGURE 7-8   T2-Weighted Imaging Features of Benign and Malignant Disease. Very high signal on T2-weighted fast spin echo images that is brighter than fat (on non–fat-suppressed sequences) and substantially brighter than glandular tissue suggests a benign lesion such as a cyst (*arrow,* **A**), intramammary lymph node (*arrows,* **B**), or fibroadenoma (**C**). Low-signal septa are particularly specific for fibroadenoma (see Fig. 7-13A). Most malignancies, unless frankly necrotic, have a signal intensity that is similar to that of fibroglandular tissue (*arrow,* **D**).

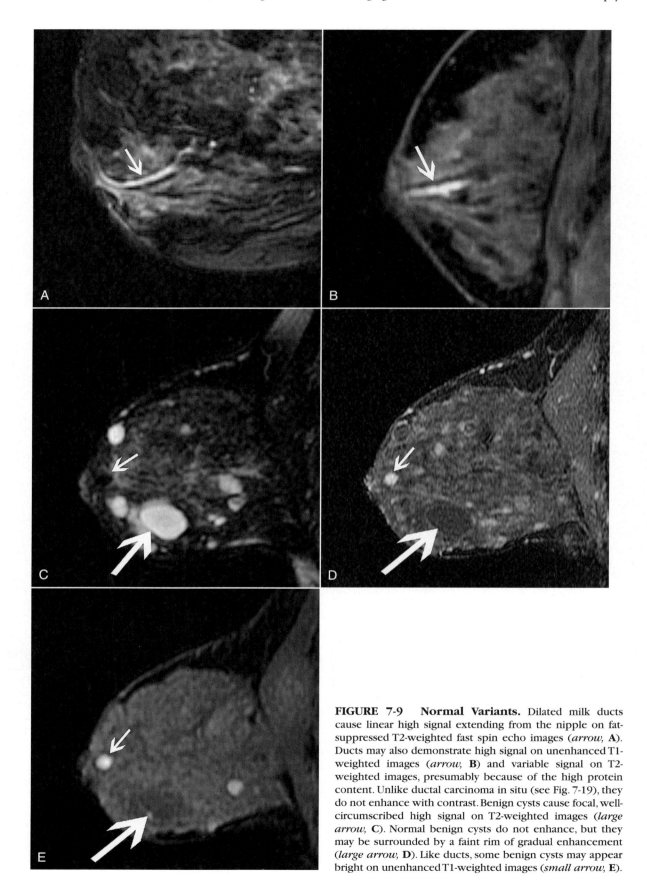

FIGURE 7-9 Normal Variants. Dilated milk ducts cause linear high signal extending from the nipple on fat-suppressed T2-weighted fast spin echo images (*arrow,* **A**). Ducts may also demonstrate high signal on unenhanced T1-weighted images (*arrow,* **B**) and variable signal on T2-weighted images, presumably because of the high protein content. Unlike ductal carcinoma in situ (see Fig. 7-19), they do not enhance with contrast. Benign cysts cause focal, well-circumscribed high signal on T2-weighted images (*large arrow,* **C**). Normal benign cysts do not enhance, but they may be surrounded by a faint rim of gradual enhancement (*large arrow,* **D**). Like ducts, some benign cysts may appear bright on unenhanced T1-weighted images (*small arrow,* **E**).

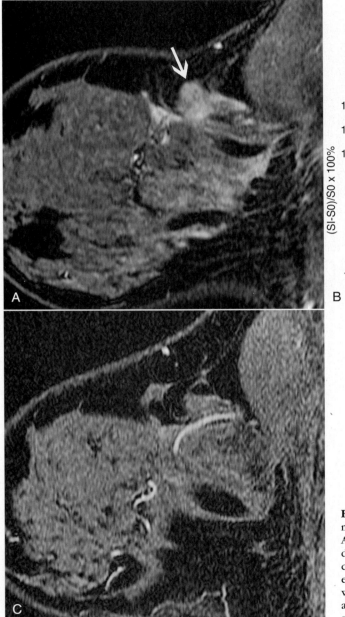

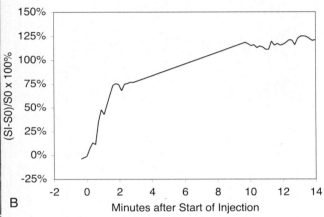

FIGURE 7-10 Hormone-Related Enhancement. Normal menstrual cycle variations may cause fibroglandular enhancement. Although hormone-related enhancement is usually mild and diffuse, it may occasionally cause focal intense enhancement that can simulate disease (*arrow*, **A**). Even though the persistent late enhancement suggested a benign etiology (**B**), repeat breast MRI was performed during the second week of the menstrual cycle (**C**) and showed that all previous findings had resolved and were hence presumably related to menstrual cycle variations.

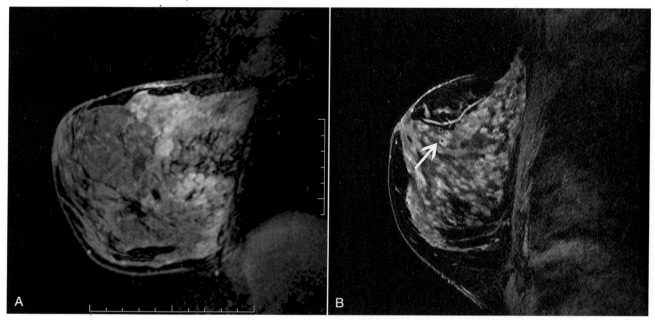

FIGURE 7-11   Fibrocystic Change. Geographic, regional, or diffuse glandular enhancement can be seen in patients with fibrocystic change (**A**). Though variable in appearance, the diagnosis is most readily established when small nonenhancing cysts are scattered throughout the lesion (*arrow,* **B**). (**A** From American College of Radiology: ACR BI-RADS—MRI, 4th ed. *In* ACR Breast Imaging Registry and Data System, Breast Imaging Atlas. Reston, VA, American College of Radiology 2003.)

gradual early enhancement, and with sustained gradual late enhancement. Occasionally, a specific diagnosis is made by the presence of tiny associated microcysts (Fig. 7-11). Adjacent cysts do not necessarily exclude carcinoma, however, so careful scrutiny of all enhancing foci remains essential to exclude concurrent malignancy.

Intramammary lymph nodes are common, especially in the upper outer quadrant (Fig. 7-12). Typically, intramammary nodes are small (5 mm or less) and have uniform high T2 signal. They are sharply circumscribed masses that may have a central fatty hilum. On dynamic imaging, they enhance avidly and rapidly, with a rapid initial enhancement and a late-phase plateau or early "washout," and hence cannot be distinguished from malignancy based on dynamic criteria alone. However, a definitive diagnosis is usually possible when lesion morphology shows their fatty hilum and close proximity to blood vessels with a "grapes on a vine" appearance. Correlation with sonography may avoid biopsy in cases in which location or morphologic criteria remain inconclusive. MRI is not as reliable as sentinel node sampling in determining the presence or absence of intranodal metastases.

Fibroadenoma is usually an oval or macrolobulated, sharply marginated, avidly and uniformly enhancing mass (Fig. 7-13). Nonenhancing internal septations are reported to be specific for benign fibroadenoma. On dynamic imaging, most fibroadenomas show early

gradual enhancement with sustained late gradual enhancement. "Young" fibroadenomas may have a more rapidly enhancing curve with sustained late-phase gradual enhancement, and they may occasionally demonstrate a late plateau of signal intensity that overlaps with the appearance of some invasive carcinomas. However, unlike many invasive carcinomas, the earliest, most avid enhancement is frequently central rather than peripheral. Among rapidly enhancing well-circumscribed masses, very high T2 signal is suggestive of benign fibroadenoma; the lack of very high T2 signal implies that malignancy cannot be excluded. The rare, well-differentiated phyllodes tumor has an appearance similar to that of fibroadenomas. Degenerating fibroadenomas, seen in older patients, do not enhance significantly and may have irregular internal signal voids that correspond to the large coarse "popcorn" calcifications seen mammographically.

Intraductal papilloma has a wide variety of appearances. Before MRI, most papillomas were identified by the presence of abnormal nipple discharge, an intraductal filling defect on galactography, or an intraductal mass on ultrasound. The analogous "classic" findings on MRI are an avidly enhancing mass at the posterior end of a fluid-filled duct (Fig. 7-14). However, papillomas have a wide variety of appearances on MRI; a fluid-filled duct is not necessarily present in all cases, and dynamic enhancement spans the entire range from "nonenhancing" to "washout" curves that mimic invasive carcinoma.

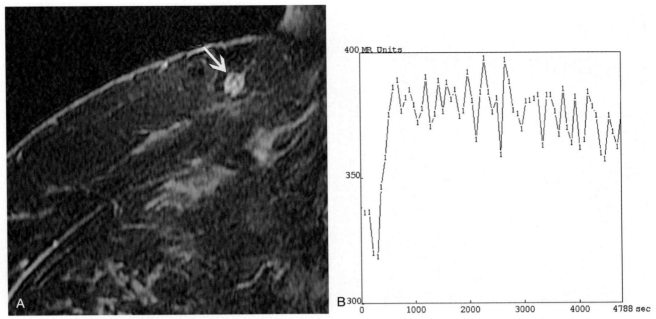

FIGURE 7-12   Intramammary Lymph Node. Usually small and located in close proximity to superficial vessels in the upper outer quadrant and axillary tail of the breast, lymph nodes demonstrate high signal on T2-weighted images (see Fig. 7-8B). All lymph nodes enhance rapidly and brightly with contrast (*arrow,* **A**), usually with a Daniel type IV or type V time course of enhancement (**B**). A normal fatty hilum can cause central low signal on fat-suppressed or subtracted images that mimics rim enhancement.

Postoperative changes include seroma, hematoma, scar, and fat necrosis. Careful history taking usually enables distinction of these lesions from primary breast lesions. Seroma and hematoma resemble cysts with variable intrinsic signal intensity, but they may have more irregular margins. Uniform rim-like enhancement occurs normally; peripheral nodular enhancement suggests residual tumor in the setting of pathologically transected margins. Scars and fat necrosis do not usually enhance beyond 2 years. Fat necrosis is typically manifested as irregular rim-like enhancement surrounding nonenhancing tissue that is identical to fat on all sequences.

Breast Cancers

Invasive ductal carcinoma (IDC) is virtually always manifested as a focal, avidly enhancing mass. Margins are usually irregular or spiculated (Fig. 7-15), but IDC may be more sharply defined in some cases. Rim enhancement and enhancing internal septations are particularly suspicious. Dynamic imaging reveals rapid initial enhancement followed by a "plateau" or early washout of signal intensity and is frequently most worrisome at the periphery of the lesion. T2 signal is similar to breast tissue; the lack of high signal distinguishes IDC from benign intramammary lymph nodes and fibroadenomas. True central nonenhancing necrosis is rare. Direct skin

or muscle invasion and architectural distortion are secondary signs of carcinoma (Fig. 7-16).

Infiltrating lobular carcinoma (ILC) has a much more variable appearance than IDC does. A particularly unique appearance is enhancement that follows the course of normal fibroglandular elements without a substantial mass effect (Fig. 7-17), which may lead to a missed diagnosis. ILC can also appear as a solitary mass or a combination of multiple masses with or without enhancing intervening fibroglandular tissue. Rarely, ILC may not enhance enough to be distinguished from surrounding breast tissue. On dynamic imaging, lobular carcinoma may have any pattern; benign patterns of dynamic curves such as either slow or rapid initial enhancement with sustained late-phase gradual enhancement do not exclude lobular carcinoma.

Mucinous carcinoma, a rare breast tumor, is a round mass that has a characteristic appearance on MRI (Fig. 7-18). The large central pool of mucin does not enhance and has very high T2 signal. Thus, mucinous carcinoma resembles a cyst, but with an irregular, thickened, avidly enhancing rim. Breast abscess may have a similar appearance.

DCIS has a very wide range of appearances on MRI. The "classic" description is enhancement in a ductal

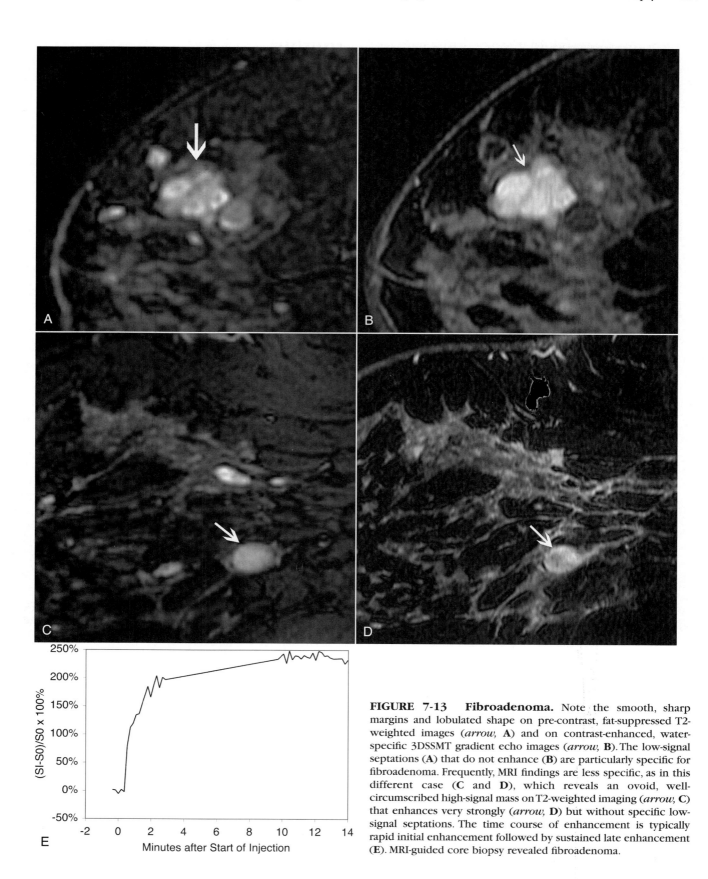

FIGURE 7-13   Fibroadenoma. Note the smooth, sharp margins and lobulated shape on pre-contrast, fat-suppressed T2-weighted images (*arrow,* **A**) and on contrast-enhanced, water-specific 3DSSMT gradient echo images (*arrow,* **B**). The low-signal septations (**A**) that do not enhance (**B**) are particularly specific for fibroadenoma. Frequently, MRI findings are less specific, as in this different case (**C** and **D**), which reveals an ovoid, well-circumscribed high-signal mass on T2-weighted imaging (*arrow,* **C**) that enhances very strongly (*arrow,* **D**) but without specific low-signal septations. The time course of enhancement is typically rapid initial enhancement followed by sustained late enhancement (**E**). MRI-guided core biopsy revealed fibroadenoma.

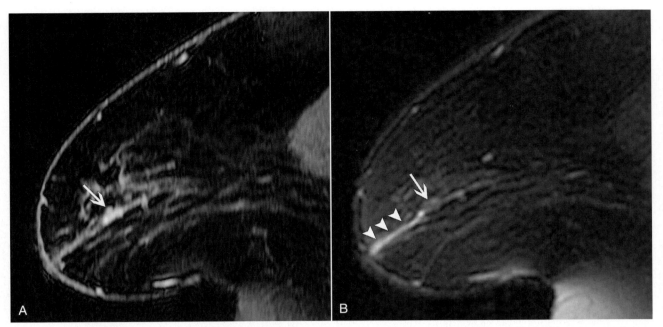

FIGURE 7-14 **Intraductal Papilloma.** Contrast-enhanced, fat-suppressed, T1-weighted, three-dimensional gradient echo (3DSSMT) MRI revealed a small, avidly enhancing retroareolar mass (*arrow*, **A**). A fluid-filled duct *(arrowheads)* extended to the mass *(arrow)* on pre-contrast, fat-suppressed T2-weighted images (**B**). Papillomas may enhance with any time course, including a rapid initial rise with a plateau mimicking invasive carcinoma. This is the classic appearance of intraductal papilloma, although not all papillomas demonstrate all these features. (From Daniel BL, Gardner RW, Birdwell RL, et al: Magnetic resonance imaging of intraductal papilloma of the breast. Magn Reson Imaging 21:887-892, 2003.)

system distribution, including segmental enhancement, or linear/branching enhancement emanating from the nipple (Fig. 7-19). Ductal enhancement per se is present in only a minority of cases. However, DCIS can be manifested as a focal mass, as geographic nonspecific enhancement, or even as enhancement indistinguishable from other breast tissue. Dynamic enhancement is also unreliable. DCIS usually enhances with a nonspecific rapid initial enhancement and a sustained gradual enhancement curve. However, any curve type can be seen, including no enhancement and suspicious rapid initial enhancement with a late-phase plateau or early "washout." Thus DCIS may resemble FCC, hormone-related enhancement, intraductal papilloma, or even invasive carcinoma. When associated with an invasive tumor, it commonly appears as a surrounding wedge of enhancing tissue that has a less worrisome dynamic enhancement curve than invasive tumor foci do. Calcifications cannot be reliably assessed with MRI, and thus mammographic correlation remains essential when attempting to determine the extent or presence of disease.

Diagnostic Limitations

Although the sensitivity of MRI is very high for invasive carcinoma, significantly higher than mammography or sonography in some settings, substantial diagnostic challenges remain (Box 7-7). Common false positives mimicking DCIS include focal fibrocystic change, hormone-related enhancement, focal fibrosis, and fibroadenomatous change. False positives occasionally mimicking invasive carcinomas include rapidly enhancing intraductal papillomas, avidly enhancing fibroadenomas lacking high T2 signal, intramammary lymph nodes without a fatty hilum, rim-enhancing fat necrosis, and enhancing spiculated surgical scars. False negatives remain rare; they are usually due to nonenhancing DCIS or ILC. Recent or ongoing chemotherapy may also reduce the sensitivity of contrast-enhanced MRI.

Small incidental enhancing lesions (IELs) are foci that are less than 5 mm, difficult to characterize, and common. Investigators vary in the level of concern that they attribute to these lesions. Regardless of size, an initial attempt should be made to characterize each

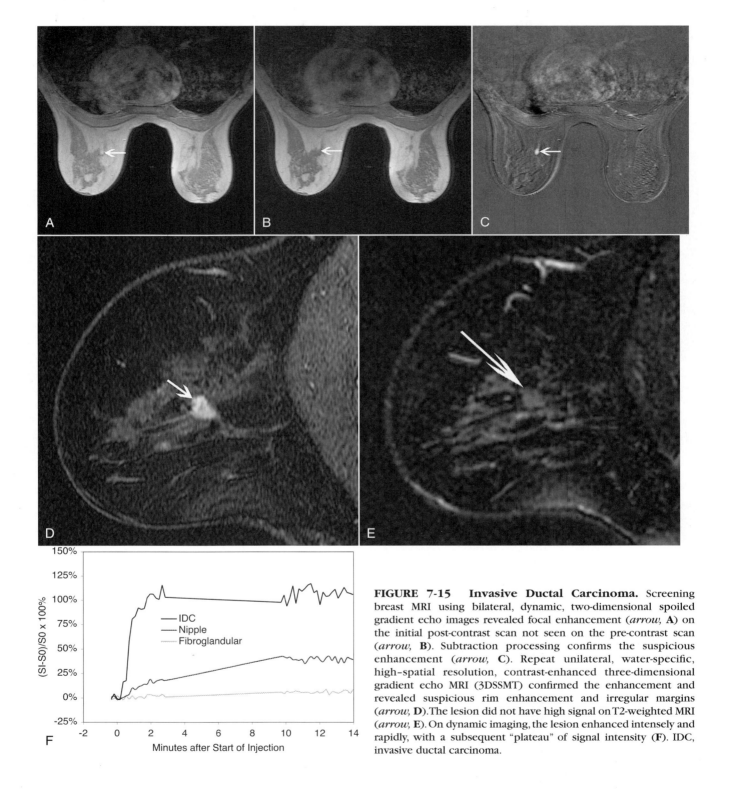

FIGURE 7-15   Invasive Ductal Carcinoma. Screening breast MRI using bilateral, dynamic, two-dimensional spoiled gradient echo images revealed focal enhancement (*arrow,* **A**) on the initial post-contrast scan not seen on the pre-contrast scan (*arrow,* **B**). Subtraction processing confirms the suspicious enhancement (*arrow,* **C**). Repeat unilateral, water-specific, high–spatial resolution, contrast-enhanced three-dimensional gradient echo MRI (3DSSMT) confirmed the enhancement and revealed suspicious rim enhancement and irregular margins (*arrow,* **D**). The lesion did not have high signal on T2-weighted MRI (*arrow,* **E**). On dynamic imaging, the lesion enhanced intensely and rapidly, with a subsequent "plateau" of signal intensity (**F**). IDC, invasive ductal carcinoma.

lesion's morphology, dynamic enhancement, and T2 signal because invasive carcinomas, fibroadenoma, or papilloma can also be very small. However, biopsy of an IEL frequently reveals no identifiable explanation. A practical approach to management is to use both the character of individual lesions along with their number and distribution and the patient's clinical setting to determine whether biopsy or follow-up MRI should be performed. In patients at very high risk for occult breast malignancy, such as those with known axillary nodal metastases and normal mammograms and physical examination, even a single relatively nonspecific IEL that is the dominant abnormality in the breast may be the index tumor and should prompt biopsy. In patients with lower risk, multiple bilateral, diffusely scattered, nonspecific small IELs have been successfully managed with serial MRI to document stability.

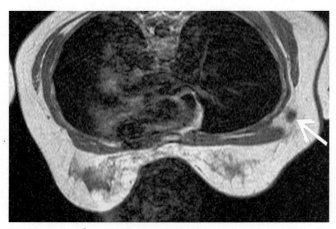

FIGURE 7-16   Enlarged Axillary Lymph Node. T1-weighted, pre-contrast spin echo images reveal a 15-mm right axillary soft tissue mass corresponding to an abnormally enlarged lymph node *(arrow)*. Note the absence of a normal fatty hilum. Although MRI may reveal grossly metastatic nodes as in this case, a normal appearance on MRI does not exclude micrometastases; the sensitivity of MRI is inferior to that of sentinel node sampling.

INDICATIONS

Large-scale randomized controlled trials, similar to the early mammography studies, have not been reported to support the widespread general use of contrast-enhanced breast MRI at this time. However, utility has been demonstrated by smaller studies in many specific situations (Box 7-8).

Screening

Improvements in genetic testing and counseling are identifying an increasing population of women who are at increased risk for the development of breast cancer. Current options include routine clinical and imaging screening with mammography or ultrasound and prophylactic mastectomy. MRI has recently been investigated as an adjunct to conventional imaging screening. In one of the largest U.S. studies, Morris et al. detected 14 tumors in 367 *BRCA1* and *BRCA2* mutation carriers, individuals with a similar risk profile and negative initial mammograms (Fig. 7-20). Optimal MRI screening intervals

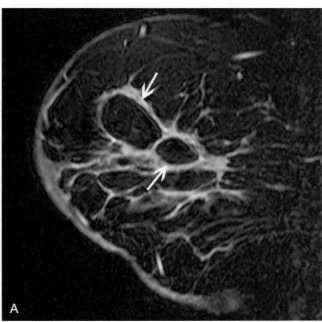

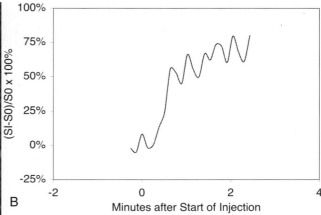

FIGURE 7-17   Infiltrating Lobular Carcinoma. Contrast-enhanced, water-selective, three-dimensional gradient echo images reveal enhancement along the normal fibroglandular elements *(arrows)*, without a significant mass effect (**A**), findings corresponding to the infiltrating pattern of spread. Initial enhancement is rapid, but followed by sustained late enhancement (**B**).

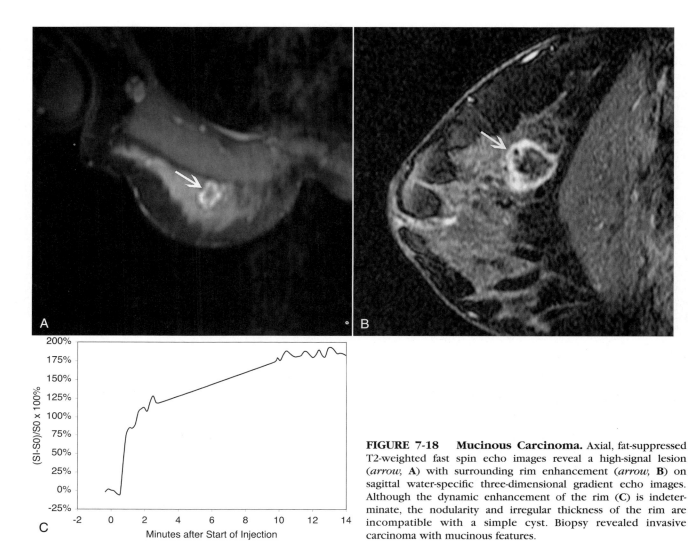

FIGURE 7-18   Mucinous Carcinoma. Axial, fat-suppressed T2-weighted fast spin echo images reveal a high-signal lesion (*arrow,* **A**) with surrounding rim enhancement (*arrow,* **B**) on sagittal water-specific three-dimensional gradient echo images. Although the dynamic enhancement of the rim (**C**) is indeterminate, the nodularity and irregular thickness of the rim are incompatible with a simple cyst. Biopsy revealed invasive carcinoma with mucinous features.

and the age at which MRI screening should be initiated have yet to be determined.

Women without a documented increased risk for breast cancer benefit less from MRI because the rate of false-positive abnormalities may substantially exceed the rate at which cancers are found and further investigation of these false-positive results may subject these women to significant morbidity. Patients with a history of direct free silicone injections of the breast for augmentation, however, cannot undergo any other type of screening (i.e., clinical breast examination, mammography, or sonography) with confidence and hence may be appropriate screening subjects when counseled accordingly about the risks associated with false-positive lesions.

Diagnosis

MRI is infrequently used to diagnose equivocal findings on mammography, sonography, or physical examination because the cost of MRI, including follow-up MRI, approaches the cost of the more traditional minimally invasive core biopsy. However, in rare instances, lesions are found that are not amenable to conventional biopsy, such as suspicious findings seen on only one mammographic view (Fig. 7-21). MRI is also used to evaluate patients with persistent bloody or cytologically abnormal nipple discharge in whom conventional galactography and ductoscopy were either unrevealing or unsuccessful. In addition, MRI is used to evaluate patients with equivocal

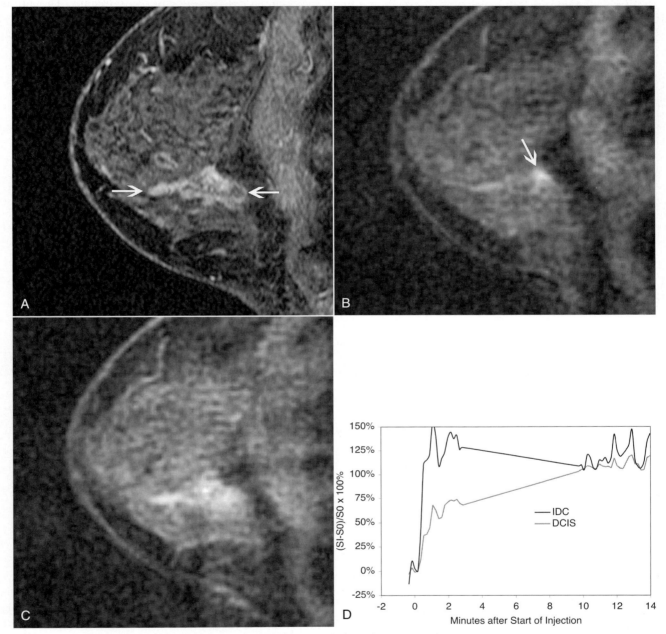

FIGURE 7-19   Ductal Carcinoma In Situ (DCIS). Sagittal high–spatial resolution water-selective three-dimensional MRI reveals enhancement in a segmental distribution corresponding to one ductal system (*arrows,* **A**). Dynamic three-dimensional spiral MRI reveals a small focus that enhanced on the initial images (*arrow,* **B**) sooner than the rest of the lesion, which enhanced on later images (**C**). This small focus, which had a "washout" curve (**D**), proved to be a 4-mm focus invasive ductal carcinoma (IDC) within the DCIS.

findings on physical examination that are mammographically and sonographically occult. However, the potential for false-positive and equivocal findings that generate biopsy or follow-up MRI must be balanced against the accuracy of simple palpation-based biopsy in this setting.

Box 7-7   Challenges in Interpretation

False Positives
Fibrocystic change
Hormone-related enhancement
Focal fibrosis, scar, fat necrosis
Fibroadenomatous change
Intraductal papilloma
Fibroadenoma
Intramammary lymph node

False Negatives
Nonenhancing ductal carcinoma in situ
Nonenhancing infiltrating lobular carcinoma
Recent/ongoing chemotherapy

Staging

MRI is frequently used preoperatively to image the extent of biopsy-proven breast cancer, especially in patients contemplating breast-conserving therapy. Though not routinely indicated as part of the local staging process in all newly diagnosed carcinomas, it is commonly used in selected subgroups, including the following:

- Patients with biopsy proven axillary lymph node metastases of breast cancer origin and normal mammograms and ultrasound (Fig. 7-22). Although the primary treatment of these patients remains systemic therapy, MRI may identify an occult primary breast tumor that can be treated with breast-conserving therapy.
- Patients with equivocal chest wall invasion on imaging or physical examination (Fig. 7-23).
- Patients with breast tissue that is suboptimally imaged by mammography, especially those with dense breast tissue, silicone implants, or silicone injections obscuring the breast.
- Patients with tumors that are poorly seen on conventional mammography, including ILC or DCIS without corresponding microcalcifications.

Box 7-8   Indications for Contrast-Enhanced Breast MRI

Screening:
  BRCA1
  BRCA2
  Family/personal history suggesting risk equivalent to that of *BRCA1/2*
  Obscured breast tissue (e.g., previous free silicone injection)
Diagnosis:
  Suspicious lesions seen on only 1 mammographic view, negative ultrasound
  Bloody nipple discharge with negative or failed galactogram
  Indeterminate palpable findings with negative mammogram and ultrasound
Staging:
  Locate the breast primary in patients with axillary metastases
  Detect chest wall invasion
  Evaluate the extent of cancer in patients with poorly evaluated breast tissue on mammography:
    Dense breasts
    Implants, free silicone injection
  Evaluate the extent of cancer in tumors poorly seen on mammography
    Infiltrating lobular carcinoma
    Ductal carcinoma in situ without corresponding microcalcifications
  Goals of breast cancer staging MRI are to
    Plan lumpectomy to reduce the rate of transected tumor at specimen margins
    Detect occult multifocal or multicentric tumor
    Detect occult contralateral tumor
    Detect residual disease when initial lumpectomy is incomplete
Management (especially patients undergoing neoadjuvant chemotherapy):
  Measure disease before initiating neoadjuvant chemotherapy
  Assess response to treatment after the initial cycle
  Localize potential residual tumor after a complete clinical response

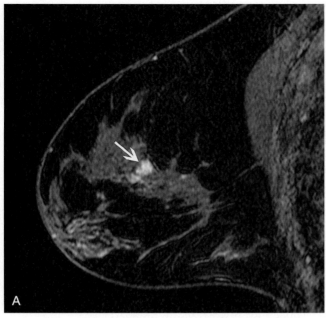

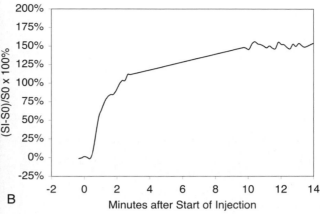

FIGURE 7-20 Ductal Carcinoma In Situ (DCIS) Detected on Screening MRI. MRI was performed after genetic testing revealed a suspicious *BRCA1* mutation. An 8-mm focal area of enhancement was noted with irregular margins on high–spatial resolution MRI (*arrow,* **A**). **B,** Dynamic imaging demonstrated a nonspecific enhancement curve. Pathologic examination revealed a 6.9-cm region of high-grade comedo DCIS.

In these patients, MRI may be used to plan the shape of the lumpectomy in an attempt to minimize the chance of transecting tumor margins. MRI may also reveal mammographically occult multifocal carcinoma (Fig. 7-24) and thereby prompt wider local excision. In addition, MRI may reveal occult multicentric or bilateral carcinoma (Fig. 7-25). Recent papers indicate that mammographically occult contralateral carcinoma is detected in 3.8% to 5.4% of patients with unilateral carcinoma. In these circumstances, preoperative biopsy is critical to pathologically confirm multicentric carcinoma or bilateral carcinoma because MRI finding can be nonspecific and may even lead to more extensive surgery than necessary in occasional patients.

Although MRI is most easily interpreted when performed in the absence of recent surgery because of the potential overlap of post-surgical healing scars and imaging findings of tumor (see earlier), it has been successfully used to map the extent of residual disease in patients with transected tumor detected at the margins of an initial excisional biopsy specimen. Asymmetric and nodular enhancement or enhancement that is non-contiguous with the biopsy site is suspicious.

Formal outcome studies demonstrating the benefit of staging MRI as an adjunct to conventional breast-conserving therapy are still in progress; however, controversy persists regarding the exact role and benefit of staging breast cancer by MRI given the high success rate of traditional breast-conserving therapy without MRI.

Management

Patients undergoing neoadjuvant chemotherapy are frequently imaged with breast MRI. Pre-treatment scans provide the most accurate nonsurgical three-dimensional measurements of the extent of tumor. Scans performed after the first one or two cycles can detect a treatment response that may predict whether completion of chemotherapy will be successful. In patients who do respond, MRI after completion of chemotherapy can be used to identify and localize residual tumor, even in patients who have had a complete clinical response (Fig. 7-26). It is important to note that in these circumstances, the dynamic enhancement of tumors may be less specific and even resemble benign disease. Indeed, any residual enhancement at the site of a previously known tumor is suspicious. Because of the poor specificity of MRI findings after chemotherapy, pre-treatment MRI is essential as a baseline for comparison.

MRI has also been investigated for its ability to detect local breast cancer recurrence. Debate persists regarding the duration of enhancement in benign post-surgical scars, although enhancement clearly decreases substantially over the first 2 years. Nevertheless, interpretation is best performed on serial MRI scans to assess whether enhancement is normally decreasing over time or suspiciously increasing over time.

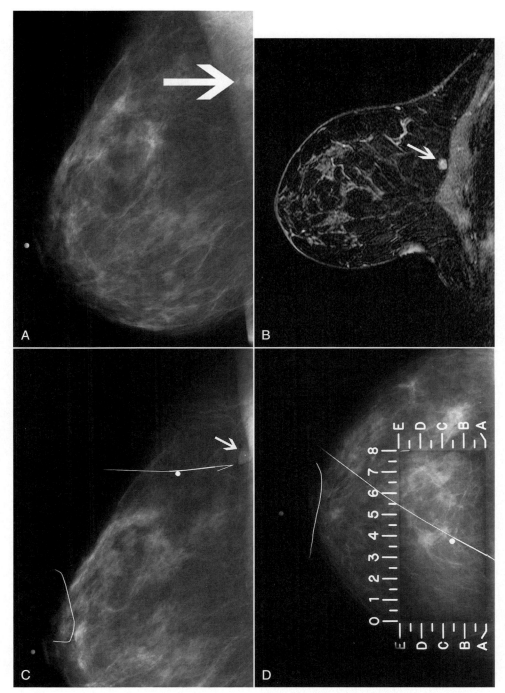

FIGURE 7-21   MRI of a Suspicious Mass Seen on One X-ray Mammographic View. A suspicious mass was noted in the superior aspect of the breast, near the chest wall on the mediolateral oblique (MLO) mammogram only (*arrow,* **A**). Water-selective three-dimensional gradient echo MRI revealed a focal enhancing mass (*arrow,* **B**). Preoperative MRI-guided wire localization was performed (not shown). After localization, an MLO mammogram (**C**) confirmed that localization was successful and the lesion was too close to the chest wall to be seen on craniocaudal views (**D**). Pathologic evaluation revealed a small fibroadenoma. (From Offodile RS, Daniel BL, Jeffrey SS, et al: MRI of suspicious breast masses seen on one mammographic view. Breast J [in press].)

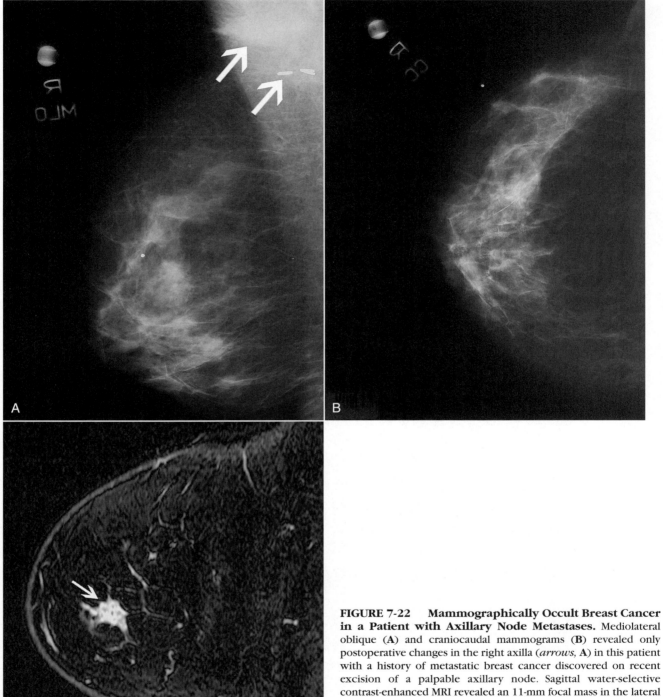

FIGURE 7-22   Mammographically Occult Breast Cancer in a Patient with Axillary Node Metastases. Mediolateral oblique (**A**) and craniocaudal mammograms (**B**) revealed only postoperative changes in the right axilla (*arrows,* **A**) in this patient with a history of metastatic breast cancer discovered on recent excision of a palpable axillary node. Sagittal water-selective contrast-enhanced MRI revealed an 11-mm focal mass in the lateral portion of the breast (*arrow,* **C**). MRI-guided, wire-localized excision revealed a 9-mm invasive ductal carcinoma that was excised with tumor-free margins.

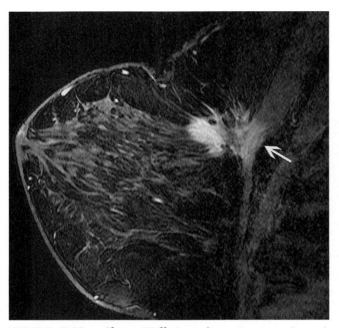

FIGURE 7-23   Chest Wall Invasion. Contrast-enhanced, three-dimensional water-specific breast MRI reveals a large spiculated mass in the posterior of the breast. The enhancing tissue traverses the normal retromammary fat plane to abut the chest wall. The focal enhancement of the pectoralis muscle *(arrow)* is consistent with invasion and indicates locally advanced disease. From American College of Radiology: ACR BI-RADS—MRI, 4th ed. *In* ACR Breast Imaging Registry and Database System, Breast Imaging Atlas. Reston, VA, American College of Radiology, 2003.

MRI-GUIDED BIOPSY (Box 7-9)

Second-Look Ultrasound

Lesions that are detected by MRI must frequently be biopsied. The easiest method of biopsy is to perform a "second-look" ultrasound examination directed toward the specific area of abnormality noted on MRI. If a corresponding lesion is seen, ultrasound-guided core needle biopsy is easily performed. Careful attention to technique is essential to ensure that the MRI abnormality corresponds to the sonographic lesion, given the difference in patient position and breast configuration between the two methods. Unfortunately, sonography fails to reveal a significant fraction of MRI-detected lesions. For these patients, biopsy must be performed under direct MRI guidance.

Preoperative Needle Localization

The simplest method of MRI-guided biopsy is preoperative MRI-guided needle localization and hookwire marking (Fig. 7-27). With the use of an open breast coil and sterile technique, an 18- or 20-gauge MRI-compatible needle is inserted in the breast and directed toward the

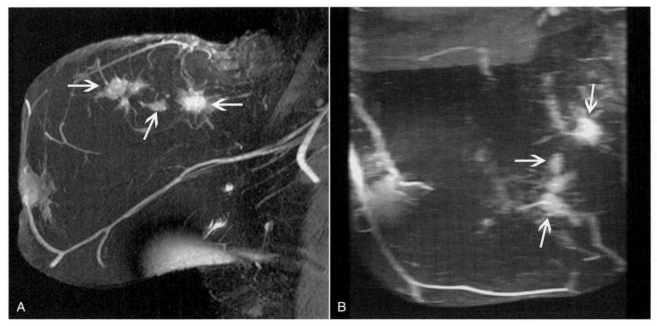

FIGURE 7-24   Multifocal Carcinoma. Water-specific, contrast-enhanced three-dimensional MRI revealed multiple suspicious enhancing masses in the upper outer quadrant *(arrows),* as shown on these 2-cm-thick slab, maximum-intensity projections in the sagittal **(A)** and axial **(B)** planes. MRI-guided lumpectomy confirmed multifocal invasive carcinoma.

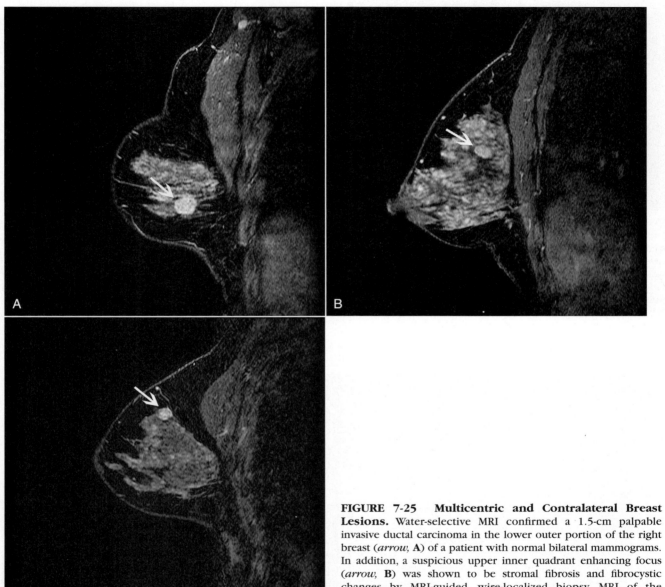

FIGURE 7-25   Multicentric and Contralateral Breast Lesions. Water-selective MRI confirmed a 1.5-cm palpable invasive ductal carcinoma in the lower outer portion of the right breast (*arrow*, **A**) of a patient with normal bilateral mammograms. In addition, a suspicious upper inner quadrant enhancing focus (*arrow*, **B**) was shown to be stromal fibrosis and fibrocystic changes by MRI-guided, wire-localized biopsy. MRI of the asymptomatic left breast also demonstrated a brightly enhancing focus (*arrow*, **C**) that proved to be an 8-mm invasive ductal carcinoma at MRI-guided biopsy.

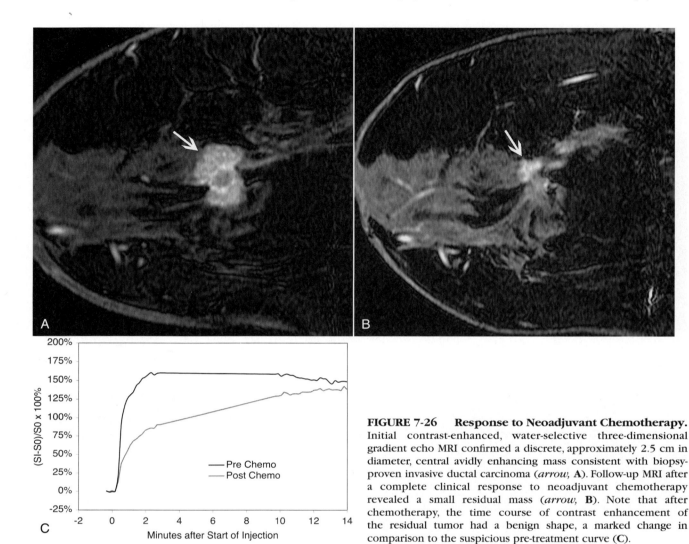

FIGURE 7-26   Response to Neoadjuvant Chemotherapy. Initial contrast-enhanced, water-selective three-dimensional gradient echo MRI confirmed a discrete, approximately 2.5 cm in diameter, central avidly enhancing mass consistent with biopsy-proven invasive ductal carcinoma (*arrow,* **A**). Follow-up MRI after a complete clinical response to neoadjuvant chemotherapy revealed a small residual mass (*arrow,* **B**). Note that after chemotherapy, the time course of contrast enhancement of the residual tumor had a benign shape, a marked change in comparison to the suspicious pre-treatment curve (**C**).

abnormality. A variety of specific methods have been proposed to determine the correct needle trajectory, including grid-coordinate positioning devices and freehand methods. Contrast-enhanced scans are critical to confirm correct localization. Procedure speed is very important because lesions commonly do not enhance preferentially over breast tissue after more than 5 to 10 minutes post-injection. A post-procedure, pre-surgery mammogram is recommended for three reasons. First, most breast surgeons are more familiar with the use of mammograms in planning the surgical approach. Second, mammography may reveal a mass or calcifications at the MRI-guided wire-localized lesion that was not previously appreciated as suspicious and can therefore be looked for on intraoperative specimen radiographs, thus maximizing the chance for accurate surgical excision. Third, mammograms document the

Box 7-9	Options for Biopsy of MRI Abnormalities

"Second-look" ultrasound-guided biopsy
MRI-guided needle localization
MRI-guided core needle biopsy

location of the MRI-guided biopsy and hence provide a critical baseline for future postoperative mammograms.

Percutaneous Core Biopsy

Percutaneous core needle biopsy (Fig. 7-28) can be performed under direct MRI guidance by both grid-

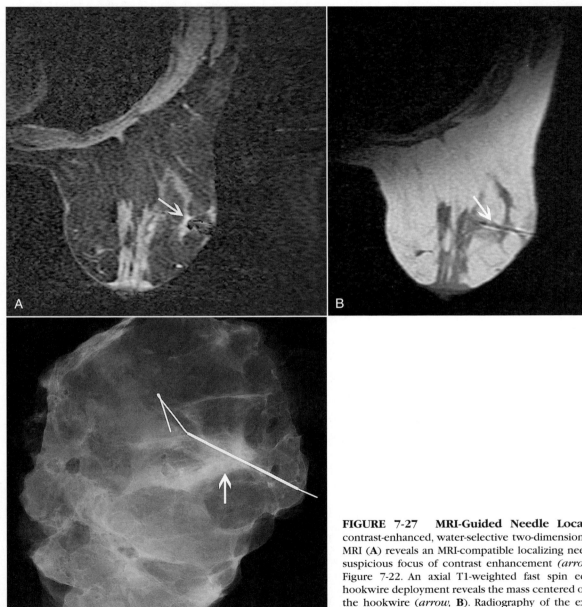

FIGURE 7-27 MRI-Guided Needle Localization. Axial, contrast-enhanced, water-selective two-dimensional gradient echo MRI (**A**) reveals an MRI-compatible localizing needle abutting the suspicious focus of contrast enhancement *(arrow)* described in Figure 7-22. An axial T1-weighted fast spin echo image after hookwire deployment reveals the mass centered on the stiffener of the hookwire *(arrow,* **B**). Radiography of the excised specimen demonstrated nonspecific glandular tissue adjacent to the hookwire *(arrow,* **C**). Pathologic examination revealed invasive ductal carcinoma.

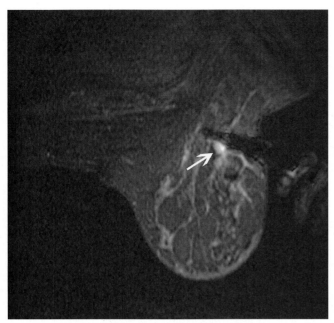

FIGURE 7-28 MRI-Guided Vacuum-Assisted Core Needle Biopsy. Axial, water-selective, two-dimensional gradient echo MRI revealed the inner trocar of a 14-gauge titanium biopsy needle extended through the focally enhancing mass *(arrow)* noted in Figure 7-13C-E. Pathologic evaluation revealed benign fibroadenoma.

coordinate and freehand methods. Devices include MRI-compatible 14-gauge titanium needles and vacuum-assisted biopsy devices. The imaging artifacts associated with core biopsy needles and the potential for breast motion remain limitations to reliable biopsy of sub-centimeter lesions given the current technology. MRI-compatible clips may be deployed after MRI-guided core needle biopsy to mark the site of biopsy. When benign results are obtained that do not specifically correspond to the expected appearance of the MRI lesion, repeat MRI-guided needle-localized surgical biopsy or follow-up MRI must be performed.

KEY ELEMENTS

Contrast enhancement in breast cancers is due to angiogenesis.

Indications for breast MRI are breast cancer screening in high-risk patients (*BRCA1, BRCA2,* or equivalent); breast cancer staging to detect mammographically occult bilateral, multicentric, multifocal, or locally extensive disease; poorly visualized tumors on mammography; diagnosis of suspicious findings that cannot be fully evaluated with conventional imaging; and before and after neoadjuvant chemotherapy.

Chemotherapy produces a potential pitfall in interpretation because it can decrease tumor conspicuity and change suspicious enhancement curves to benign persistent curves despite the persistence of viable, residual cancer.

Proper technique includes a dedicated breast coil, a contrast bolus followed by a saline flush, fat suppression, or subtraction.

Both morphology and enhancement curves are important in interpretation of MRI.

Abnormal enhancement is defined as enhancement brighter than normal surrounding glandular tissue on the first post-contrast scan or early in the initial enhancement phase.

ACR BI-RADS terms for morphologic features of abnormal enhancement include focus, focal area, mass, linear, ductal, segmental, regional, multiple regions, and diffuse enhancement.

Suspicious morphologic findings on MRI include an irregular shape, irregular or spiculated margins, rim enhancement, and enhancing internal septations.

Associated findings of focal skin thickening, satellite lesions, lymphadenopathy, and skin or chest wall invasion are suspicious for cancer in the appropriate clinical setting.

Suspicious enhancement curves include a rapid initial rise and abrupt transition to a late-phase plateau or washout; the curve shape is also called a "square root sign" or a "cancer corner."

Benign enhancement curves include a slow initial rise and a late persistent enhancement phase.

Fibroadenomas are usually bright on T2-weighted images if myxoid and dark on T2-weighted images if sclerotic and may have dark internal septations and a persistent late enhancement phase.

DCIS may be difficult to distinguish from fibrocystic changes.

Classic patterns for DCIS include clumped enhancement in a ductal, linear, or segmental distribution, particularly if it is asymmetric.

DCIS does not always display rapid initial enhancement with a plateau or washout.

Pitfalls in interpreting rim enhancement include fat necrosis and inflamed cysts; pre-contrast T2-weighted images can reduce false positives.

Pitfalls in interpreting benign-appearing masses include cancers with a benign morphology and a suspicious enhancement curve.

Mastitis and inflammatory cancer both produce breast edema and abnormal enhancement.

Papillomas and lymph nodes may have rapid initial rise and plateau or washout patterns and can thus be a cause of false-positive findings that generate biopsy.

MRI-guided preoperative needle localization and MRI-guided core biopsy must be performed rapidly because the signal intensity of the tumor may be indistinguishable from surrounding enhancing breast tissue within 10 minutes.

SUGGESTED READINGS

Agoston AT, Daniel BL, Herfkens RJ, et al: Intensity-modulated parametric mapping for simultaneous display of rapid dynamic and high–spatial-resolution breast MR imaging data. Radiographics 21:217-226, 2001.

American College of Radiology: ACR Breast Imaging Reporting and Data System, Breast Imaging Atlas. Reston, VA, American College of Radiology, 2003.

Balu-Maestro C, Chapellier C, Bleuse A, et al: Imaging in evaluation of response to neoadjuvant breast cancer treatment benefits of MRI. Breast Cancer Res Treat 72:145-152, 2002.

Bedrosian I, Mick R, Orel SG, et al: Changes in the surgical management of patients with breast carcinoma based on preoperative magnetic resonance imaging. Cancer 98:468-473, 2003.

Bedrosian I, Schlencker J, Spitz FR, et al: Magnetic resonance imaging–guided biopsy of mammographically and clinically occult breast lesions. Ann Surg Oncol 9:457-461, 2002.

Boetes C, Mus RD, Holland R, et al: Breast tumors: Comparative accuracy of MR imaging relative to mammography and US for demonstrating extent. Radiology 197:743-747, 1995.

Brenner RJ: Needle localization of breast lesions: Localizing data. AJR Am J Roentgenol 179:1643, author reply 1644, 2002.

Brinck U, Fischer U, Korabiowska M, et al: The variability of fibroadenoma in contrast-enhanced dynamic MR mammography. AJR Am J Roentgenol 168:1331-1334, 1997.

Brown J, Buckley D, Coulthard A, et al: Magnetic resonance imaging screening in women at genetic risk of breast cancer: Imaging and analysis protocol for the UK multicentre study. UK MRI Breast Screening Study Advisory Group. Magn Reson Imaging 18:765-776, 2000.

Brown J, Smith RC, Lee CH: Incidental enhancing lesions found on MR imaging of the breast. AJR Am J Roentgenol 176:1249-1254, 2001.

Buadu LD, Murakami J, Murayama S, et al: Breast lesions: Correlation of contrast medium enhancement patterns on MR images with histopathologic findings and tumor angiogenesis. Radiology 200:639-649, 1996.

Chenevert TL, Helvie MA, Aisen AM, et al: Dynamic three-dimensional imaging with partial k-space sampling: Initial application for gadolinium-enhanced rate characterization of breast lesions. Radiology 196:135-142, 1995.

Cohen EK, Leonhardt CM, Shumak RS, et al: Magnetic resonance imaging in potential postsurgical recurrence of breast cancer: Pitfalls and limitations. Can Assoc Radiol J 47:171-176, 1996.

Daniel BL, Birdwell RL, Black JW, et al: Interactive MR-guided, 14-gauge core-needle biopsy of enhancing lesions in a breast phantom mode. Acad Radiol 4:508-512, 1997.

Daniel BL, Birdwell RL, Butts K, et al: Freehand iMRI-guided large-gauge core needle biopsy: A new minimally invasive technique for diagnosis of enhancing breast lesions. J Magn Reson Imaging 13:896-902, 2001.

Daniel BL, Birdwell RL, Ikeda DM, et al: Breast lesion localization: A freehand, interactive MR imaging–guided technique. Radiology 207:455-463, 1998.

Daniel B, Herfkens R: Intraoperative MR imaging: Can image guidance improve therapy? Acad Radiol 9:875-877, 2002.

Daniel BL, Yen YF, Glover GH, et al: Breast disease: Dynamic spiral MR imaging. Radiology 209:499-509, 1998.

Degani H, Chetrit-Dadiani M, Bogin L, Furman-Haran E: Magnetic resonance imaging of tumor vasculature. Thromb Haemost 89:25-33, 2003.

Degani H, Gusis V, Weinstein D, et al: Mapping pathophysiological features of breast tumors by MRI at high spatial resolution. Nat Med 3:780-782, 1997.

Esserman L, Hylton N, Yassa L, et al: Utility of magnetic resonance imaging in the management of breast cancer: Evidence for improved preoperative staging. J Clin Oncol 17:110-119, 1999.

Harms SE, Flamig DP, Hesley KL, et al: MR imaging of the breast with rotating delivery of excitation off resonance: Clinical experience with pathologic correlation. Radiology 187:493-501, 1993.

Heywang SH, Wolf A, Pruss E, et al: MR imaging of the breast with Gd-DTPA: Use and limitations. Radiology 171:95-103, 1989.

Hochman MG, Orel SG, Powell CM, et al: Fibroadenomas: MR imaging appearances with radiologic-histopathologic correlation. Radiology 204:123-129, 1997.

Hrung JM, Langlotz CP, Orel SG, et al: Cost-effectiveness of MR imaging and core-needle biopsy in the preoperative work-up of suspicious breast lesions. Radiology 213:39-49, 1999.

Hrung JM, Sonnad SS, Schwartz JS, Langlotz CP: Accuracy of MR imaging in the work-up of suspicious breast lesions: A diagnostic meta-analysis. Acad Radiol 6:387-397, 1999.

Hwang ES, Kinkel K, Esserman LJ, et al: Magnetic resonance imaging in patients diagnosed with ductal carcinoma-in-situ: Value in the diagnosis of residual disease, occult invasion, and multicentricity. Ann Surg Oncol 10:381-388, 2003.

Ikeda DM, Baker DR, Daniel BL: Magnetic resonance imaging of breast cancer: Clinical indications and breast MRI reporting system. J Magn Reson Imaging 12:975-983, 2000.

Ikeda DM, Hylton NM, Kinkel K, et al: Development, standardization, and testing of a lexicon for reporting contrast-enhanced breast magnetic resonance imaging studies. J Magn Reson Imaging 13:889-895, 2001.

Kelcz F, Santyr GE, Cron GO, Mongin SJ: Application of a quantitative model to differentiate benign from malignant breast lesions detected by dynamic, gadolinium-enhanced MRI. J Magn Reson Imaging 6:743-752, 1996.

Kinkel K, Helbich TH, Esserman LJ, et al: Dynamic high–spatial-resolution MR imaging of suspicious breast lesions: Diagnostic criteria and interobserver variability. AJR Am J Roentgenol 175:35-43, 2000.

Kinoshita T, Odagiri K, Andoh K, et al: Evaluation of small internal mammary lymph node metastases in breast cancer by MRI. Radiat Med 17:189-193, 1999.

Kinoshita T, Yashiro N, Yoshigi J, et al: Inflammatory intra-mammary lymph node mimicking the malignant lesion in dynamic MRI: A case report. Clin Imaging 26:258-262, 2002.

Kuhl CK: Interventional breast MRI: Needle localisation and core biopsies. J Exp Clin Cancer Res 21(3 Suppl):65-68, 2002.

Kuhl CK: High-risk screening: Multi-modality surveillance of women at high risk for breast cancer (proven or suspected carriers of a breast cancer susceptibility gene). J Exp Clin Cancer Res 21(3 Suppl):103-106, 2002.

Kuhl CK, Bieling HB, Gieseke J, et al: Healthy premenopausal breast parenchyma in dynamic contrast-enhanced MR imaging of the breast: Normal contrast medium enhancement and cyclical-phase dependency. Radiology 203:137-144, 1997.

Kuhl CK, Elevelt A, Leutner CC, et al: Interventional breast MR imaging: Clinical use of a stereotactic localization and biopsy device. Radiology 204:667-675, 1997.

Kuhl CK, Klaschik S, Mielcarek P, et al: Do T2-weighted pulse sequences help with the differential diagnosis of enhancing lesions in dynamic breast MRI? J Magn Reson Imaging 9:187-196, 1999.

Kuhl CK, Mielcareck P, Klaschik S, et al: Dynamic breast MR imaging: Are signal intensity time course data useful for differential diagnosis of enhancing lesions? Radiology 211:101-110, 1999.

Kuhl CK, Schild HH: Dynamic image interpretation of MRI of the breast. J Magn Reson Imaging 12:965-974, 2000.

Kuhl CK, Schmutzler RK, Leutner CC, et al: Breast MR imaging screening in 192 women proved or suspected to be carriers of a breast cancer susceptibility gene: Preliminary results. Radiology 215:267-279, 2000.

Leong CS, Daniel BL, Herfkens RJ, et al: Characterization of breast lesion morphology with delayed 3DSSMT: An adjunct to dynamic breast MRI. J Magn Reson Imaging 11:87-96, 2000.

Liberman L, Morris EA, Benton CL, et al: Probably benign lesions at breast magnetic resonance imaging: Preliminary experience in high-risk women. Cancer 98:377-388, 2003.

Liberman L, Morris EA, Dershaw DD, et al: Ductal enhancement on MR imaging of the breast. AJR Am J Roentgenol 181:519-525, 2003.

Liberman L, Morris EA, Dershaw DD, et al: MR imaging of the ipsilateral breast in women with percutaneously proven breast cancer. AJR Am J Roentgenol 180:901-910, 2003.

Liberman L, Morris EA, Dershaw DD, et al: Fast MRI-guided vacuum-assisted breast biopsy: Initial experience. AJR Am J Roentgenol 181:1283-1293, 2003.

Liberman L, Morris EA, Kim CM, et al: MR imaging findings in the contralateral breast of women with recently diagnosed breast cancer. AJR Am J Roentgenol 180:333-341, 2003.

Liberman L, Morris EA, Lee MJ, et al: Breast lesions detected on MR imaging: Features and positive predictive value. AJR Am J Roentgenol 179:171-178, 2002.

Morris EA: Illustrated breast MR lexicon. Semin Roentgenol 36:238-249, 2001.

Morris EA, Liberman L, Ballon DJ, et al: MRI of occult breast carcinoma in a high-risk population. AJR Am J Roentgenol 181:619-626, 2003.

Morris EA, Liberman L, Dershaw DD, et al: Preoperative MR imaging–guided needle localization of breast lesions. AJR Am J Roentgenol 178:1211-1220, 2002.

Morris EA, Schwartz LH, Drotman MB, et al: Evaluation of pectoralis major muscle in patients with posterior breast tumors on breast MR images: Early experience. Radiology 214:67-72, 2000.

Muller-Schimpfle M, Ohmenhauser K, Sand J, et al: Dynamic 3D-MR mammography: Is there a benefit of sophisticated evaluation of enhancement curves for clinical routine? J Magn Reson Imaging 7:236-240, 1997.

Nunes LW, Englander SA, Charafeddine R, Schnall MD: Optimal post-contrast timing of breast MR image acquisition for architectural feature analysis. J Magn Reson Imaging 16:42-50, 2002.

Nunes LW, Schnall MD, Orel SG: Update of breast MR imaging architectural interpretation model. Radiology 219:484-494, 2001.

Obdeijn IM, Brouwers-Kuyper EM, Tilanus-Linthorst MM, et al: MR imaging–guided sonography followed by fine-needle aspiration cytology in occult carcinoma of the breast. AJR Am J Roentgenol 174:1079-1084, 2000.

Offodile RS, Daniel BL, Jeffrey SS, et al: MRI of suspicious breast masses seen on one mammographic view. Breast J (in press).

Orel SG, Dougherty CS, Reynolds C, et al: MR imaging in patients with nipple discharge: Initial experience. Radiology 216:248-254, 2000.

Partridge SC, Gibbs JE, Lu Y, et al: Accuracy of MR imaging for revealing residual breast cancer in patients who have undergone neoadjuvant chemotherapy. AJR Am J Roentgenol 179:1193-1199, 2002.

Partridge SC, McKinnon GC, Henry RG, Hylton NM: Menstrual cycle variation of apparent diffusion coefficients measured in the normal breast using MRI. J Magn Reson Imaging 14:433-438, 2001.

Perlet C, Schneider P, Amaya B, et al: MR-guided vacuum biopsy of 206 contrast-enhancing breast lesions. Rofo Fortschr Geb Rontgenstr Neuen Bildgeb Verfahr 174:88-95, 2002.

Qayyum A, Birdwell RL, Daniel BL, et al: MR imaging features of infiltrating lobular carcinoma of the breast: Histopathologic correlation. AJR Am J Roentgenol 178:1227-1232, 2002.

Ralleigh G, Walker AE, Hall-Craggs MA, et al: MR imaging of the skin and nipple of the breast: Differentiation between tumour recurrence and post-treatment change. Eur Radiol 11:1651-1658, 2001.

Rieber A, Zeitler H, Rosenthal H, et al: MRI of breast cancer: Influence of chemotherapy on sensitivity. Br J Radiol 70:452-458, 1997.

Rodenko GN, Harms SE, Pruneda JM, et al: MR imaging in the management before surgery of lobular carcinoma of the breast: Correlation with pathology. AJR Am J Roentgenol 167:1415-1419, 1996.

Schnall MD, Rosten S, Englander S, et al: A combined architectural and kinetic interpretation model for breast MR images. Acad Radiol 8:591-597, 2001.

Slanetz PJ, Edmister WB, Yeh ED, et al: Occult contralateral breast carcinoma incidentally detected by breast magnetic resonance imaging. Breast J 8:145-148, 2002.

Soderstrom CE, Harms SE, Farrell RS Jr, et al: Detection with MR imaging of residual tumor in the breast soon after surgery. AJR Am J Roentgenol 168:485-488, 1997.

Stoutjesdijk MJ, Boetes C, Jager GJ, et al: Magnetic resonance imaging and mammography in women with a hereditary risk of breast cancer. J Natl Cancer Inst 93:1095-1102, 2001.

Talele AC, Slanetz PJ, Edmister WB, et al: The lactating breast: MRI findings and literature review. Breast J 9:237-240, 2003.

Teifke A, Lehr HA, Vomweg TW, et al: Outcome analysis and rational management of enhancing lesions incidentally detected on contrast-enhanced MRI of the breast. AJR Am J Roentgenol 181:655-662, 2003.

Tilanus-Linthorst MM, Bartels CC, Obdeijn AI, Oudkerk M: Earlier detection of breast cancer by surveillance of women at familial risk. Eur J Cancer 36:514-519, 2000.

Tilanus-Linthorst MM, Obdeijn AI, Bontenbal M, Oudkerk M: MRI in patients with axillary metastases of occult breast carcinoma. Breast Cancer Res Treat 44:179-182, 1997.

Trecate G, Tess JD, Vergnaghi D, et al: Lobular breast cancer: How useful is breast magnetic resonance imaging? Tumori 87:232-238, 2001.

Tsuboi N, Ogawa Y, Inomata T, et al: Changes in the findings of dynamic MRI by preoperative CAF chemotherapy for patients with breast cancer of stage II and III: Pathologic correlation. Oncol Rep 6:727-732, 1999.

Viehweg P, Heinig A, Lampe D, et al: Retrospective analysis for evaluation of the value of contrast-enhanced MRI in patients treated with breast conservative therapy. MAGMA 7:141-152, 1998.

Viehweg P, Lampe D, Buchmann J, Heywang-Kobrunner SH: In situ and minimally invasive breast cancer: Morphologic and kinetic features on contrast-enhanced MR imaging. MAGMA 11:129-137, 2000.

Viehweg P, Paprosch I, Strassinopoulou M, Heywang-Kobrunner SH: Contrast-enhanced magnetic resonance imaging of the breast: Interpretation guidelines. Top Magn Reson Imaging 9:17-43, 1998.

Warner E, Plewes DB, Shumak RS, et al: Comparison of breast magnetic resonance imaging, mammography, and ultrasound for surveillance of women at high risk for hereditary breast cancer. J Clin Oncol 19:3524-3531, 2001.

The Postoperative Breast and Breast Cancer Treatment–Related Imaging

DEBRA M. IKEDA

FREDERICK M. DIRBAS

Introduction
Normal Postoperative Changes
Breast Cancer Treatment
Sentinel Lymph Node Biopsy
Breast Conservation: Preoperative, Perioperative, and
Radiation Therapy Changes
    Preoperative Imaging
    Specimen Radiography
    Perioperative Imaging
    Imaging after Radiation Therapy
Treatment Failure
Mastectomy Sites
Key Elements

INTRODUCTION

It is important to understand the natural history of postoperative imaging findings and their evolution in the breast because postoperative alterations can mimic cancer even when the pathology is benign. This chapter will describe the normal appearance of the breast after surgery for benign or malignant disease, as well as the appearance of the breast after sentinel lymph node (SLN) biopsy, systemic adjuvant therapy, and radiation therapy for women with breast cancer.

NORMAL POSTOPERATIVE CHANGES

Normal postoperative findings on mammography include architectural distortion, increased density, and parenchymal scarring in at least 50% of patients (Box 8-1). These findings diminish in severity over time (Fig. 8-1). After 3 to 5 years, the findings should be stable on subsequent mammograms. About 50% to 55% of cases have complete resolution of all biopsy changes on the mammogram. The remaining 45% to 50% of patients have variable mammographic findings ranging from spiculated mass–like scars to slight architectural distortion (Fig. 8-2A).

As a rule, mammograms are not often obtained immediately after diagnostic surgical excisional biopsy. However, in the rare cases in which a radiograph is obtained within a few days of the procedure, the mammogram will show a round or oval mass in the postoperative site representing a seroma or hematoma, with or without air in the biopsy cavity (Fig. 8-2B). The adjacent breast tissue displays increased density caused by local edema and/or hemorrhage, and there is usually skin thickening at the incision and thickening of trabeculae in subcutaneous fat.

Over the subsequent weeks, the air and fluid collection is resorbed and replaced by fibrosis and scarring. Sometimes, retraction of skin from the scar is noted. In 50% to 55% of cases, the biopsy cavity resolves so completely that it leaves no scar or distortion in the underlying breast parenchyma, and only comparison with pre-biopsy mammograms indicates that breast tissue is missing. In other cases, the scar appears as a chronic architectural distortion or a spiculated mass more evident on one projection than the other. In still other but more rare cases, seroma cavities persist and appear as a round or oval mass.

Fat necrosis is common after a breast biopsy and usually appears as a radiolucent lipid-filled mass. Symptomatic patients with fat necrosis usually have a palpable breast mass and a history of a biopsy or blunt trauma. If acute, bruising may be present on physical examination, and if chronic, palpable lumps may form in the region of fat necrosis. Mammography is pathognomonic if it shows lipid cysts or typical calcified eggshell-type rims around a radiolucent center (Fig. 8-3A).

In still other cases, the spiculation from the scar has such a mass-like appearance that it simulates cancer, and the true nature of the scar is not recognized unless one knows that a biopsy has been performed in this location

Box 8-1   Normal Postoperative Findings for Benign Disease

Focal skin change (early)
Increased focal density (edema) near the biopsy site (early)
Oval fluid or fluid/air collection (early)
Complete resolution of biopsy findings (late—50% to 55% of all cases)
Time when findings resolve: 3 to 5 years after biopsy
Postoperative findings seen after 3 to 5 years (45% to 50% of all cases)
    Architectural distortion (48%)
    Skin thickening/deformity (17%)
    Parenchymal scarring (15%)
Scars: poorly defined masses with spiculation

Modified from Brenner RJ, Pfaff JM: Mammographic changes after excisional breast biopsy for benign disease. AJR Am J Roentgenol 167:1047-1052, 1996; and Sickles EA, Herzog KA: Mammography of the postsurgical breast. AJR Am J Roentgenol 136:585-588, 1981.

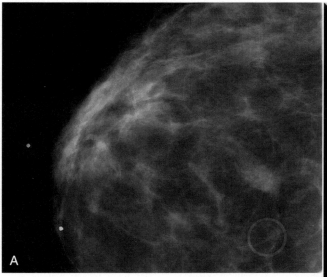
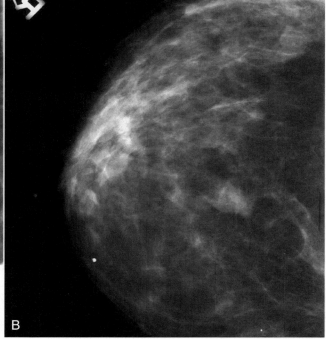

FIGURE 8-1   Pre-biopsy Mammogram and Normal Post-biopsy Changes. Mediolateral oblique (MLO) (**A**) and craniocaudal (CC) (**B**) mammograms show a slightly spiculated mass in the midportion of the breast. Biopsy revealed focal fibrosis.

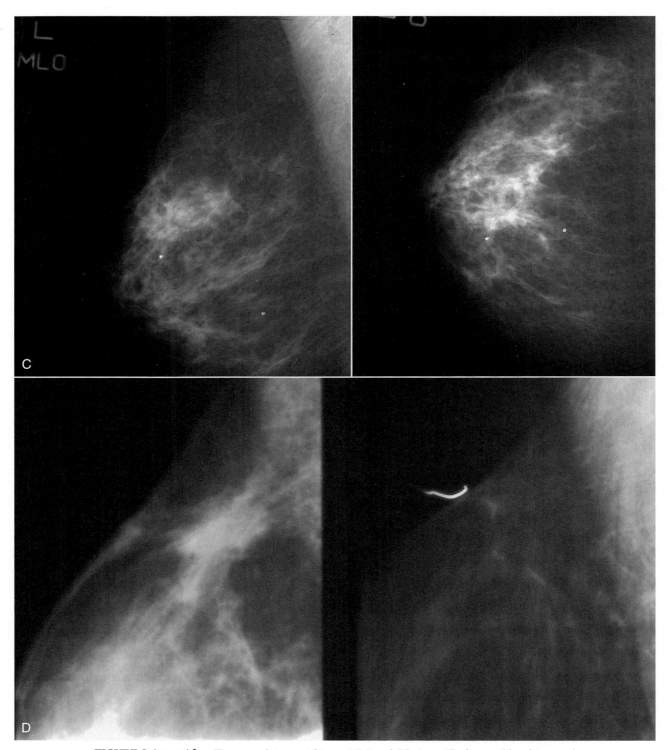

FIGURE 8-1 cont'd   Two years later, post-biopsy MLO and CC views (**C**) show mild architectural distortion where the mass was removed. Notice the difficulty in identifying the distortion against the heterogeneous breast background. **D,** In another patient, cropped MLO views of the upper part of the breast show immediate post-biopsy and post-radiation change with scarring in the biopsy site *(left).* The *right* image shows that the edema and scarring have almost completely resolved at 2 years in this case.

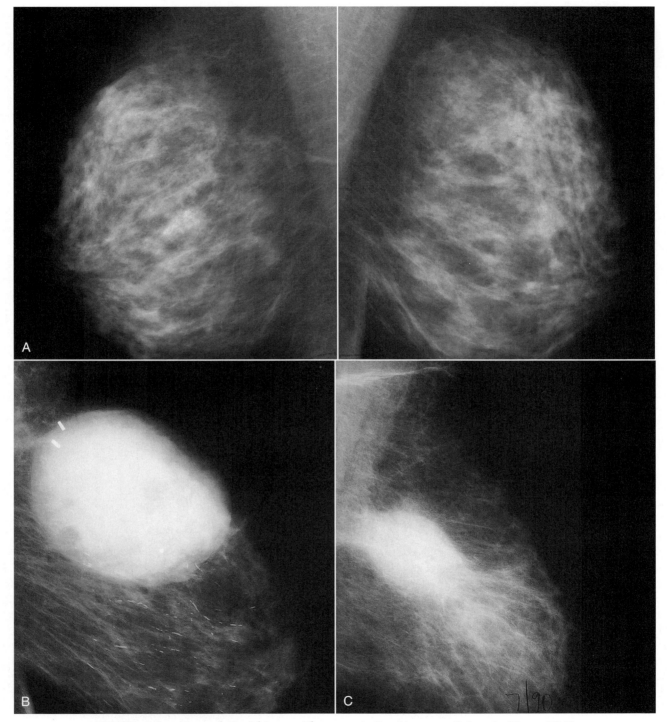

FIGURE 8-2   Normal Post-biopsy Changes. A, Post-biopsy mediolateral oblique (MLO) views show mild architectural distortion representing a normal post-biopsy scar in the upper part of the left breast. Note that without the history of a benign biopsy, the architectural distortion should prompt a work-up to exclude cancer or radial scar. **B,** In another patient, a post-biopsy MLO view shows a large oval mass representing a huge seroma/hematoma after biopsy for cancer. Two surgical clips are seen in the superior portion of the hematoma. **C,** Four years later, an MLO view shows a persistent, but smaller seroma/hematoma. The two surgical clips have moved inferiorly and are obscured by the residual fluid collection.

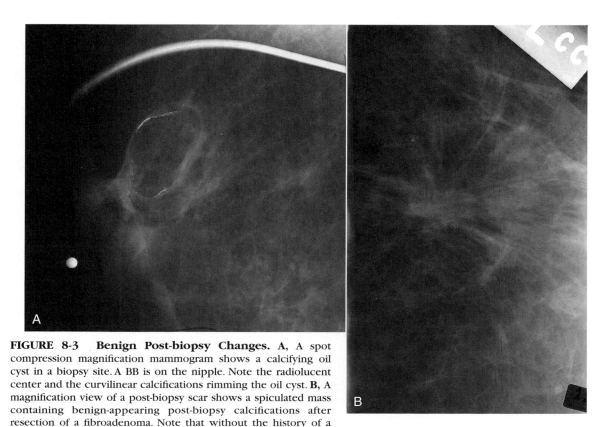

FIGURE 8-3   Benign Post-biopsy Changes. A, A spot compression magnification mammogram shows a calcifying oil cyst in a biopsy site. A BB is on the nipple. Note the radiolucent center and the curvilinear calcifications rimming the oil cyst. **B,** A magnification view of a post-biopsy scar shows a spiculated mass containing benign-appearing post-biopsy calcifications after resection of a fibroadenoma. Note that without the history of a previous biopsy, cancer would be strongly considered.

(Fig. 8-3B). For this reason, documentation of the date and location in the breast of previous biopsies on the breast history sheet is important. Some facilities also use a linear metallic scar marker over the biopsy scar to indicate the site of a previous biopsy before mammography. On the mammogram, the linear metallic scar marker on the skin will be near, but not immediately adjacent, to the scar marker because the skin is pressed away from the underlying breast parenchyma. If a spiculated mass is found far from the metallic scar marker, the preoperative mammograms should be reviewed to determine whether the spiculated mass is cancer rather than a scar.

On ultrasound, the immediate postoperative site shows a fluid collection. The collection may contain air in the immediate postoperative period, but more commonly it is completely filled with fluid, sometimes containing septa or debris (Fig. 8-4A-C). The incision can occasionally be traced from the biopsy cavity up to the skin, which is thickened.

Usually, the fluid in the biopsy cavity resolves and only the fibrotic scar remains. In these cases, ultrasound reveals the scar as a hypoechoic spiculated mass that simulates breast cancer, but it should correlate with the post-

operative site (Fig. 8-5). Correlation of the history and the physical finding of a scar on the skin can distinguish this normal postoperative finding from cancer.

On magnetic resonance imaging (MRI), the immediate post-biopsy cavity is a fluid-filled structure with surrounding tissue enhancement (Fig. 8-6). Post-biopsy scarring enhancement persists for up to 18 months and should then subside (Box 8-2). The usefulness of immediate post-biopsy MRI in cancer staging lies in depicting cancer at the biopsy margin and cancer foci away from the initial biopsy site that still require surgical excision.

BREAST CANCER TREATMENT

Breast cancer treatment consists of the initial cancer diagnosis, surgery and/or radiation therapy to establish staging and local/regional control, and systemic treatment. The initial diagnosis is often established by percutaneous biopsy with or without image guidance. In other cases, surgical biopsy, again with or without image guidance, is performed. Breast tumors are staged by the TNM (*t*umor, lymph *n*ode, *m*etastasis) classification of breast cancer from the American Joint Committee on Cancer (Table 8-1).

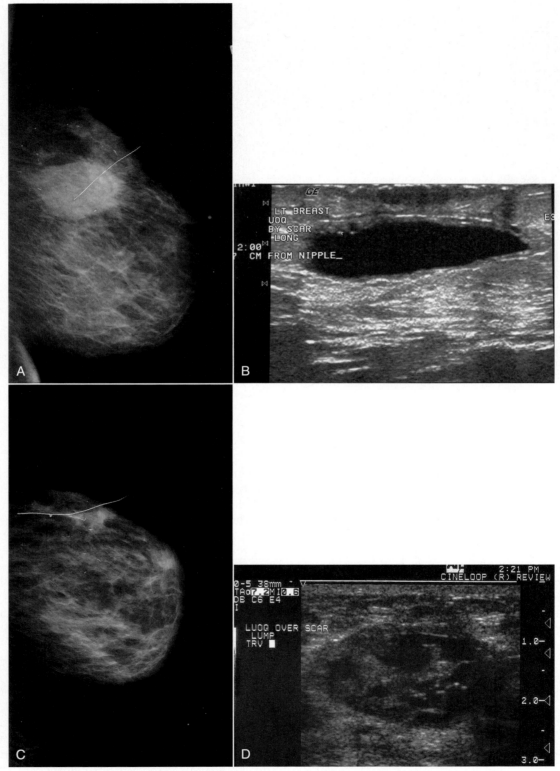

FIGURE 8-4   Seroma after Biopsy. A, A mediolateral oblique mammogram after biopsy shows a mass in the biopsy site under the scar marker. **B,** Ultrasound under the scar shows a typical fluid collection representing the seroma. The collection was aspirated. Two years later, the fluid collection has resolved, with only scarring remaining (**C**). A septated seroma is seen in another patient (**D**).

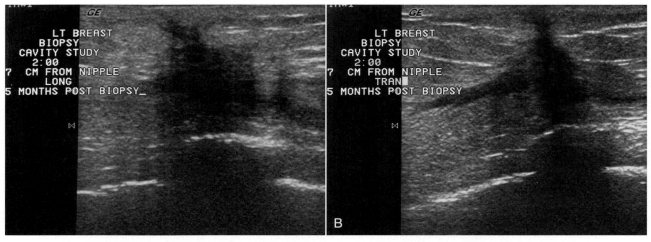

FIGURE 8-5   Biopsy Scars on Ultrasound. Five months after biopsy and radiation therapy, longitudinal (**A**) and transverse (**B**) scans show a hypoechoic triangular-shaped scar containing fluid extending to the skin surface. Note the skin thickening and acoustic shadowing at the scar correlating with scarring on the skin.

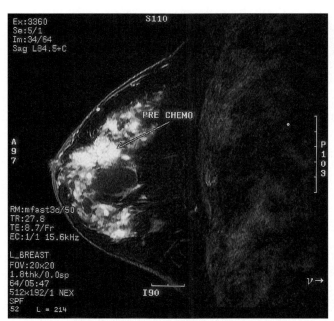

FIGURE 8-6   Postoperative Biopsy Site on Magnetic Resonance Imaging. A sagittal 3DSSMT scan (3DSSMT combines a water-selective spectral-spatial excitation and an on-resonance magnetization transfer pulse with three-dimensional spoiled gradient echo imaging) shows a post-biopsy seroma after removal of invasive ductal cancer. Enhancing masses superior to the biopsy cavity and elsewhere in the breast represent other foci of breast cancer that are distinguishable from scarring by their lumpy appearance.

Box 8-2   Enhancement on MRI after Biopsy

Up to 9 months after biopsy and radiation therapy there is strong enhancement in the biopsy site. Ten to 18 months after therapy, the enhancement slowly subsides, with no significant enhancement in 94% of cases.

From Heywang-Kobrunner SH, Schlegel A, Beck R, et al: Contrast enhanced MRI of the breast after limited surgery and radiation therapy. J Comput Assist Tomogr 17:891-900, 1993.

Once a cancer diagnosis is established, local control of malignancy requires surgical eradication of tumor in the breast with microscopically clear margins. This objective is achieved by lumpectomy followed by radiotherapy or mastectomy. Both approaches yield equivalent local control of disease and identical survival in women with tumors 4 cm or smaller in diameter and positive or negative axillary lymph nodes, as shown by Protocol B-06 conducted by the National Surgical Adjuvant Breast and Bowel Project (NSABP).

Breast-conserving surgery achieves local tumor control by surgical removal of the cancer with a margin of normal breast tissue, usually followed by whole-breast irradiation. Breast-conserving therapy is used when the entire tumor can be removed with a good cosmetic result, and the decision to proceed with such therapy should take into account the incision, breast size, and cancer location.

The breast imager helps select candidates for breast-conserving surgery or mastectomy by determining the extent of the tumor, and aids the surgeon in planning the optimal approach to eradicate all gross tumor. Because whole-breast irradiation usually follows surgery, relative contraindications to radiation therapy are taken into con-

Table 8-1   TNM Staging Classification for Breast Cancer

Tumor (T)

TX	Primary tumor not assessable
T0	No evidence of primary tumor, chemotherapy, mastectomy, radiotherapy
Tis	Carcinoma in situ
Tis (DCIS)	Ductal carcinoma in situ
Tis (LCIS)	Lobular carcinoma in situ
Tis (Paget)	Paget's disease of the nipple with no tumor
T1	Tumor ≤ 2 cm in greatest dimension
T1mic	Microinvasion ≤ 0.1 cm in greatest dimension
T1a	Tumor .01 cm but not >0.5 cm in greatest dimension
T1b	Tumor >0.5 cm but not >1 cm
T1c	Tumor >1 cm but not >2 cm
T2	Tumor >2 cm but <5 cm in greatest dimension
T3	Tumor more than 5 cm in greatest dimension
T4	Tumor of any size with direct extension to the chest wall or skin
T4a	Extension to the chest wall (ribs, intercostal muscles, or serratus anterior)
T4b	Peau d'orange, ulceration, or satellite skin nodules
T4c	T4a plus T4b
T4d	Inflammatory

Regional Lymph Node Status (N)*

NX	Regional lymph nodes not assessable (removed)
N0	No regional lymph node involvement
N1	Metastasis to movable ipsilateral axillary node(s)
N2	Metastasis to ipsilateral axillary lymph node(s) fixed or matted
N2a	Metastasis in nodes fixed to each other or to other structures
N2b	Metastasis in clinically apparent ipsilateral internal mammary nodes without axillary lymph node metastasis
N3	Metastases to ipsilateral supraclavicular or infraclavicular nodes or clinically apparent ipsilateral internal mammary lymph nodes with or without clinically evident axillary lymph node involvement

Distant Metastases (M)

MX	Distant metastases cannot be assessed
M0	No distant metastases
M1	Distant metastases

Stage Groupings

Stage 0	Tis	N0	M0
Stage I	T1	N0	M0
Stage IIA	T0	N1	M0
	T1	N1	M0
	T2	N0	M0
Stage IIB	T2	N1	M0
	T3	N0	M0
Stage IIIA	T0	N2	M0
	T1	N2	M0
	T2	N2	M0
	T3	N1, N2	M0
Stage IIIB	T4	Any N	M0
Stage IIIC	Any T	N3	M0
Stage IV	Any T	Any N	M1

*Additional lymph node staging classifications for sentinel lymph node status and micrometastasis.

TNM, *t*umor size, status of lymph *n*odes, distant *m*etastases.

From Singletary S, Allred C, Ashley P, et al: Revision of the American Joint Committee on Cancer Staging System for Breast Cancer. J Clin Oncol 20:3628-3636, 2002. The original source material is the AJCC Cancer Staging Manual, 6th ed. New York, Springer-Verlag, 2002.

<table>
<tr><td>

Box 8-3   Contraindications to Whole-Breast Radiation Therapy

Pregnancy
Previous breast radiation therapy
Multicentric or diffuse disease
Collagen vascular disease
Poor cosmetic result (relative contraindication)

</td></tr>
</table>

<table>
<tr><td>

Box 8-4   Factors Affecting the Frequency of In-Breast Tumor Recurrence after Radiation Therapy

Invasive ductal cancer with an extensive intraductal component
Residual tumor in the breast
Younger women
Large ductal carcinoma in situ tumors
Lymphatic or vascular invasion
Multicentricity

</td></tr>
</table>

sideration when selecting breast conservation candidates. Relative contraindications to radiation therapy include previous radiation therapy, pregnancy, collagen vascular disease, and multicentric or diffuse disease (Box 8-3). Axillary adenopathy is not a contraindication.

After breast-conserving surgery, whole-breast irradiation achieves control of residual microscopic disease. Six randomized trials of lumpectomy and radiation therapy showed the frequency of local recurrence and overall survival rates to be generally comparable to mastectomy. In-breast tumor recurrences (IBTRs) are reported in 5% of patients at 5 years and in 10% to 15% at 10 years after completion of therapy. Treatment failures are treated by salvage mastectomy.

Local treatment failures consisting of ductal carcinoma in situ (DCIS) or invasive tumors smaller than 2 cm may have a better prognosis; accordingly, some believe that it is important to diagnose recurrences or new cancers early. Invasive IBTR usually occurs in the lumpectomy site or quadrant within the first 7 years, but rarely earlier than 18 months after treatment. IBTR after 7 years will more likely occur in any quadrant, not necessarily at the original site, and is usually a new cancer. IBTR is more likely in women who have invasive cancer with an extensive intraductal component, residual disease in the breast, younger age, a large DCIS tumor, lymphatic or vascular invasion, or multicentricity (Box 8-4).

Mastectomy and axillary lymph node dissection (ALND) are performed when it is not possible to excise the entire breast tumor with a good cosmetic result, if the woman has a contraindication to radiotherapy, or if it is the patient's desire. Unless a medical contraindication to reconstruction exists, patients are always offered breast reconstruction with an autologous tissue flap or a tissue expander after mastectomy. Because many women undergo mastectomy, it is important to know the radiologic appearance of the mastectomy site after reconstruction with an autologous tissue flap. Moreover, the contralateral breast is often larger than the reconstructed breast, and reduction mammaplasty may be required on the contralateral side. Reduction mammaplasty and breast reconstruction have a characteristic appearance

<table>
<tr><td colspan="2">

Table 8-2   Location of Lymph Nodes Draining the Breast

</td></tr>
<tr><td>Level I nodes</td><td>Infralateral to lateral edge of the pectoralis minor</td></tr>
<tr><td>Level II nodes</td><td>Behind the pectoralis minor muscle</td></tr>
<tr><td>Level III nodes</td><td>Between the pectoralis minor and subclavius muscle (Halsted's ligament)</td></tr>
</table>

and should not be mistaken for cancer. These procedures are presented in Chapter 9.

SENTINEL LYMPH NODE BIOPSY

Although breast cancer cell type and size influence the prognosis, axillary staging is the most important predictor of overall survival. Traditionally, such staging was established by ALND with removal of at least 10 axillary lymph nodes, including all of level I and some level II lymph nodes (Table 8-2). To potentially avoid ALND in women with clinically and pathologically normal nodes, the SLN biopsy technique was developed to identify lymph nodes most likely to harbor metastases. Completion ALND with removal of level I/II nodes is usually carried out if an SLN biopsy is positive or in centers that do not perform SLN dissection. SLNs are identified by isosulfan blue dye, radioisotope tracers, palpation, or a combination of these techniques (Box 8-5). The most common radioisotope tracer used is technetium Tc 99m sulfur colloid. Clinical trials are in progress to study the long-term safety, accuracy, and effectiveness of SLN biopsy.

Because lymph node metastases are the most important prognostic factor for patients with breast cancer, axillary lymph node sampling is a critical part of staging for breast cancer. However, a standard level I/II ALND is a morbid procedure associated with numbness, paresthesias, range-of-motion difficulties, and arm swelling. To preserve axillary staging but minimize the impact of ALND, the SLN biopsy technique was adapted from methods used for melanoma to identify the lymph node(s) most likely harboring breast cancer metastases. As with melanoma, radionuclide tracers or blue dye are injected into the breast and carried to the breast lymphatics draining the tumor or biopsy cavity. The lymph node(s) that collects the tracer or dye is called the "sentinel lymph node" under the supposition that this node would have the highest yield of occult metastases. Once identified by radiotracer, blue dye, or palpation, the SLN undergoes more rigorous sectioning than do other nodes. In some facilities, the SLN also undergoes immunohistochemistry staining for low-molecular-weight cytokeratins (IHC). Some facilities also use intraoperative frozen section, extensive frozen section, or imprint cytology to identify metastases in SLNs at the time of surgery, and the surgeon will proceed with ALND if the SLN is positive. By focusing only on positive SLNs, axillary dissection can be avoided in the roughly 65% to 70% of women with negative axillae.

When the SLN is positive for cancer, standard level I/II ALND is performed because chemotherapy treatment options may change with the absolute number of positive lymph nodes and because ALND may improve regional control of disease. Survival rates decrease as more nodes are positive.

Because of the limited axillary dissection required for SLN biopsy, the SLN technique is associated with substantially less morbidity than is traditional ALND. Numerous validation series of the SLN technique show a small false-negative rate, high accuracy, and high SLN identification in experienced hands. In general, SLN identification rates exceed 92%. As shown by Turner et al., when the SLN is negative, most non-SLNs will also be negative with a small (1.7%) non-SLN positive rate. Other authors quote higher false-negative rates of 4% to 7%.

Various techniques may be used to identify the SLN with radionuclide or dye. Subareolar, intradermal, and intraparenchymal injection sites appear to drain to the same lymphatic pathways for SLN identification. Martin

et al. reported only slightly higher SLN identification rates for intradermal (98%) versus intraparenchymal (89%) injection of mapping agents, with comparable false-negative rates (4.8% versus 4.4%). Interestingly, SLNs identified by intradermal agents did not have 100% concordance with SLNs identified by intraparenchymal agents. Similar findings were reported by Bauer et al., who showed that subareolar injections went to many of the same nodes identified by agents injected into the breast parenchyma, again with 90% concordance. Martin et al. showed that in 463 women with more than one SLN, the hottest SLN contained a metastasis in 80% of cases, the metastasis was found in 20% of cases in which the SLN was not the most radioactive, and in 27% of cases, blue dye did not identify the positive SLN. This study resulted in recommending removal of radioactive, blue, or clinically suspicious lymph nodes.

The radioisotope technique involves injection of a radionuclide tracer into breast tissue surrounding the previous biopsy cavity or tumor, into subcutaneous tissue or dermis over the tumor, or into the subareolar region before surgery. The surgeon identifies the "hot" SLN node in the operating room with a hand-held gamma probe. Alternatively or in conjunction with radionuclide tracers, the surgeon injects isosulfan blue dye in the operating room into tissue surrounding the breast biopsy cavity or tumor, into subcutaneous or subdermal tissue over the tumor, or into the retroareolar region minutes before the "blue" SLN is harvested. Injection of the blue dye is timed according to the location of the tumor, with the transit time of blue dye from an upper outer quadrant injection taking between 3 and 5 minutes and 7 minutes for lower inner quadrant injections. Delay between injection and identification of the SLN may allow the dye to traverse the SLN, drain into regional lymph nodes, and produce multiple blue axillary lymph nodes. McMasters et al. showed that dual agents halved the false-negative rate for SLNs (11.8% versus 5.8%).

The role of the radiologist is to understand the rationale for SLN biopsy and facilitate its performance. First, the radiologist must *not* inject radionuclide tracers *into* the tumor or biopsy cavity because radionuclide injected into a tumor is likely to sit there rather than be transported to the lymphatics. Tumor lymphatics are abnormal and inefficient in radionuclide uptake. Similarly, radionuclide injected into a biopsy cavity cannot be transported to the lymphatics.

Preoperative lymphoscintigraphy is used in some facilities to assist in preoperative localization of SLNs in the axilla or in extra-axillary sites (Fig. 8-7). Most commonly, these sentinel nodes will be in the supraclavicular, infra-clavicular, or internal mammary groups. SLNs in an internal mammary chain location might undergo thoracic dissection or radiation therapy. Knowledge of a medial SLN location allows the surgeon an opportunity to plan

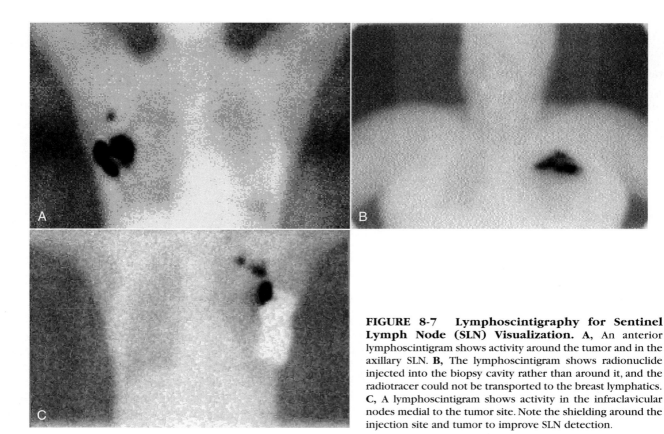

FIGURE 8-7 Lymphoscintigraphy for Sentinel Lymph Node (SLN) Visualization. A, An anterior lymphoscintigram shows activity around the tumor and in the axillary SLN. **B,** The lymphoscintigram shows radionuclide injected into the biopsy cavity rather than around it, and the radiotracer could not be transported to the breast lymphatics. **C,** A lymphoscintigram shows activity in the infraclavicular nodes medial to the tumor site. Note the shielding around the injection site and tumor to improve SLN detection.

internal mammary node biopsy, possibly thoracotomy, and/or radiation therapy. Although the use of radiation in these patients is somewhat controversial, it is important to note that both medial and lateral breast tumors drain to the internal mammary lymph nodes. Some facilities do not perform lymphoscintigraphy because of the very low frequency of isolated positive biopsy findings in an internal mammary SLN and the relatively few cases that would result in meaningful changes in prognosis or therapy.

Non-visualization of the SLN on lymphoscintigraphy does not preclude identification of the SLN by the surgeon in the operating room. The SLN may be within thick adipose tissue and can be identified only by the gamma probe in the operating room. Identification of SLNs in the operating room in the setting of non-visualization on lymphoscintigraphy can be increased if blue dye is also used.

Palpable axillary adenopathy may be due to a true SLN being replaced by tumor. Lymphatics carrying radioisotope or dye may be blocked by tumor in the true SLN and drain to other lymph nodes, thereby resulting in a secondary node falsely identified as the "sentinel" node.

The SLN technique was originally used only for small tumors or post-biopsy sites, but the indications for case selection are expanding. Some facilities are using the technique for prophylactic mastectomy or DCIS because SLN biopsy has the potential to detect invasion, but currently, too few cases are available to determine the need for SLN biopsy for these indications. Other potential indications include breast cancer in men, multicentric disease, or a clinically positive axilla. In the latter case, some patients with breast cancer have a clinical false-positive examination from existing implants or reactive adenopathy from the biopsy. Alternatively, neoadjuvant chemotherapy may increase the false-negative rate, as shown by numerous studies.

Micrometastases are defined as metastases 0.2 to 2.0 mm in size. Because the SLN technique evaluates a single node with rigorous methods, IHC stains may show micrometastases in 11% to 36% not identified by hematoxylin and eosin staining; such micrometastases range from single cells, cell clusters, or masses smaller than 2 mm but larger than .2 mm. Retrospective series show that micrometastases in lymph nodes are associated with lower overall survival rates and higher disease recurrence, but the actual clinical significance of single cells, cell clusters, or micrometastases smaller than 2 mm is unknown. Specifically, the benefit of systemic therapy in these cases is currently unknown.

Table 8-3   Breast Imaging Relating to Breast-Conserving Therapy

Timing	Reason	Technique(s)
Preoperative	Ipsilateral tumor extent and contralateral tumor	Bilateral mammography
		US or MRI as warranted
Preoperative	Establish diagnosis	Percutaneous biopsy
Perioperative	Tumor excision	Preoperative needle localization (as needed)
		Specimen radiography
	SLN identification	Radionuclide injection
		Lymphoscintigraphy (as needed)
Pre-radiation	Check for residual tumor	Ipsilateral unilateral mammogram; US or MRI as needed
Post-radiation	Baseline/tumor recurrence	Ipsilateral unilateral mammogram (initial one at 6 mo, then 6-12 mo)
	Evaluate ipsilateral and contralateral breast	Bilateral mammogram (12 mo)
	Clinical problem	Ipsilateral unilateral mammogram
		US or MRI as needed

MRI, magnetic resonance imaging; SLN, sentinel lymph node; US, ultrasound.
(Modified from Dershaw DD: The conservatively treated breast. *In* Diagnosis of Diseases of the Breast. Philadelphia, WB Saunders, 1997, p. 553.)

BREAST CONSERVATION: PREOPERATIVE, PERIOPERATIVE, AND RADIATION THERAPY CHANGES

Preoperative Imaging

Mammographic evaluation of the extent of tumor is an important tool for selecting appropriate breast conservation therapy candidates and planning surgery (Table 8-3, Fig. 8-8). Either alone or with ultrasound, mammography helps identify any suspicious foci of tumor for preoperative localization in an effort to resect all gross tumor with a rim of normal breast tissue. Mammography can also identify diffuse or multicentric disease, a finding that precludes breast conservation therapy. Extensive, innumerable benign calcifications may hinder follow-up by mammography and limit early detection of tumor recurrence in the treated breast.

MRI has been especially useful in predicting the extent of tumor before the first surgical procedure (Fig. 8-9), and some have claimed particular effectiveness in women with invasive lobular cancer or invasion of tumor into the pectoralis muscle or chest wall (Fig. 8-10). Bedrosian et al. (2003) reported a 95% tumor detection rate with MRI and a change in surgical management in 26% (69/267) of patients requiring wider/separate excision or mastectomy, with pathologic verification in 71% (49/69). With respect to invasive lobular carcinoma, several studies have suggested that MRI may be more effective in detecting the extent of disease than physical examination, mammography, and ultrasound are. However, false-negative studies in these series have led to mixed opinion regarding the routine use of MRI in staging invasive lobular carcinoma

or in cases with extensive DCIS. Morris et al. reported chest wall involvement in five of five cases at surgery when MRI suggested posterior breast tumor obliteration of the fat plane with muscle enhancement. No muscle involvement was seen at surgery in 14 of 14 cases when muscle enhancement was absent. Overall, these studies show that MRI may be helpful in surgical planning, but they also indicate a number of unnecessary biopsies because of a relative lack of specificity and false-negative results in the case of invasive lobular cancer or DCIS.

Specimen Radiography

If preoperative needle localization has been performed, specimen radiography or specimen sonography is used to determine whether the suspicious finding has been removed. If not, the surgeon can be guided to the incompletely resected area if the lesion has been transected by using architectural landmarks in the specimen and on the preoperative mammogram. Investigators have documented the benefit of performing specimen imaging. The adequacy of margins, however, is most reliably evaluated by histologic section.

Perioperative Imaging

As needed, post-biopsy mammograms are obtained to determine the completeness of tumor excision (Fig. 8-11). These studies are particularly appropriate before the initiation of breast irradiation, but they should be performed before beginning any suggested further treatment if residual tumor is suspected.

Magnification views may be necessary if routine views of the lumpectomy site fail to visualize the biopsied region

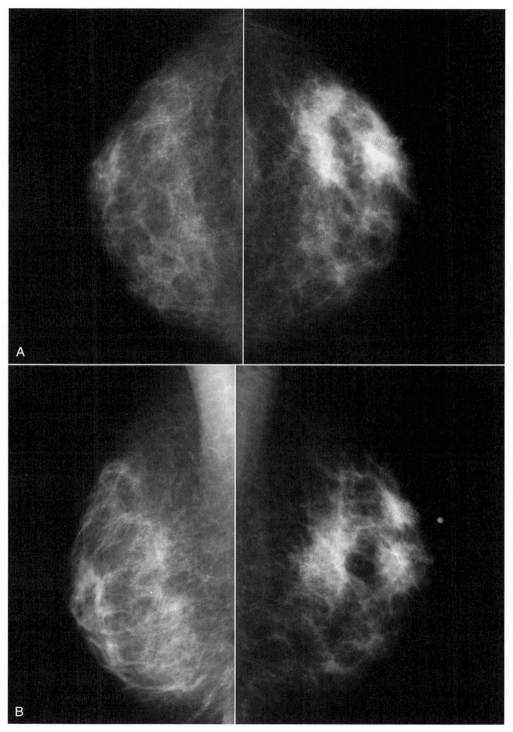

FIGURE 8-8   Mammography Showing a Poor Candidate for Breast Conservation.
Although this patient felt only one mass in her left breast, craniocaudal (**A**) and mediolateral oblique
(**B**) mammograms show three spiculated masses over a large region, thus rendering this patient a
poor candidate for breast conservation.

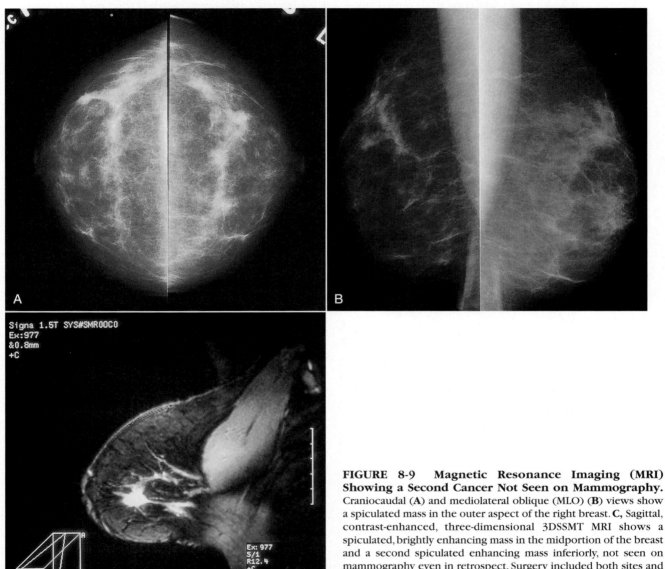

FIGURE 8-9   Magnetic Resonance Imaging (MRI) Showing a Second Cancer Not Seen on Mammography. Craniocaudal (**A**) and mediolateral oblique (MLO) (**B**) views show a spiculated mass in the outer aspect of the right breast. **C,** Sagittal, contrast-enhanced, three-dimensional 3DSSMT MRI shows a spiculated, brightly enhancing mass in the midportion of the breast and a second spiculated enhancing mass inferiorly, not seen on mammography even in retrospect. Surgery included both sites and showed two separate foci of invasive ductal cancer. Note that the "upper" right breast mass on the upright MLO mammogram moves to the "midportion" of the breast on the prone MRI scans because of the configuration of the breast tissue.

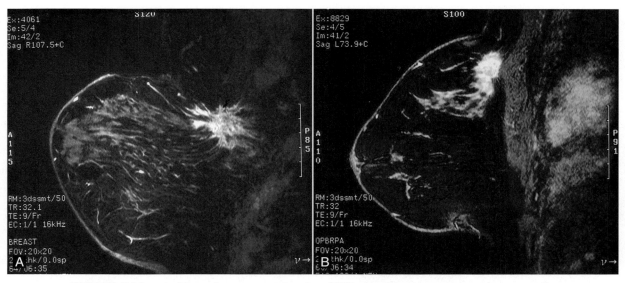

FIGURE 8-10   **A,** Magnetic resonance imaging (MRI) showing extension into the pectoralis muscle. Sagittal, contrast-enhanced, three-dimensional 3DSSMT MRI shows a spiculated posterior enhancing mass extending into and enhancing the pectoralis muscle. **B,** MRI showing tumor on top of the pectoralis muscle. In contrast to **A,** sagittal, contrast-enhanced, 3DSSMT MRI shows an irregular enhancing mass abutting the pectoralis muscle but without enhancing it, thus suggesting no tumor invasion. Although the surgeon may take some of the pectoralis muscle at surgery to achieve clear margins, the tumor does not extend into the muscle or chest wall.

sufficiently or if calcifications are suspected. Residual microcalcifications are not always due to residual tumor. Dershaw et al. found the positive predictive value of residual microcalcifications representing residual tumor to be 69%, with the likelihood that they represent residual tumor being greatest in cases with DCIS and more than five microcalcifications. However, the absence of calcifications does not invariably indicate the absence of tumor.

Imaging after Radiation Therapy

Recommendations for follow-up mammography after radiation therapy vary by institution. Most facilities obtain a unilateral mammogram immediately after the conclusion of radiation therapy, with further follow-up bilateral mammograms at 6- to 12-month intervals. Obtaining a mammogram relatively soon after completion of radiation therapy establishes a baseline for future reference (Fig. 8-12).

Normal lumpectomy and radiation therapy alterations apparent on the mammogram include the usual post-biopsy changes in the surgical site plus diffuse skin thickening and breast edema (Box 8-6; see Fig. 8-12). Unlike normal focal postoperative edema, breast edema from radiation therapy encompasses the entire breast and not just the region around the postoperative site. On physical examination, the breast commonly shows peau

d'orange, a large swollen areola or nipple, occasional brownish or red skin, and occasional breast tenderness and swelling. Skin thickening in the immediate post–radiation therapy period is due to breast edema from small-vessel damage and, later, is due to fibrotic change. Findings of breast edema are most obvious when compared with the contralateral side or older mammograms.

On the mammogram, the findings of breast edema are skin and stromal thickening, diffuse increased breast density, and trabecular thickening in subcutaneous fat. The usual changes of the post-biopsy scar are superimposed on the findings of whole-breast edema. The biopsy cavity, seen initially as a fluid-filled mass, may be partially obscured by surrounding breast edema from radiation therapy. These changes usually decrease somewhat over a period of $2\frac{1}{2}$ to 3 years or may remain stable. With resolution of the surrounding breast edema, the biopsy cavity may become more apparent but should not grow in size.

Progression of breast edema is abnormal and should be investigated. Other etiologies of unilateral breast edema outside the radiation therapy setting are inflammatory breast cancer, mastitis, lymphoma, and obstructed breast lymphatic or venous drainage.

After completion of whole-breast irradiation, many facilities use an electron beam boost to sterilize the operative site. Some facilities line the cavity with radiopaque markers to guide the electron beam boost and use

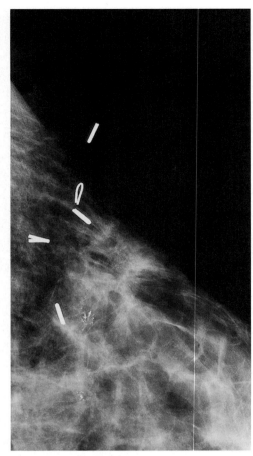

FIGURE 8-11   Residual Tumor. After biopsy of pleomorphic calcifications showing invasive ductal cancer, the post-biopsy mammogram shows residual calcifications in the biopsy site surrounded by metallic clips in the cavity.

x-ray imaging for guidance (Fig. 8-13). Other facilities use breast ultrasound to delineate and mark the skin over the breast biopsy cavity for the electron beam boost.

In about 25% of women, calcifications develop in the treated breast at the biopsy site. Although most will be due to benign dystrophic calcification, fat necrosis, or calcifying suture material, magnification views of calcifications in the biopsy site are required to distinguish them from the pleomorphic calcifications of cancer recurrence (Fig. 8-14). Fat necrosis may be evident if it has dystrophic appearance or forms around a radiolucent center. The dystrophic calcifications in fat necrosis can simulate malignancy, but magnification orthogonal projections may show the beginnings of the typical curvilinear shape of fat necrosis not evident on only one view. Careful inspection of the previous mammogram may also help by showing that the calcifications are forming around a radiolucent center of fat. Sometimes,

dystrophic calcifications cannot be distinguished from cancer and prompt biopsy.

Biopsy should be performed on suspicious pleomorphic calcifications. Some suspicious calcifications represent incompletely resected tumor, especially in the absence of a post-biopsy, pre–radiation therapy mammogram. Comparison to the original pre-biopsy mammograms is important to determine whether the original microcalcifications were not totally excised and should undergo re-excision.

Nonspecific microcalcifications in or near the biopsy site are a problem. Such calcifications may be benign or malignant. Calcifications that diminish or disappear may represent resolving benign calcifications as a result of changes in the calcium phosphate product in the breast, or they may represent residual tumor that has responded to therapy. Disappearing calcifications are worrisome if a suspicious mass replaces the disappearing calcifications.

Unchanging nonspecific calcifications should be monitored or biopsied because they may represent benign changes or incompletely resected tumor. Increasing microcalcifications are suggestive of breast cancer recurrence and should prompt biopsy unless they are specific for dystrophic calcifications or fat necrosis.

The postoperative cavity produces a mass in the location of the original tumor, and as the scar evolves, the mass representing the scar disappears or may become spiculated (Fig. 8-15). In the latter case, the scar may become smaller and less apparent over time, with stabilization at 2 to 3 years. Central fat necrosis may produce a radiolucent center in the biopsy cavity. However, if the scar grows in size or becomes denser or more mass-like in comparison to the baseline study, recurrent carcinoma should be suspected and prompt biopsy (Fig. 8-16).

On MRI, the breast biopsy scar enhances for up to 18 months. Recurrent invasive cancers usually appear as a mass in or near the biopsy site in the first few years. Cancers recurring as DCIS are more difficult to identify because DCIS may not produce the characteristic rapid enhancement and late-phase plateau or washout kinetic curve types and may show a nonspecific segmental or regional pattern of enhancement. Moreover, chemotherapy changes the enhancement pattern of the breast in that it diminishes enhancement of normal breast parenchyma and tumor alike.

With chemotherapy, suspicious kinetic late-phase plateau or washout curve patterns can change to a late-phase benign persistent pattern. The change in the kinetic curve pattern should not be mistaken for total tumor destruction by chemotherapy in the face of abnormal enhancement morphology. Investigators have shown viable biopsy-proven invasive breast cancers displaying change to a benign kinetic curve pattern after chemotherapy. If one has any doubt regarding a controversial

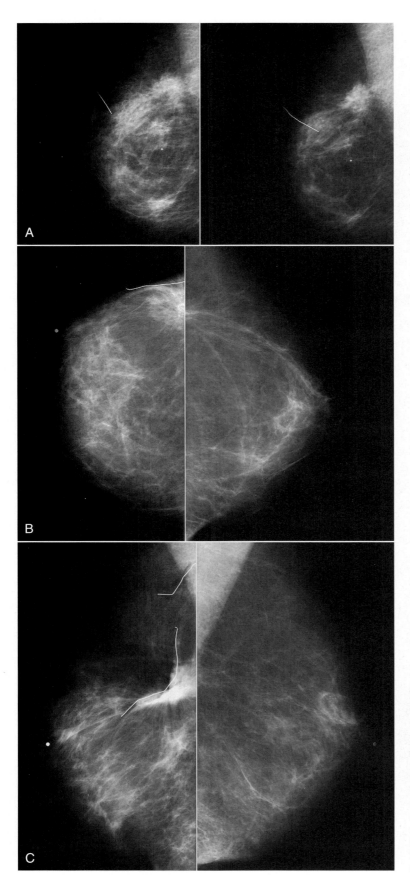

FIGURE 8-12   Normal Post-biopsy/Radiation Therapy Changes over Time. A, Mediolateral oblique (MLO) views immediately after biopsy and radiation therapy for cancer *(left)* and 2 years later *(right)* show initial distortion in the biopsy site and edema with skin thickening in the rest of the breast. Later *(right)*, the edema resolves and the biopsy scar is more apparent. (**B** and **C**) Linear scar markers show the biopsy site and the axillary node dissection on craniocaudal (**B**) and MLO (**C**) views in a different patient 1 year after biopsy and radiation therapy with distortion and skin deformity in the biopsy site. The biopsied right breast is smaller than the left and shows persistent skin thickening and density from radiation therapy.   *Continued*

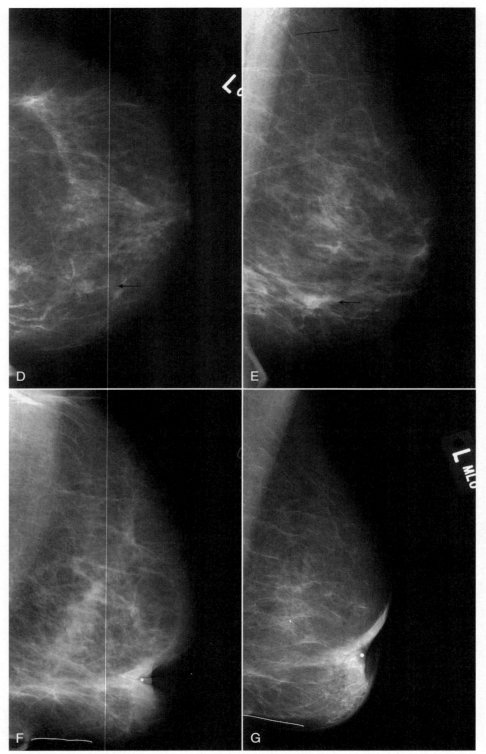

FIGURE 8-12 cont'd   Craniocaudal (**D**) and MLO (**E**) views show a round invasive ductal cancer *(arrow)* in the lower inner aspect of the left breast. One year after biopsy and radiation therapy, note the skin deformity, edema, and skin thickening in the lower portion of the breast on an MLO view (**F**). At 3 years the edema has diminished, but the skin thickening and deformity persist (**G**). This mammogram is the new baseline appearance for the rest of this woman's life.

Box 8-6   Mammographic Findings after Breast Conservation and Radiation Therapy*

Whole-breast edema
Post-biopsy scar
Skin retraction/deformity (variable)
Axillary node dissection distortion (if performed)
Metallic clips outlining the biopsy cavity (variable)

*The findings are worst at 6 months, diminish, and then stabilize at 2 to 3 years.

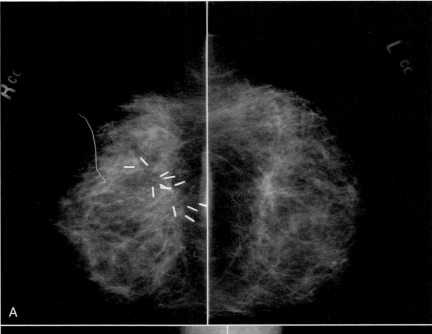

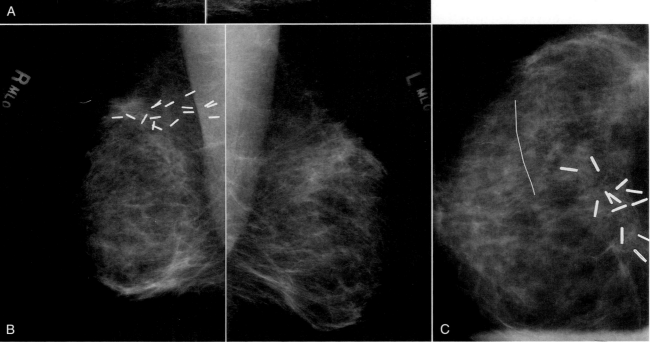

FIGURE 8-13   Markers in the Biopsy Site for Electron Beam Boost. Craniocaudal (**A**) and mediolateral oblique (**B**) mammograms show post-biopsy change in the upper outer portion of the right breast, with metallic markers lining the biopsy site. The markers are used as a guide for radiation therapy ports. **C,** A magnification craniocaudal view shows the markers, which are partly obscuring the architectural distortion in the biopsy site.

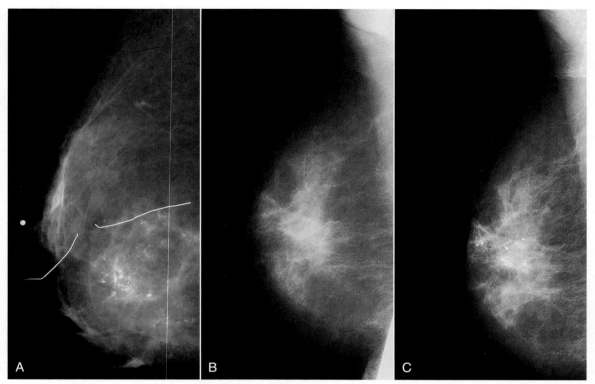

FIGURE 8-14   Calcifications after Radiation Therapy. A, After radiation therapy for ductal carcinoma in situ, new calcifications formed in the lower part of the left breast in the biopsy site and prompted biopsy, which showed fat necrosis. **B,** In another patient, a mediolateral oblique view after radiation therapy shows scarring in the upper portion of the breast. **C,** Three years later, new calcifications suddenly formed in the biopsy site. Biopsy revealed cancer.

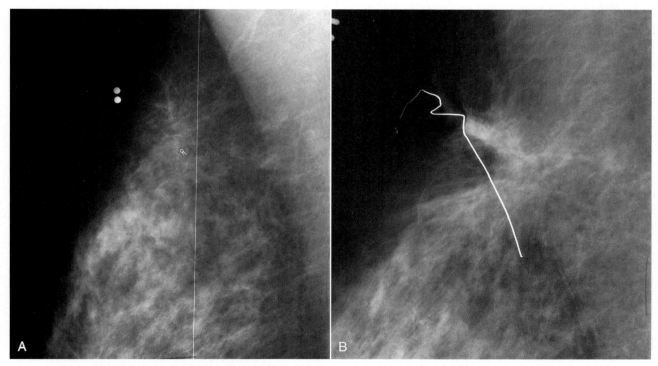

FIGURE 8-15   Scarring at a Biopsy Site. A, A pre-biopsy cropped mediolateral oblique (MLO) view shows a clip where cancer was biopsied by stereotaxis; two BBs show the previous needle entry site. **B,** A post-biopsy cropped MLO view shows architectural distortion and skin deformity at the biopsy scar. The normal biopsy scars have a little central density. Cancer recurrences display pleomorphic calcifications, increasing density, or mass-like change in the scar, which are not present here. Contrast **B** to the cancer recurrence in Figure 8-16A.

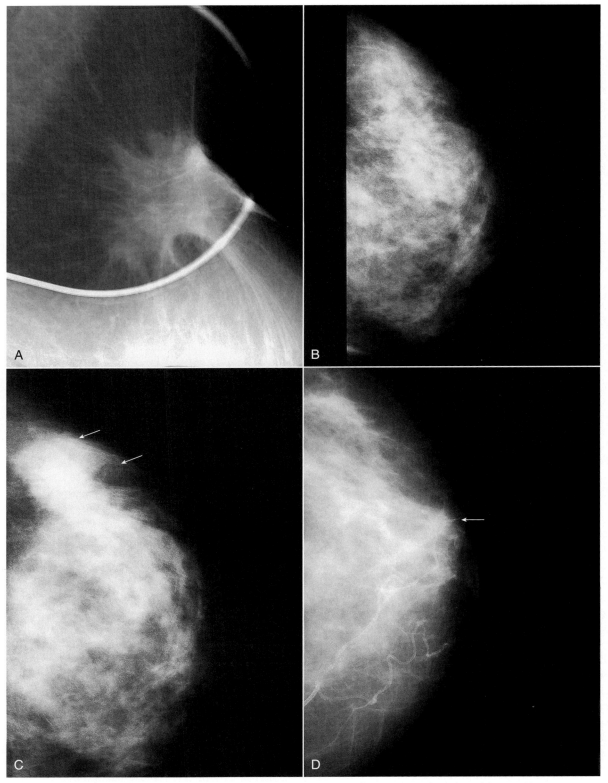

FIGURE 8-16   Breast Cancer Occurring at a Biopsy Site. A, A post-biopsy spot mediolateral oblique view shows architectural distortion, skin retraction, and deformity at a biopsy scar. Unlike normal biopsy scars, which have a little density in their central part, this spot view shows a moderately mass-like area in the scar which was invasive ductal cancer. Contrast this tumor with the normal post-biopsy scar in Figure 8-15B. **B,** In another patient, a post-biopsy craniocaudal (CC) view shows architectural distortion in the outer portion of the breast after biopsy and radiation therapy for cancer. **C,** Five years later, a developing density *(arrows)* is present in the outer part of the breast. Biopsy showed recurrent cancer. **D,** In a third patient, a post-biopsy CC view shows minimal architectural distortion near the nipple after biopsy and radiation therapy for cancer *(arrow)*.

Continued

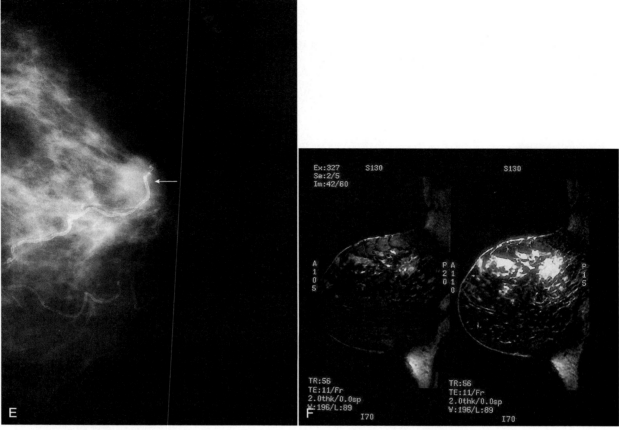

FIGURE 8-16 cont'd   The next year a developing mass *(arrow)* was noted in the biopsy site (**E**). Biopsy showed recurrent cancer. **F,** Sagittal 3DSSMT non-contrast–enhanced *(left)* and contrast-enhanced *(right)* magnetic resonance images show segmental enhancement in a cancer recurrence in the upper part of the breast long after biopsy and radiation therapy.

finding on MRI in the post-chemotherapy setting, biopsy should be considered.

TREATMENT FAILURE

The incidence of treatment failure is about 1% per year. Women who receive adequate therapy and are at greatest risk for failure include those younger than 35 years and especially those younger than 30 years, women treated for infiltrating ductal carcinoma with a large intraductal component, women with intraductal carcinoma of the comedo type, women with intraductal cancer measuring 2.5 cm or greater in diameter, and those treated for more than one synchronous cancer in the same breast. Gross residual tumor also has a poor prognosis, but microscopic residual disease may not.

Recurrent disease may be diagnosed by mammography and/or physical examination. About half of the recurrences are detected by mammography and half by physical examination. Those that are mammographically

Box 8-7	Benign and Suspicious Mammographic Findings Developing in the Biopsy Site after Breast Conservation and Radiation Therapy

Pleomorphic calcifications (cancer recurrence or residua)
Nonspecific calcifications (benign or malignant)
Dystrophic calcifications (benign)
Suture calcifications (benign)
Oil cyst (benign)
Developing density or mass (suspicious)

detected usually contain pleomorphic microcalcifications or masses (Box 8-7). Palpable recurrences are usually manifested as masses, are more frequently invasive cancer, and may be displayed on the mammogram as developing densities or masses and on ultra-

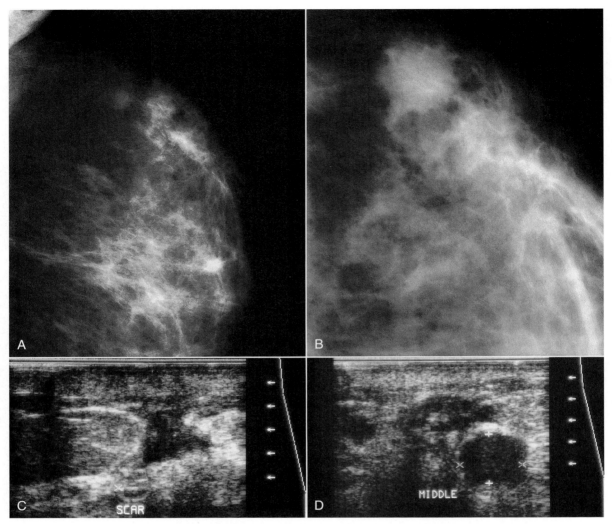

FIGURE 8-17   Treatment Failure. Mediolateral oblique views 1 year (**A**) and 1.5 years (**B**) after radiation therapy show a palpable mass in the biopsy site in the upper part of the breast. Ultrasound at 1.5 years shows a fluid-filled scar at the biopsy site (**C**) and a round hypoechoic solid mass (*calipers*) corresponding to the palpable mass adjacent to the fluid collection that represents recurrence of invasive ductal cancer (**D**).

sound as a mass separate from or in continuity with the biopsy scar (Fig. 8-17).

Recurrent tumor in the irradiated breast may arise at the site of the original tumor or elsewhere in the breast (Fig. 8-18). Recurrences at the original tumor site are usually due to failure to eradicate the original cancer and represent true treatment failures; they occur sooner than tumor developing elsewhere in the breast. Tumors developing outside the treated area occur at the same rate as tumor forming in the contralateral breast and represent new cancers. Breast irradiation does not lead to an increased incidence of breast cancer in the opposite breast or the boosted area of the treated breast.

Recurrent tumor is usually treated with salvage mastectomy.

Treatment failure within 2 years may be simulated by palpable granulomas or fat necrosis in the biopsy site that may show no change on the mammogram. Because it is difficult to differentiate these benign entities from recurrent cancer, biopsy is inevitable unless pathognomonic findings suggestive of fat necrosis are present.

MASTECTOMY SITES

After mastectomy, breast reconstruction options include an implant, a latissimus dorsi flap with a tissue expander when significant breast skin has been lost, or a transverse rectus abdominis myocutaneous (TRAM) flap. In the case of subcutaneous mastectomy, the breast

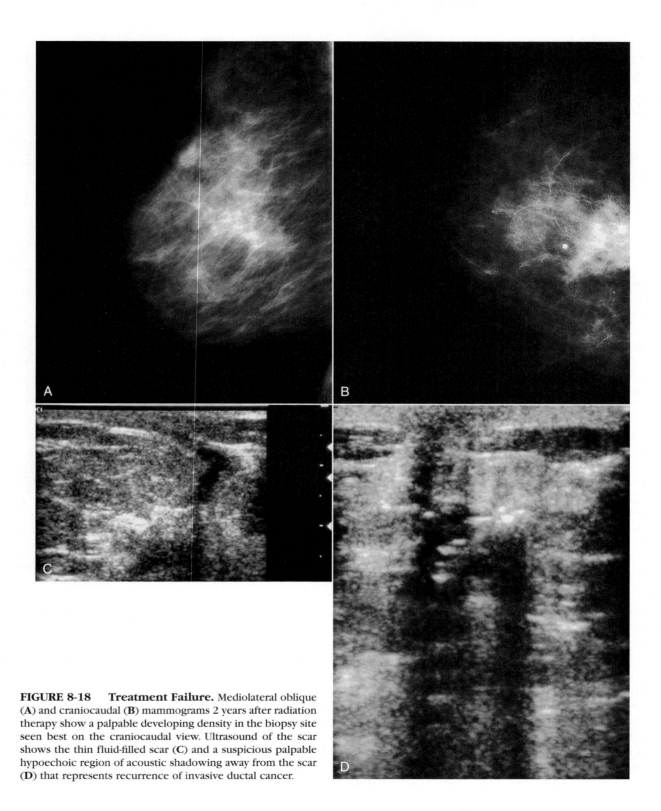

FIGURE 8-18   Treatment Failure. Mediolateral oblique (**A**) and craniocaudal (**B**) mammograms 2 years after radiation therapy show a palpable developing density in the biopsy site seen best on the craniocaudal view. Ultrasound of the scar shows the thin fluid-filled scar (**C**) and a suspicious palpable hypoechoic region of acoustic shadowing away from the scar (**D**) that represents recurrence of invasive ductal cancer.

tissue is removed as for simple (total) mastectomy, except that the nipple-areolar complex is preserved and an implant is inserted.

Breast cancer recurrence in an unreconstructed mastectomy site is usually detected by physical examination. The yield of imaging for breast cancer detection is low because of the small amount of breast tissue remaining, so surveillance mammography of the mastectomy site is not usually performed.

KEY ELEMENTS

Immediate post-surgical breast changes on mammography include increased density (local edema), oval or round masses (seroma/hematoma) with or without air, and skin thickening.

The fluid in the surgical site resolves over the next few weeks and months in most cases.

Post-surgical changes diminish in severity over time and are stable at 3 to 5 years.

Fifty percent to 55% of patients undergoing surgical breast biopsy for benign disease have no mammographic findings at 3 years.

The remaining 45% to 50% of patients show architectural distortion, parenchymal changes (scarring) that may be spiculated, or increased density that can simulate breast cancer.

To determine whether a spiculated density on the mammogram is a post-biopsy scar or cancer, it is important to correlate the post-surgical site with the location of the spiculated finding.

Fat necrosis occurring in a biopsy site is visualized as radiolucent lipid-filled masses, with occasional curvilinear calcifications forming around the lucent center.

On ultrasound, the immediate post-surgical site appears as a fluid-filled mass representing the seroma; it occasionally displays septa, debris, or fluid tracking up to the skin incision.

If only the fibrotic scar remains, ultrasound reveals a hypo-echoic spiculated mass that simulates breast cancer, but it should correlate with the postoperative site.

On MRI, the immediate post-biopsy cavity is a fluid-filled structure with surrounding tissue enhancement.

Post-biopsy scarring enhancement persists for up to 18 months and should then subside.

Breast tumors are staged by the TNM (tumor, lymph node, metastasis) classification of breast cancer from the American Joint Committee on Cancer.

Local control of breast cancer requires surgical eradication of tumor by mastectomy or lumpectomy, followed by radiotherapy.

The breast imager aids the surgeon in selecting candidates for breast-conserving surgery by determining the extent of tumor.

Relative contraindications to radiation therapy include previous radiation therapy, pregnancy, collagen vascular disease, and multicentric or diffuse disease.

In-breast tumor recurrences are reported in 5% of women at 5 years and in 10% to 15% at 10 years after completion of therapy.

Treatment failures after breast conservation are managed by salvage mastectomy.

The sentinel lymph node biopsy technique identifies the lymph node most likely to harbor metastasis. Radionuclide tracers or blue dye is injected into the breast and later carried into the breast lymphatics draining the tumor or biopsy cavity.

A "hot" node, a blue node, or an abnormal palpable node identified at surgery is a sentinel lymph node.

The sentinel lymph node may be examined by hematoxylin and eosin staining, as well as by immunohistochemistry staining for low-molecular-weight cytokeratins (IHC).

The sentinel lymph node may be identified at surgery even with non-visualization of a sentinel lymph node at lymphoscintigraphy.

MRI has been used for predicting the extent of tumor before the initial breast cancer surgical procedure, with some false-negatives results in women with invasive lobular carcinoma and ductal carcinoma in situ.

If preoperative needle localization has been performed, specimen radiography or specimen sonography is used to determine whether the suspicious finding has been removed.

As needed, post-biopsy mammograms determine the completeness of tumor excision, are particularly appropriate before the initiation of breast irradiation, and should be performed if residual tumor is suspected.

Most facilities obtain a unilateral mammogram immediately after the conclusion of radiation therapy, with further follow-up bilateral mammograms at 6- to 12-month intervals.

Breast edema from radiation therapy encompasses the entire breast and is manifested as diffuse increased parenchymal density, skin thickening, and trabecular thickening in subcutaneous fat.

Post-surgical and post–radiation therapy changes usually decrease somewhat over a period of $2\frac{1}{2}$ to 3 years or may remain stable.

Calcifications in the biopsy site in an irradiated breast represent fat necrosis, dystrophic calcifications, calcifying suture material, or breast cancer recurrence.

Chemotherapy changes the MRI enhancement pattern of the breast by diminishing enhancement of normal breast parenchyma and tumor alike.

On MRI, suspicious post-chemotherapy kinetic late-phase plateau or washout curve patterns can change to a benign persistent late-phase pattern despite the presence of viable breast cancer.

Recurrent cancer on mammography shown by pleomorphic microcalcifications is frequently ductal carcinoma in situ.

Palpable recurrences are usually manifested as mammographic masses and are more frequently invasive cancers.

Breast reconstruction includes an implant, a latissimus dorsi flap, or a transverse rectus abdominis myocutaneous flap.

Breast cancer recurrence in an unreconstructed mastectomy site is usually detected by physical examination.

SUGGESTED READINGS

Alazraki NP, Styblo T, Grant SF, et al: Sentinel node staging of early breast cancer using lymphoscintigraphy and the intraoperative gamma-detecting probe. Semin Nucl Med 30:56-64, 2000.

American Joint Committee on Cancer: AJCC Cancer Staging Manual, 6th ed. New York, Springer-Verlag, 2002.

Bauer TW, Spitz FR, Callans LS, et al: Subareolar and peritumoral injection identify similar sentinel nodes for breast cancer. Ann Surg Oncol 9:169-176, 2002.

Bedrosian I, Mick R, Orel SG, et al: Changes in the surgical management of patients with breast carcinoma based on preoperative magnetic resonance imaging. Cancer 98:468-473, 2003.

Bedrosian I, Reynolds C, Mick R, et al: Accuracy of sentinel lymph node biopsy in patients with large primary breast tumors. Cancer 88:2540-2545, 2000.

Bevilacqua JL, Gucciardo G, Cody HS, et al: A selection algorithm for internal mammary sentinel lymph node biopsy in breast cancer. Eur J Surg Oncol 28:603-614, 2002.

Birdwell RL, Smith KL, Betts BJ, et al: Breast cancer: Variables affecting sentinel lymph node visualization at preoperative lymphoscintigraphy. Radiology 220:47-53, 2001.

Brenner RJ, Pfaff JM: Mammographic features after conservation therapy for malignant breast disease: Serial findings standardized by regression analysis. AJR Am J Roentgenol 167:171-178, 1996.

Brenner RJ, Pfaff JM: Mammographic changes after excisional breast biopsy for benign disease. AJR Am J Roentgenol 167:1047-1052, 1996.

Cody HS 3rd, Fey J, Akhurst T, et al: Complementarity of blue dye and isotope in sentinel node localization for breast cancer: Univariate and multivariate analysis of 966 procedures. Ann Surg Oncol 8:13-19, 2001.

Cody HS 3rd, Urban JA: Internal mammary node status: A major prognosticator in axillary node–negative breast cancer. Ann Surg Oncol 2:32-37, 1995.

Cote RJ, Peterson HF, Chaiwun B, et al: Role of immunohistochemical detection of lymph-node metastases in management of breast cancer. International Breast Cancer Study Group. Lancet 354:896-900, 1999.

Crivellaro M, Senna G, Dama A, et al: Anaphylaxis due to patent blue dye during lymphography, with negative skin prick test. J Investig Allergol Clin Immunol 13:71-72, 2003.

Denison CM, Ward VL, Lester SC, et al: Epidermal inclusion cysts of the breast: Three lesions with calcifications. Radiology 204:493-496, 1997.

Dershaw DD, Shank B, Reisinger S: Mammographic findings after breast cancer treatment with local excision and definitive irradiation. Radiology 164:455-461, 1987.

Dowlatshahi K, Fan M, Anderson JM, Bloom KJ: Occult metastases in sentinel nodes of 200 patients with operable breast cancer. Ann Surg Oncol 8:675-681, 2001.

Dowlatshahi K, Fan M, Snider HC, Habib FA: Lymph node micrometastases from breast carcinoma: Reviewing the dilemma. Cancer 80:1188-1197, 1997.

Dupont EL, Kuhn MA, McCann C, et al: The role of sentinel lymph node biopsy in women undergoing prophylactic mastectomy. Am J Surg 180:274-277, 2000.

Fischer U, Kopka L, Grabbe E: Breast carcinoma: Effect of preoperative contrast-enhanced MR imaging on the therapeutic approach. Radiology 213:881-888, 1999.

Fisher B, Dignam J, Wolmark N, et al: Lumpectomy and radiation therapy for the treatment of intraductal breast cancer: Findings from National Surgical Adjuvant Breast and Bowel Project B-17. J Clin Oncol 16:441-452, 1998.

Freedman GM, Fowble BL, Nicolaou N, et al: Should internal mammary lymph nodes in breast cancer be a target for the radiation oncologist? Int J Radiat Oncol Biol Phys 46:805-814, 2000.

Golshan M, Martin WJ, Dowlatshahi K: Sentinel lymph node biopsy lowers the rate of lymphedema when compared with standard axillary lymph node dissection. Am Surg 69:209-211, discussion 212, 2003.

Heywang SH, Hilbertz T, Beck R, et al: Gd-DTPA enhanced MR imaging of the breast in patients with postoperative scarring and silicon implants. J Comput Assist Tomogr 14:348-356, 1990.

Hill AD, Tran KN, Akhurst T, et al: Lessons learned from 500 cases of lymphatic mapping for breast cancer. Ann Surg 229:528-535, 1999.

Huvos AG, Hutter RV, Berg JW: Significance of axillary macrometastases and micrometastases in mammary cancer. Ann Surg 173:44-46, 1971.

Jannink I, Fan M, Nagy S, et al: Serial sectioning of sentinel nodes in patients with breast cancer: A pilot study. Ann Surg Oncol 5:310-314, 1998.

Karamlou T, Johnson NM, Chan B, et al: Accuracy of intraoperative touch imprint cytologic analysis of sentinel lymph nodes in breast cancer. Am J Surg 185:425-428, 2003.

Keshtgar MR, Ell PJ: Clinical role of sentinel-lymph-node biopsy in breast cancer. Lancet Oncol 3:105-110, 2002.

Krag D, Weaver D, Ashikaga T, et al: The sentinel node in breast cancer—a multicenter validation study. N Engl J Med 339:941-946, 1998.

Lacour J, Le M, Caceres E, et al: Radical mastectomy versus radical mastectomy plus internal mammary dissection. Ten year results of an international cooperative trial in breast cancer. Cancer 51:1941-1943, 1983.

Lagios MD: Clinical significance of immunohistochemically detectable epithelial cells in sentinel lymph node and bone marrow in breast cancer. J Surg Oncol 83:1-4, 2003.

Liberman L: Lymphoscintigraphy for lymphatic mapping in breast carcinoma. Radiology 228:313-315, 2003.

Liberman L, Van Zee KJ, Dershaw DD, et al: Mammographic features of local recurrence in women who have undergone breast-conserving therapy for ductal carcinoma in situ. AJR Am J Roentgenol 168:489-493, 1997.

Mamounas EP: Sentinel lymph node biopsy after neoadjuvant systemic therapy. Surg Clin North Am 83:931-942, 2003.

Mariani L, Salvadori B, Marubini E, et al: Ten year results of a randomised trial comparing two conservative treatment strategies for small size breast cancer. Eur J Cancer 34:1156-1162, 1998.

Martin RC, Derossis AM, Fey J, et al: Intradermal isotope injection is superior to intramammary in sentinel node biopsy for breast cancer. Surgery 130:432-438, 2001.

McCarter MD, Yeung H, Fey J, et al: The breast cancer patient with multiple sentinel nodes: When to stop? J Am Coll Surg 192:692-697, 2001.

McCarter MD, Yeung H, Yeh S, et al: Localization of the sentinel node in breast cancer: Identical results with same-day and day-before isotope injection. Ann Surg Oncol 8:682-686, 2001.

McMasters KM, Chao C, Wong SL, et al: Sentinel lymph node biopsy in patients with ductal carcinoma in situ: A proposal. Cancer 95:15-20, 2002.

McMasters KM, Tuttle TM, Carlson DJ, et al: Sentinel lymph node biopsy for breast cancer: A suitable alternative to routine axillary dissection in multi-institutional practice when optimal technique is used. J Clin Oncol 18:2560-2566, 2000.

McMasters KM, Wong SL, Martin RC 2nd, et al: Dermal injection of radioactive colloid is superior to peritumoral injection for breast cancer sentinel lymph node biopsy: Results of a multiinstitutional study. Ann Surg 233:676-687, 2001.

Mendelson EB: Evaluation of the postoperative breast. Radiol Clin North Am 30:107-138, 1992.

Montague ED: Conservation surgery and radiation therapy in the treatment of operable breast cancer. Cancer 53(Suppl): 700-704, 1984.

Montague ED, Fletcher GH: Local regional effectiveness of surgery and radiation therapy in the treatment of breast cancer. Cancer 55(Suppl):2266-2272, 1985.

Morris EA, Schwartz LH, Drotman MB, et al: Evaluation of pectoralis major muscle in patients with posterior breast tumors on breast MR images: Early experience. Radiology 214:67-72, 2000.

Mumtaz H, Hall-Craggs MA, Davidson T, et al: Staging of symptomatic primary breast cancer with MR imaging. AJR Am J Roentgenol 169:417-424, 1997.

Nathanson SD, Wachna DL, Gilman D, et al: Pathways of lymphatic drainage from the breast. Ann Surg Oncol 8:837-843, 2001.

Orel SG, Schnall MD, Powell CM, et al: Staging of suspected breast cancer: Effect of MR imaging and MR-guided biopsy. Radiology 196:115-122, 1995.

Orel SG, Troupin RH, Patterson EA, Fowble BL: Breast cancer recurrence after lumpectomy and irradiation: Role of mammography in detection. Radiology 183:201-206, 1992.

Pendas S, Dauway E, Giuliano R, et al: Sentinel node biopsy in ductal carcinoma in situ patients. Ann Surg Oncol 7:15-20, 2000.

Philpotts LE, Lee CH, Haffty BG, et al: Mammographic findings of recurrent breast cancer after lumpectomy and radiation therapy: Comparison with the primary tumor. Radiology 201:767-771, 1996.

Sandrucci S, Mussa A: Sentinel lymph node biopsy and axillary staging of T1-T2 N0 breast cancer: A multicenter study. Semin Surg Oncol 15:278-283, 1998.

Schwartz GF, Giuliano AE, Veronesi U: Proceeding of the consensus conference of the role of sentinel lymph node biopsy in carcinoma of the breast, April 19-22, 2001, Philadelphia, PA, USA. Breast J 8:124-138, 2002.

Shen P, Glass EC, DiFronzo LA, Giuliano AE: Dermal versus intraparenchymal lymphoscintigraphy of the breast. Ann Surg Oncol 8:241-248, 2001.

Sickles EA, Herzog KA: Mammography of the postsurgical breast. AJR Am J Roentgenol 136:585-588, 1981.

Singletary SE, Greene FL: Revision of breast cancer staging: The 6th edition of the TNM Classification. Semin Surg Oncol 21:53-59, 2003.

Steinhoff MM: Axillary node micrometastases: Detection and biologic significance. Breast J 5:325-329, 1999.

Turner RR, Ollila DW, Krasne DL, Giuliano AE: Histopathologic validation of the sentinel lymph node hypothesis for breast carcinoma. Ann Surg 226:271-276, discussion 276-278, 1997.

Veronesi U, Paganelli G, Viale G, et al: Sentinel lymph node biopsy and axillary dissection in breast cancer: Results in a large series. J Natl Cancer Inst 91:368-373, 1999.

Veronesi U, Paganelli G, Viale G, et al: A randomized comparison of sentinel-node biopsy with routine axillary dissection in breast cancer. N Engl J Med 349:546-553, 2003.

Veronesi U, Zurrida S, Mazzarol G, Viale G: Extensive frozen section examination of axillary sentinel nodes to determine selective axillary dissection. World J Surg 25:806-808, 2001.

Yarbro JW, Page DL, Fielding LP, et al: American Joint Committee on Cancer prognostic factors consensus conference. Cancer 86:2436-2446, 1999.

Zafrani B, Fourquet A, Vilcoq JR, et al: Conservative management of intraductal breast carcinoma with tumorectomy and radiation therapy. Cancer 57:1299-1301, 1986.

Breast Implants

DEBRA M. IKEDA

YVONNE KARANAS

Introduction
Implant Types
Implant Complications
Implant Rupture
Implant Imaging for Rupture
    Mammography
    Ultrasound
    Magnetic Resonance Imaging
Breast Reconstruction
Reduction Mammaplasty
Key Elements

INTRODUCTION

Silicone breast implants were introduced in 1962. An estimated 2 million women in the United States have silicone breast implants, with approximately 80% placed for breast augmentation and the remainder for breast reconstruction after mastectomy. On April 16, 1992, the U.S. Food and Drug Administration (FDA) restricted the use of silicone implants to women undergoing breast reconstruction for mastectomy because of concern about implant rupture and a possible association with connective tissue disease.

Addressing these concerns, an article by Tugwell et al. discussed a U.S. District Court order establishing a National Science Panel to assess whether existing scientific studies show an association between silicone breast implants and connective tissue disease. They concluded that there was no scientific evidence to show a relationship between silicone breast implants and connective tissue disease or breast cancer. Currently, silicone gel breast implants may be used for breast reconstruction after mastectomy in the United States. Saline-filled implants may be used for breast augmentation. Some forms of silicone gel and other implants are under review by the FDA for approval.

IMPLANT TYPES

The basic design of silicone gel–filled implants is silicone gel contained in an envelope composed of a silicone elastomer (Box 9-1) (Fig. 9-1A-D). Silicone is a synthetic polymer of cross-linked chains of dimethylsiloxane and can be solid, liquid, or gel. Breast implants are filled with silicone gel, which makes them soft and movable. The outer envelope can be textured or smooth, polyurethane coated, or uncoated. A single-lumen implant is composed of an outer shell filled with silicone gel. Double- or triple-lumen implants have two or more inside envelopes containing saline or silicone gel, depending on the implant type. Some implants contain only saline and can be visualized on mammography because they are relatively radiolucent. Some implants are covered with a finely textured mesh-like surface over the outer envelope that is composed of a polyurethane-coated material to prevent fibrous capsular formation. This type of implant was banned because of the release of 2, 4 toluene-diamine (TDA), a byproduct suspected to cause cancer in laboratory animals. Other less common implants include those filled with a polyvinyl alcohol sponge or a lipid substance (called the "Trilucent" implant), the latter of which may show a serous/lipid level on magnetic resonance imaging (MRI) if ruptured. "Stacked" implants are two single-lumen implants that are placed one on top of the other in the breast for aesthetic purposes.

IMPLANT COMPLICATIONS

Munker et al. reported on Trilucent implants in 27 patients who elected to exchange their implants for a fourth-generation cohesive silicone implant. Of these 27 patients, 14 had a change in the volume of their implants but not all were aware of the change, and capsular contraction was not present (Baker grade II (see Table 9-1). Fifty-five percent of the implants had thickening or color changes caused by peroxidation of the triglyceride contents, and the implant capsule was adherent to breast tissues, in particular, the pectoralis muscle, which led to prolonged operative times. Rizkalla et al. reported similar results, with a reoperation rate of 20% (10/50) and an implant deflation rate of 10% (5/50). The Medical Devices Agency withdrew the Trilucent implant from the market in March 1999 with a subsequent recommendation in June 2000 that the implants be removed. A new

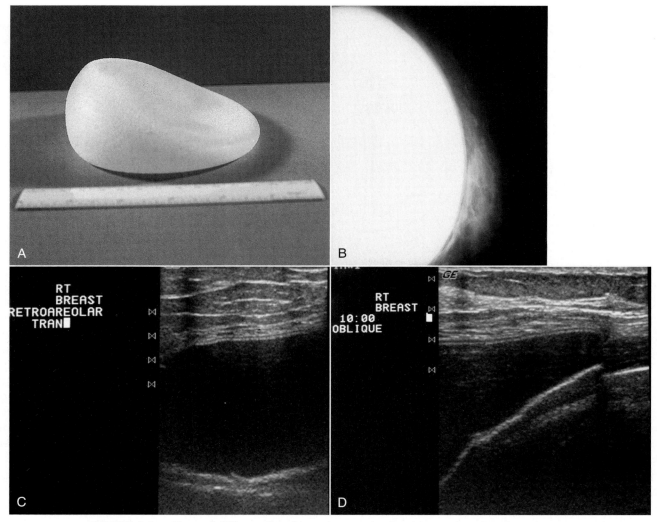

FIGURE 9-1   Normal Silicone Implant. Photograph of a silicone gel implant from the side (**A**). The implant will be placed underneath the breast tissue and either on top of or underneath the pectoralis muscle at surgery. The corresponding mammogram (**B**) shows a dense structure near the chest wall and a little breast tissue around it. **C,** Ultrasound of a typical intact silicone implant shows the breast tissue in the near field and the oval hypoechoic implant near the chest wall. Note that the appearance of a normal silicone implant is almost anechoic and simulates a very, very large cyst. **D,** Ultrasound of an intact silicone implant shows a typical normal edge artifact causing shadowing where the edge of the implant meets breast tissue. Typical normal reverberation artifact is seen in the near field of the implant, similar to artifacts seen in a normal urinary bladder.   *Continued*

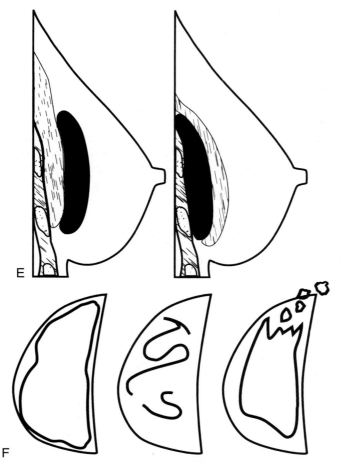

E

F

FIGURE 9-1 cont'd   **E,** Schematic of implant placement: on the *left*, subglandular implant placement; on the *right*, subpectoral implant placement. **F,** Schematic of implant complications. On the *left*, a fibrous capsule forms around an intact implant. In the *middle*, the implant shell may rupture, but the silicone is contained in the fibrous capsule—called "intracapsular rupture." On the *right*, the implant capsule and the fibrous capsule are ruptured, with silicone outside the fibrous capsule—called "extracapsular rupture."

	Table 9-1 Baker Classification		
Grade	**Breast Firmness**	**Implant**	**Implant Visibility**
I	Soft	Nonpalpable	Nonvisible
II	Minimal	Palpable	Nonvisible
III	Moderate	Easily palpable	Distortion visible
IV	Severe	Hard, tender, cold	Distortion may be marked

From: Baker JL Jr: Augmentation mammaplasty. *In* Owsley JQ Jr, Peterson RA (eds): Symposium on Aesthetic Surgery of the Breast, 1978. St. Louis, CV Mosby, 1978.

Box 9-2   Untoward Effects of Breast Implants

Rupture
Contraction of the fibrous capsule
Hematoma
Infection
Silicone gel "bleed"
Calcification of the fibrous capsule

type of alloplastic material for implants that contains carboxymethylcellulose, called Hydrogel, was introduced into the European market. Of 12 patients with 20 implants placed between 1996 and 1997 reported by Cicchetti et al., none showed immediate complications and had Baker I or II capsular contraction at 3.5 years of follow-up.

Direct injection of various materials, including paraffin and liquid silicone, has also been used for breast augmentation. Complications from direct injection include granulomatous reactions, which may result in hard breast masses simulating malignant tumors on physical examination and obscuring underlying breast tissue on mammography.

Silicone gel–filled implants are surgically placed in either the subglandular or subpectoral position (Fig. 9-1E).

In either case, the body generally forms a fibrous capsule around the implant. The fibrous capsule is usually soft, nonpalpable, and undetectable, but it can undergo capsular contraction and become hard and resistant, with a suboptimal appearance and feel of the implant. The Baker classification describes the types of capsular formation on implants (Table 9-1). The incidence of capsular contracture may be diminished by the use of textured submuscular implants, although the use of such implants remains controversial. Other reports attribute implant failure to a subpectoral location and implant age, especially implants manufactured in the late 1970s and early 1980s (second-generation implants). Closed capsulotomy, or manual breaking of the fibrous capsule, was used to make a hard implant more soft and movable and is associated with implant rupture. Open surgical capsulotomy in which the hardened implant capsule is removed is an alternative.

Untoward complications associated with silicone gel–filled breast implants include contracture of the fibrous capsule, calcification of the fibrous capsule, hematoma, infection, implant rupture, and the controversial silicone gel "bleed" in which silicone gel leaks outside the implant through an intact envelope (Box 9-2). Capsular contracture is the most common complication, with a reported incidence of more than 70% in some older series and only about a 20% incidence in more recent series.

Table 9-2	Implant Rupture Types	
Intracapsular rupture	Fibrous capsule contains silicone gel	Envelope ruptured
Extracapsular rupture	Silicone gel outside fibrous capsule	Envelope ruptured
Gel bleed (controversial)	Silicone outside envelope	Envelope intact

IMPLANT RUPTURE

Implant integrity is classified as intact, intact with gel bleed, intracapsular rupture, or extracapsular rupture (Table 9-2). Breast implant rupture is defined as loss of integrity of the implant shell and is divided into two types: (1) intracapsular, defined as implant envelope rupture with silicone gel contained within the fibrous capsule, and (2) extracapsular, defined as implant envelope rupture with silicone gel extruded outside the fibrous capsule (Fig. 9-1F). The complication of gel bleed is defined as silicone gel leakage through an intact implant envelope, although the existence of gel bleed versus small, undetected ruptures remains controversial.

A clinical diagnosis of implant rupture is often difficult to make. Feng and Amini reported significant risk factors for implant rupture: implant age, retroglandular location, capsular contracture, local symptoms, implant type (double-lumen and polyurethane-covered implants rupture less frequently than smooth gel implants), and manufacturer. The clinical history, signs, and symptoms may be helpful but are frequently nonspecific; in one series of 19 symptomatic patients with ruptured implants, women complained of palpable axillary, breast, or chest wall masses, pain, or changes in the size, shape, or texture of the breast. In one surgical series, 3 of the 32 patients reviewed were asymptomatic. Because physical examination misses about 50% of ruptures, clinicians turned to imaging to help diagnose ruptured implants when the clinical findings were questionable.

IMPLANT IMAGING FOR RUPTURE

Mammography

The normal silicone implant is quite dense and completely opaque, obscures and displaces much of the surrounding breast tissue, and produces a smooth white oval opacity near the chest wall (Fig. 9-2). The pectoralis muscle curves over the implant in subpectoral implants

and is underneath the implant in subglandular implants. A silicone gel–filled implant is not as compressible as breast tissue and can be ruptured if compressed too hard during mammography or closed capsulotomy. Because limited compression decreases visualization of the surrounding breast tissue for breast cancer screening, the Mammography Quality Standards Assurance Act recommends four views of each implanted breast, including two views that exclude as much of the implant as possible, known as implant-displaced views, and two views that include the implant (Box 9-3). Implant integrity is evaluated on limited-compression mammograms in which the implant is surrounded by noncompressed breast tissue, and breast tissue is evaluated on the implant-displaced views.

This technique does not completely resolve the problem of imaging small breast cancers but optimizes the amount of breast tissue displayed on the mammogram. Various reports suggest using both physical examination and breast ultrasound as an adjunct to mammography in evaluating mammographically detected breast masses or palpable findings. Ultrasound can be especially helpful in determining whether a true mass exists when the mammogram is equivocal or in the setting of a palpable mass. Ultrasound can evaluate the entire breadth of the breast tissue down to the implant and distinguishes breast masses from the snowstorm appearance of silicone granulomas caused by ruptured implants (Fig. 9-2C).

Unlike opaque silicone implants, saline implants are radiolucent structures surrounded by a dense silicone outer envelope in which small wrinkles may be seen. When a saline implant ruptures, the saline diffuses into the breast tissue and the envelope shrinks back against the chest wall (Fig. 9-2D). Saline outer/silicone inner double-lumen implants have an outer envelope containing saline surrounding a dense inner silicone implant filling. All these implants become surrounded by a fibrous capsule, which is not usually visible unless it calcifies. A calcified fibrous capsule shows dystrophic sheet-like calcifications along the implant surface and appears slightly bumpy on the nondisplaced implant views (Fig. 9-2E). If one is concerned that the calcifications are in breast parenchyma rather than in the implant capsule, spot magnification mammograms may be used to distinguish the calcified capsule, which should stay closely applied to the implant, from intraparenchymal calcifications, which may be displaced from the implant capsule (Fig. 9-3A-D).

When evaluating breast tissue for cancer in women with implants, it is important to inspect both the implant-displaced views and the breast tissue adjacent to the implant on the non–implant-displaced views. The implant-displaced views may display a mass near the implant or the fibrous capsule (Fig. 9-4A-G). Spot compression mammograms or other fine-detail views for

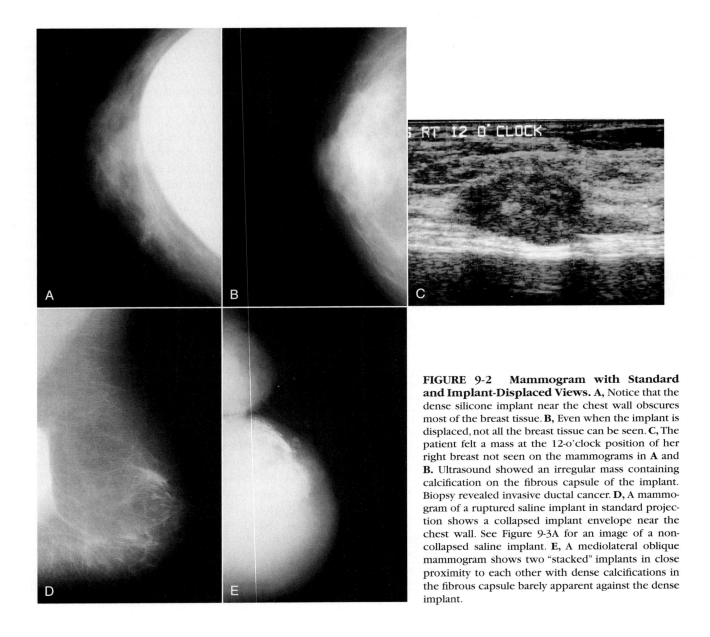

FIGURE 9-2   Mammogram with Standard and Implant-Displaced Views. A, Notice that the dense silicone implant near the chest wall obscures most of the breast tissue. **B,** Even when the implant is displaced, not all the breast tissue can be seen. **C,** The patient felt a mass at the 12-o'clock position of her right breast not seen on the mammograms in **A** and **B.** Ultrasound showed an irregular mass containing calcification on the fibrous capsule of the implant. Biopsy revealed invasive ductal cancer. **D,** A mammogram of a ruptured saline implant in standard projection shows a collapsed implant envelope near the chest wall. See Figure 9-3A for an image of a non-collapsed saline implant. **E,** A mediolateral oblique mammogram shows two "stacked" implants in close proximity to each other with dense calcifications in the fibrous capsule barely apparent against the dense implant.

Box 9-3   Mammography of Implants

Four views of each breast:
　　CC and ML or MLO with the implant
　　CC and ML or MLO implant-displaced views
Magnification, spot, and other fine-detail views can be performed in the implanted breast
Five percent of screenings show asymptomatic rupture

CC, craniocaudal; MLO, mediolateral oblique.

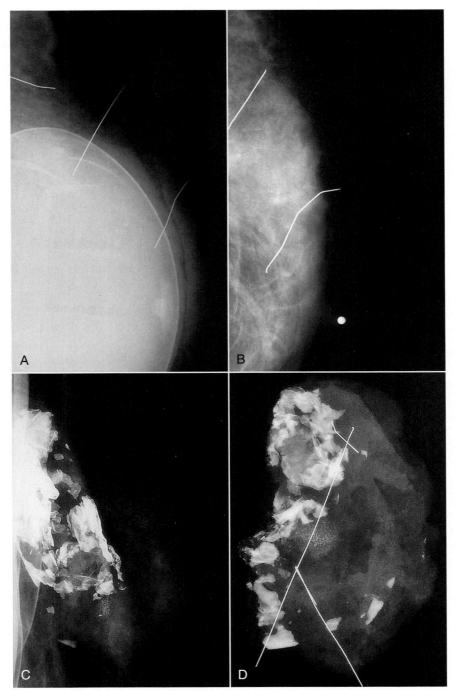

FIGURE 9-3   Calcifications near Implants. A, A mediolateral oblique (MLO) mammogram shows a saline implant with metallic linear scar markers near calcifications close to the implant. Note that the implant is less dense than the silicon implant and that the little wrinkles in the implant and an anterior valve can be seen. **B,** A magnification implant-displaced view of **A** shows pleomorphic calcifications in the breast tissue. Biopsy revealed ductal carcinoma in situ. **C,** An implant-displaced MLO mammogram shows a subpectoral saline implant in another patient and a calcified fibrous capsule from a previously removed subglandular polyurethane-covered implant. Notice the dystrophic sheet-like calcifications around the previous implant cavity. **D,** Tiny mesh-like microcalcifications were seen near the dystrophic implant capsule and were removed by preoperative needle localization, as seen on specimen radiography; these microcalcifications represented the calcifying mesh of the outer polyurethane coating.

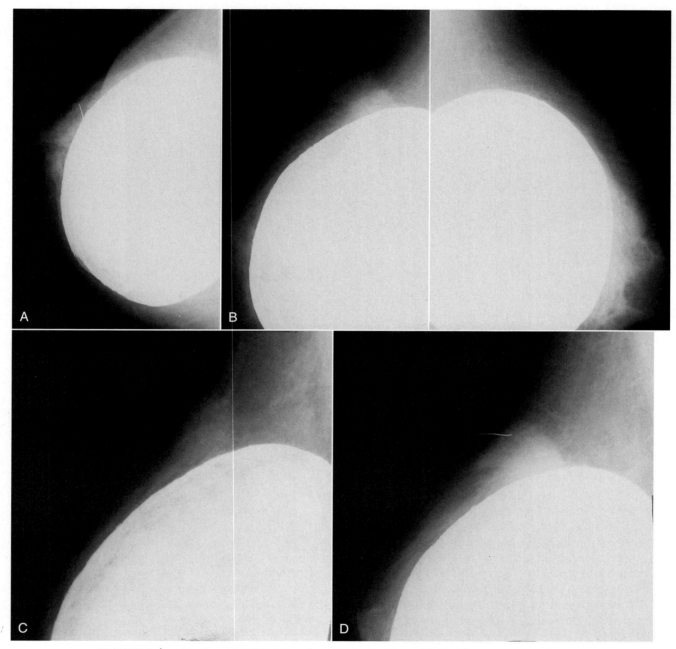

FIGURE 9-4   Craniocaudal (CC) (**A**) and mediolateral oblique (MLO) (**B**) mammograms show a dense mass near the implant in the upper portion of the right breast on the MLO view only. The mass is obscured by the implant on the CC view. **C** and **D**, Photographically magnified views of the upper portion of the right breast in 1999 (**C**) and 2002 (**D**) show that the mass is new and developing in a previous biopsy site; the mass was seen on implant-displaced views because it was pushed away with the implant, thus showing the importance of analyzing mammograms that include the implant as well as the implant-displaced view.

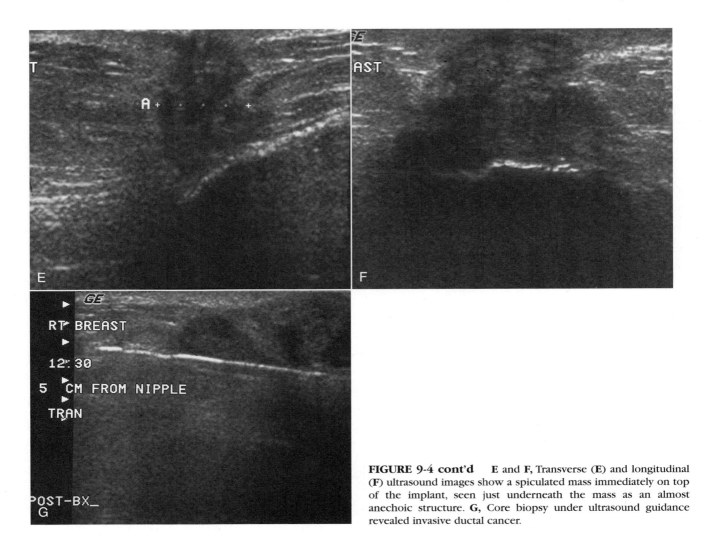

FIGURE 9-4 cont'd   **E** and **F,** Transverse (**E**) and longitudinal (**F**) ultrasound images show a spiculated mass immediately on top of the implant, seen just underneath the mass as an almost anechoic structure. **G,** Core biopsy under ultrasound guidance revealed invasive ductal cancer.

masses or suspicious calcifications can be used in women with implants, just as any other woman. Needle localization, ultrasound-guided core biopsy, and stereotactic core biopsy can all be performed in women with implants.

A retrospective review of screening mammograms in 350 asymptomatic women with breast implants suggested that the asymptomatic implant rupture rate is 5%. On mammography, extracapsular rupture is diagnosed by extravasation of silicone gel outside the implant envelope either as blobs of silicone in breast tissue or within implant ducts or as extruded silicone in contiguity with the implant contour (Fig. 9-5A-C) (Table 9-3). After implant rupture, removal of all extravasated silicone is often impossible without removing much of the breast tissue, and the extravasated silicone is therefore left in the breast. If residual silicone is left within breast tissue after removal of a ruptured implant and a new silicone implant is placed, evaluation of rupture of the new implant becomes even more difficult. Silicone within

axillary lymph nodes implies extravasation of silicone and extracapsular rupture (Fig. 9-5D).

Lobulation of the silicone implant or other contour changes in the envelope indicate capsular contraction, herniation of an intact implant envelope through a break in the surrounding fibrous capsule, or a contained implant leak (Table 9-4). Because both implant lobulation and a contained leak have the same mammographic appearance, ultrasound is needed to make the diagnosis of a rupture (Fig. 9-5E and F). Mammography cannot identify posterior ruptures of the implant near the chest wall or intracapsular ruptures when the contour of the implant is normal.

Direct silicone or paraffin injections result in multiple tiny round eggshell-type calcifications that obscure the underlying breast tissue. Because silicone granulomas may become quite hard, both physical examination and mammography of the underlying tissue are nearly impossible (Fig. 9-6). Ultrasound of patients with silicone

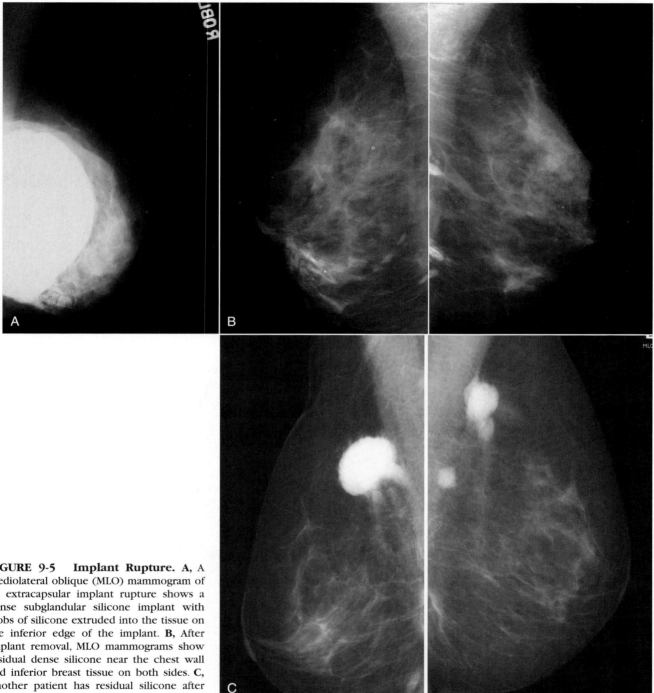

FIGURE 9-5 Implant Rupture. A, A mediolateral oblique (MLO) mammogram of an extracapsular implant rupture shows a dense subglandular silicone implant with globs of silicone extruded into the tissue on the inferior edge of the implant. **B,** After implant removal, MLO mammograms show residual dense silicone near the chest wall and inferior breast tissue on both sides. **C,** Another patient has residual silicone after removal of an implant because of rupture.

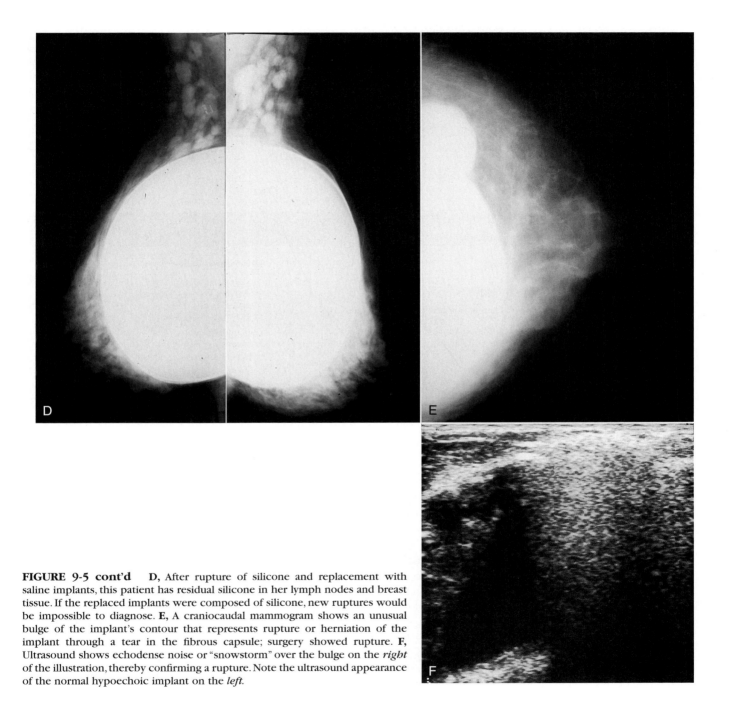

FIGURE 9-5 cont'd   D, After rupture of silicone and replacement with saline implants, this patient has residual silicone in her lymph nodes and breast tissue. If the replaced implants were composed of silicone, new ruptures would be impossible to diagnose. **E,** A craniocaudal mammogram shows an unusual bulge of the implant's contour that represents rupture or herniation of the implant through a tear in the fibrous capsule; surgery showed rupture. **F,** Ultrasound shows echodense noise or "snowstorm" over the bulge on the *right* of the illustration, thereby confirming a rupture. Note the ultrasound appearance of the normal hypoechoic implant on the *left*.

Table 9-3   Imaging Findings with Rupture

	Intracapsular	Extracapsular	Gel Bleed
Mammography	(−)	Silicone globs in breast tissue Silicone in lymph nodes Silicone in ducts Implant contour deformity (+/−)	(+/−)
Ultrasound	Stepladder sign	Snowstorm or echodense noise	Snowstorm or echodense noise
MRI	Linguine sign Teardrop/keyhole sign Subcapsular lines Water droplets (+/−)	Silicone outside the envelope Signs of intracapsular rupture	Teardrop/keyhole sign Subcapsular lines

Table 9-4   False-Positive Imaging Findings for Rupture

	Sign	Differential Diagnosis
Mammography	Implant contour deformity	Contained rupture Capsular contraction Herniation through a capsule tear
	Intraparenchymal silicone	Previous leak with the ruptured implant removed
Ultrasound	Stepladder	Intracapsular rupture Intact multilumen implant
MRI	Linguine	Intracapsular rupture
	Water droplets (+/−)	Intact multilumen implant

injections shows multiple areas of "snowstorm" or "echodense noise" that casts shadows throughout the breast and obscures the breast tissue, thus rendering evaluation for breast cancer difficult with this modality as well.

Some women have their implants removed and not replaced. After implant removal, the mammogram shows architectural distortion centrally in the breast near the chest wall from the implant cavity. The implant cavity may become inapparent on mammography, may scar, or may fill with fluid and give rise to a mass (Fig. 9-7). The fibrous capsule is not always removed with the implant. If the fibrous capsule has calcified, the mammogram shows dystrophic calcifications in the retained fibrous capsule that are distributed in a curvilinear pattern of sheet-like calcifications near the chest wall. Calcifying polyurethane-covered implants produce a typical fine mesh-like appearance representing calcification of the sponge-like covering. This appearance can be mistaken for cancer and will sometimes prompt biopsy.

Ultrasound

Ultrasound is an adjunct to mammography in the diagnosis of ruptured breast implants. The normal single-lumen implant has a smooth echogenic edge, and the inside of the implant is anechoic, similar to a cyst. Minor contour abnormalities and short radial folds are noted as incidental findings. Reverberation artifacts are normal echogenic features in an intact implant; they are the same width as the breast tissue anterior to the implant and are easily distinguished from ruptures (Fig. 9-8). Ultrasound signs of rupture have varying sensitivities of 25% to 65% and specificities of 57% to 98%. Ultrasound is less expensive than MRI and is thought to be more cost-effective than MRI in diagnosing ruptures.

Extracapsular rupture is diagnosed by the classic "snowstorm" sign or echodense noise, a characteristic echogenic finding caused by the slow velocity of sound in silicone with respect to the surrounding breast parenchyma. Silicone or paraffin injections will have an

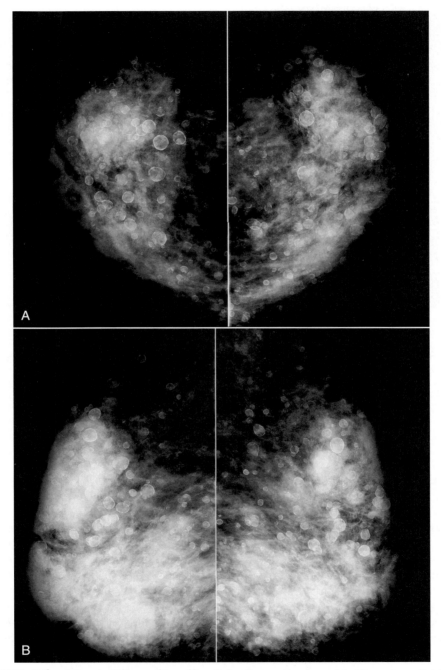

FIGURE 9-6   Direct Silicone/Paraffin Injections. Craniocaudal (**A**) and mediolateral oblique (**B**) mammograms show dense tissue and multiple eggshell-type calcifications compatible with paraffin or silicone injections.

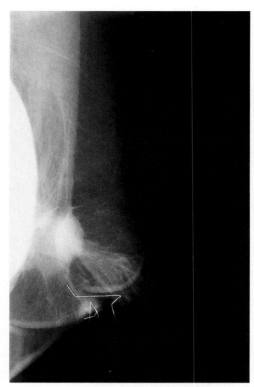

FIGURE 9-7 After removal of a subglandular implant and placement of a subpectoral implant, this patient has a characteristic "removed-implant cavity" distortion on top of her chest wall, now filled with fluid; this fluid-filled distortion is producing a small smooth oval mass projecting on the pectoralis muscle. Note the metallic linear scar markers showing the scars in the lower part of the breast associated with skin distortion and deformity.

appearance similar to extracapsular rupture and are characterized by echodense noise. "Snowstorm" or echodense noise looks like air in the bowel wall, has an intense echogenic appearance, and obscures all findings beneath it (Fig. 9-9A-C). It can be distinguished from edge artifact by scanning at different angles, which will produce the same echogenic appearance. Another sign of extracapsular rupture is a hypoechoic mass corresponding to large globules of silicone extruded away from the implant (Fig. 9-9D). In this situation, so much silicone is extruded that the silicone glob appears as a hypoechoic mass similar to the intact implant rather than echodense noise. To ensure the correct diagnosis, a skin marker can be placed on the hypoechoic mass and a repeat mammogram obtained to correlate silicone on the radiograph with the ultrasound finding.

"Gel bleed" is defined as silicone gel outside an intact implant envelope and is shown as "snowstorm" or echodense noise. By definition, gel bleed indicates extracapsular silicone surrounding an intact implant, but this definition is controversial because some investigators believe that there will always be a tiny rupture accompanying "gel bleed." Given that ultrasound examinations demonstrating echodense noise can be caused by severe gel bleed, it is controversial whether the scan should be classified as a true- or false-positive examination, especially because silicone is outside the implant and in direct contact with human tissue.

Intracapsular rupture is diagnosed by the "stepladder" sign, which represents the collapsing ruptured implant shell within the fibrous capsule. The stepladder sign is characterized by multiple thin echogenic lines within the implant that do not extend to the periphery of the implant; the thin lines represent echoes of the collapsing implant wall folding in on itself. The stepladder sign is seen with both intracapsular and extracapsular rupture (Fig. 9-10). False-positive "stepladder" signs are caused by intact multilumen implants producing multiple linear echoes in the implant, similar to an intracapsular rupture.

Diffuse linear echoes, debris, or diffuse low-level echoes within the implant may also indicate intracapsular rupture, but they are less definitive. In a small percentage of studies, ultrasound produces false-negative results.

Magnetic Resonance Imaging

In a meta-analysis of implants imaged by MRI for rupture by Cher et al., the summary MRI sensitivity for rupture was 78% and the summary specificity was 91%, with an odds ratio for overall test accuracy of 40.1 (range, 18.8 to 85.4) when receiver operating characteristics meta-analysis methodology was used.

In the setting of ruptured implants, MRI distinguishes breast tissue from leaking silicone, contrasting fat and water in glandular tissue from silicone, and the dark silicone envelope containing the silicone gel (Fig. 9-11). MRI techniques that evaluate silicone breast implants include T1-weighted spin-echo imaging, gradient echo imaging, T2-weighted fast spin echo imaging, short tau inversion recovery (STIR) imaging, and the modified three-point Dixon technique, which yield sensitivities and specificities of 95% to 98% and 50% to 93%, respectively (Box 9-4). The modified three-point Dixon chemical shift technique has the distinct advantage of allowing selective imaging of silicone by separation of the signal of silicone from that of fat and water based on the chemical shift of silicone (1.3 to 1.6 parts per million lower than that of lipid). Inversion recovery fast spin echo (IRFSE) sequences combines the speed of a T2-weighted fast spin echo sequence with homogeneous fat suppression.

Patients are scanned prone in a dedicated breast coil to diminish breathing artifacts from chest wall movement. The implant is usually scanned in the axial and sagittal/oblique planes. MRI of a normal single-lumen silicone

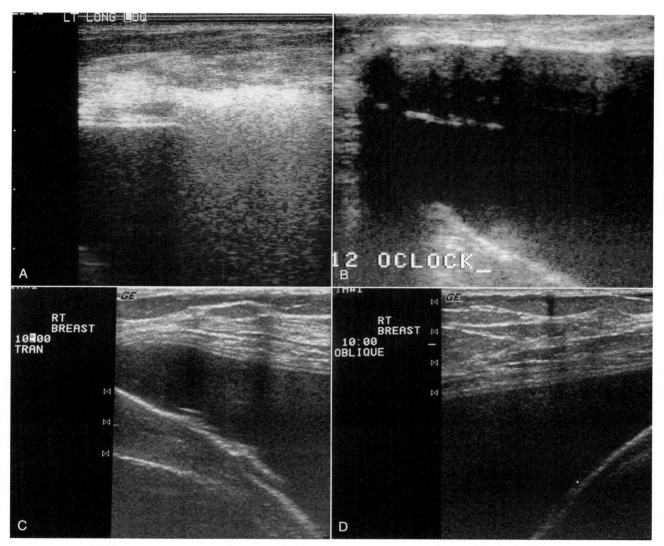

FIGURE 9-8   "Snowstorm or Echodense Noise" versus Reverberation Artifact on Ultrasound. A, Ultrasound shows breast tissue in the near field, the normal anechoic implant with normal reverberation artifacts in the near field, and echodense noise or "snowstorm" artifact representing extracapsular silicone. Compare the normal reverberation artifact on the *left* with rupture on the *right*. **B,** Ultrasound shows a normal anechoic implant with normal reverberation artifacts in the near field of the implant that are as thick as the breast tissue above it and a bright line within the implant representing a normal radial fold that extends to the periphery of the implant when scanned from multiple angles. **C,** Reverberation artifact is shown as gray speckles in the near field of a normal silicone implant with normal radial folds on its inferior aspect. Contrast the reverberation artifact with findings of "snowstorm" or "echodense noise" from the rupture in **A.** Note that rupture in **A** produces a bright shadow that obscures all features of structures deep to the extruded silicone whereas reverberation artifact occurs only in the near field and does not obscure deeper structures in **C. D,** Normal intact implant on ultrasound.

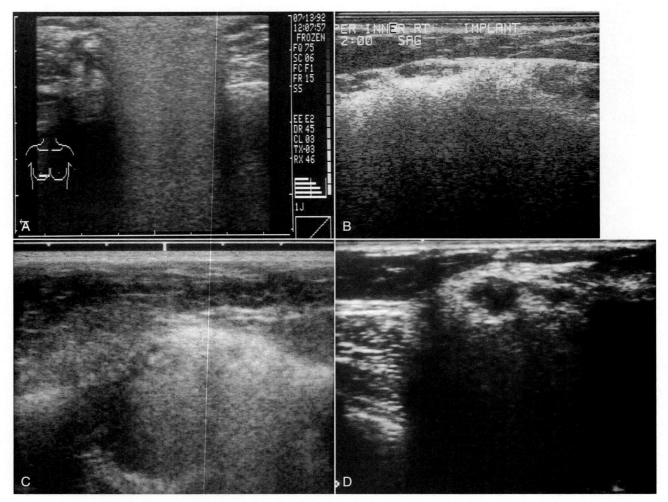

FIGURE 9-9   Implant Rupture on Ultrasound. A, Ultrasound of a breast with extracapsular silicone shows the bright gray "echodense noise" or "snowstorm" artifact that obscures the implant below. **B,** The "snowstorm" appearance on ultrasound in another patient with a large extracapsular rupture fills the image and obscures all adjacent structures, including the breast tissue and implant below. **C,** The snowstorm appearance on ultrasound is seen in the breast parenchyma on the right side and is almost obscuring the implant below. **D,** An extracapsular rupture in a patient who had a glob of silicone is producing a hypoechoic mass in the breast tissue above the implant, but surrounded by echodense noise. The extruded glob of silicone was confirmed by placing a marker over the finding and obtaining a mammogram, which showed silicone. Note that the larger silicone glob produces a mass similar to the intact implant in the lower right-hand corner of the image.

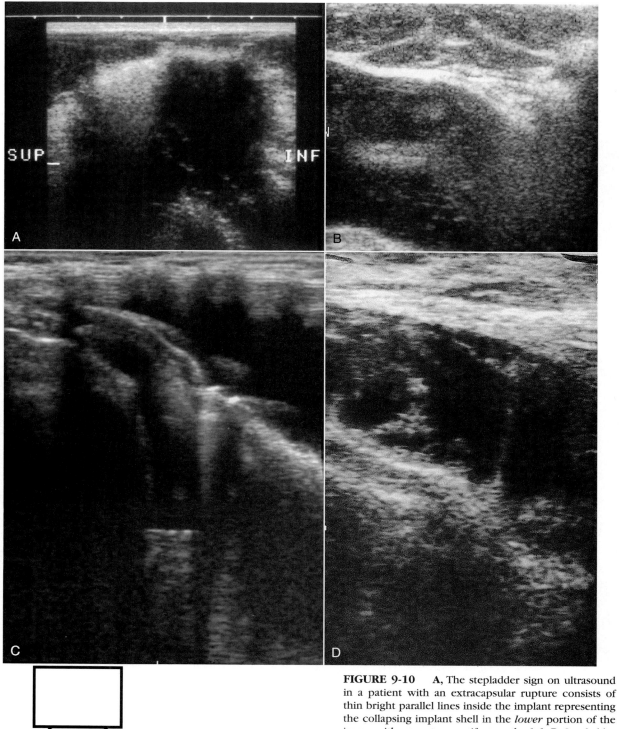

FIGURE 9-10 **A,** The stepladder sign on ultrasound in a patient with an extracapsular rupture consists of thin bright parallel lines inside the implant representing the collapsing implant shell in the *lower* portion of the image with snowstorm artifact on the *left*. **B,** Stepladder sign and multiple tiny linear echoes in the implant in a patient with an extracapsular rupture and a snowstorm artifact on the *right*. **C,** False-positive stepladder sign in a multilumen saline implant in which multiple lines represent the multiple envelopes in this intact multilumen implant. **D,** A true stepladder sign in intracapsular rupture consists of multiple thick and thin linear echoes in the implant that do not always extend to the periphery. **E,** Schematic of scanning an intracapsular rupture showing a "stepladder." The transducer shows the collapsing implant envelope, which is producing multiple lines, or a "stepladder," on ultrasound.

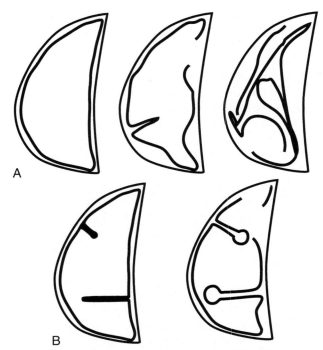

FIGURE 9-11   Schematic of Intracapsular Rupture. A, On the *left* is an intact implant in a fibrous capsule. When the implant shell breaks, the shell pulls away from the fibrous capsule and produces the "subcapsular line" *(middle)*. Later, when the entire shell collapses into the fibrous capsule, the "linguine sign" is produced, which looks like a loose thread *(right)*. **B,** Schematic of radial folds versus keyholes. As seen on the *left,* an intact implant can fold on itself and produce dark lines called "radial folds" that extend to the periphery of the implant but are totally black inside *(left)*. With a rupture, silicone intersperses between the collapsing envelope and the fibrous capsule and produces a white center inside the fold called a "keyhole" or an "inverted teardrop," indicative of intracapsular rupture *(right)*.

implant shows high signal from the silicone with a smooth oval border (Fig. 9-12A). Minor implant bulges or herniations and short and long radial folds are noted as incidental findings. Radial folds are dark lines in the bright silicone that extend to the periphery of the implant and represent folds in the implant envelope (Fig. 9-12B). Reactive fluid around the implant and water droplets are classified as nonspecific findings but are noted in the report, particularly if the findings are marked or implant infection is suspected.

Extracapsular rupture is diagnosed by detecting silicone outside the fibrous capsule, within the breast parenchyma or axilla (Fig. 9-13). Signs of intracapsular rupture will always be present with the finding of extracapsular rupture. Severe gel bleed is diagnosed if a thin coating of silicone is identified around the periphery of the implant.

Intracapsular rupture is diagnosed by detection of the "linguine" sign, which consists of dark lines inside the implant that do not extend to the periphery. The dark lines represent the collapsing ruptured implant shell

Box 9-4	MRI Techniques for Implants
T1 weighted spin echo	
Gradient echo	
T2 weighted fast spin echo	
Short tau inversion recovery (STIR)	
Modified three-point Dixon	

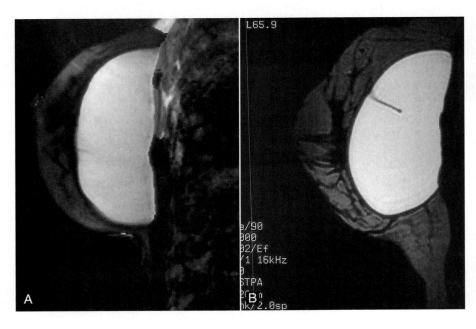

L65.9

FIGURE 9-12   A, Normal silicone implant on magnetic resonance imaging (MRI). **B,** Normal silicone implant on MRI with a normal radial fold.

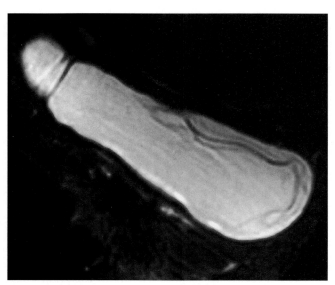

FIGURE 9-13   Axial magnetic resonance imaging of an extracapsular rupture shows extravasated silicone seen as a bulge in the axillary portion of the implant and the linguine sign.

contained within an intact fibrous capsule (Fig. 9-14). Other signs of intracapsular rupture are the "teardrop" or keyhole sign, which represents silicone within a short radial fold. Other signs of intracapsular rupture include an intracapsular mottled appearance of the silicone or a dark subcapsular line paralleling the implant shell that cannot be traced to the periphery of the implant; this line represents incomplete shell collapse.

In an early series of 143 patients with 281 silicone implants, MRI showed a sensitivity of 76% and a specificity of 97% for implant rupture. This series used a T2-weighted fast spin echo technique, a T2-weighted fast spin echo technique with water suppression, and a T1-weighted spin echo technique with fat suppression.

In another series of 30 patients with 59 implants, MRI had a sensitivity of 100%, a specificity of 63%, a positive predictive value of 71%, a negative predictive value of 100%, and an accuracy of 81% in the detection of rupture/bleed. The "linguine" sign was the most sensitive (93%) and specific (65%) finding for rupture. The "non-specific" sign of water droplets within the implant had a sensitivity of 92% and a low specificity of 44% (Box 9-5). Linear extension of silicone along the chest wall and the presence of reactive fluid were neither sensitive nor specific for rupture. Nonspecific signs such as contour deformity (77%, 10/13), water droplets (54%, 7/13), and

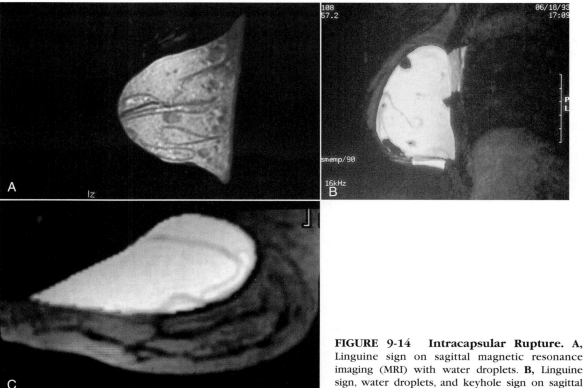

FIGURE 9-14   Intracapsular Rupture. A, Linguine sign on sagittal magnetic resonance imaging (MRI) with water droplets. **B,** Linguine sign, water droplets, and keyhole sign on sagittal MRI. **C,** Linguine sign on axial MRI.

reactive fluid (23%, 3/13) were common. In this series, MRI was shown to be more sensitive and accurate than mammography and ultrasound in detecting breast implant rupture or bleed.

The modest MRI specificity noted in most series was predominantly due to pitfalls in imaging interpretation, namely, misinterpreting contour abnormalities and overinterpreting findings within the implant. Knowledge of the type of implant before imaging is crucial for accurate interpretation (Fig. 9-15) because of the possibility of overdiagnosing ruptures in women with complex multi-lumen implants, stacked implants, or a history of previous ruptures (see Table 9-4).

Finally, patients should understand that breast MRI for the diagnosis of implant rupture is not the same as for the diagnosis of breast cancer. Specifically, implant MRI examinations do not use intravenous contrast, which is essential for the diagnosis of breast cancers (Box 9-6).

BREAST RECONSTRUCTION

After mastectomy, the breast may be reconstructed with a tissue expander followed by an implant, autologous tissue, or a combination of the two. Implant reconstruction usually requires placement of a tissue expander at the time of mastectomy and subsequent expansion of the skin to replace the skin removed during mastectomy. At a subsequent surgery the tissue expander is removed and a permanent implant placed. The transverse rectus

---

Box 9-5	Nonspecific Findings on MRI

Water droplets
Reactive fluid around the implant
Bulges in contour
Radial folds (normal finding)

Box 9-6	Reducing False-Positive MRI Studies

Know the history (previous ruptures)
Know the implant type
Beware of cancer

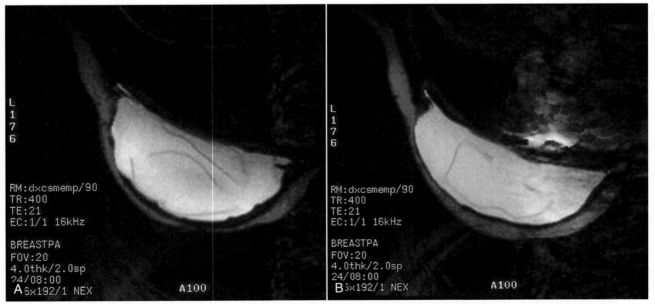

FIGURE 9-15   Complex Silicone-Silicone Double-Lumen Implant Simulating Intracapsular Rupture. Multiple lines simulating the linguine sign are seen in the implant on axial magnetic resonance imaging (MRI) (**A**), but other axial images (**B**) show the multiple lumens in this silicone outer lumen, silicone inner lumen, custom complex implant. This case illustrates the importance of knowing the implant type before MRI interpretation.

abdominis myocutaneous (TRAM) flap remains the most common form of autologous tissue reconstruction, and it may be performed as a pedicle or free flap. Finally, a latissimus dorsi myocutaneous flap with an implant may be used when additional skin is needed to close the wound or additional soft tissue is required. Although other flaps are used for breast reconstruction, these three methods remain the most popular. The reconstructive method selected depends on the patient's goals, medical history, body habitus, physical examination, and potential need for adjuvant therapy.

In the case of subcutaneous mastectomy, the breast tissue is excised with a small shell of tissue left under the skin, and an implant is placed in the cavity. A small amount of breast tissue is left underneath the skin to maintain skin vascularity, and the nipple may or may not be resected. Because of high rates of recurrence, this operation is not routinely performed for cancer treatment or prophylactic prevention of cancer in high-risk patients. In patients undergoing tissue expansion after mastectomy, very little if any breast tissue has been left in the mastectomy site, and the breast is left with little or no glandular tissue to image on mammography. Usually, a saline expander is left in the mastectomy site and gradually enlarged until the space is adequate to hold an appropriately sized implant. Patients with subcutaneous mastectomies or mastectomies with implant placement may undergo mammography if there is enough breast tissue to compress around the implant, but frequently, too little tissue is left to compress for an adequate view of the surrounding breast tissue. Breast cancer recurrences appear as suspicious calcifications or masses when breast tissue is adequately seen.

In the case of TRAM, latissimus dorsi, and free flap reconstructions, fat and muscle are transferred to the mastectomy site with attachments to vascular structures and shaped to form a breast. A nipple can be reconstructed out of skin and tattooed to provide color similar to the contralateral side.

Traditionally, autologous flaps were not imaged by mammography, but mammography can be helpful in evaluating these structures. The most common findings are relative radiolucency centrally, with or without density from muscle fibers around the edges of the area of tissue transfer. Most findings on mammography were consistent with normal fat and muscle within the TRAM or latissimus dorsi flaps (Fig. 9-16A and B). Common mammographic findings included calcifications from fat necrosis, benign dermal calcifications, calcified hematoma, and clustered microcalcifications. Areas of increased or decreased density without calcifications are also identified and appear to be related to post-surgical changes and fat necrosis.

Mammography is a useful diagnostic tool in patients who have undergone TRAM flap breast reconstruction and have suspicious physical findings postoperatively. In a 2001 article by Shaikh et al., breast cancer recurrence in TRAM flaps often occurred as masses that must be distinguished from granulomas or fat necrosis. The diagnosis is usually established by fine-needle aspiration or biopsy. In another study, Helvie et al. found six breast cancers in women undergoing TRAM flap reconstruction; they appeared as four suspicious masses and two suspicious microcalcification clusters.

REDUCTION MAMMAPLASTY

Reduction mammaplasty is performed most commonly for macromastia. Often, a breast reduction or mastopexy (breast lift) is performed to match the "normal" breast to a reconstructed breast or to match a breast that has undergone breast conservation therapy. Reduction mammaplasty and mastopexy are also performed solely for aesthetic purposes. During surgery, skin and breast parenchyma are removed from the breast and the nipple is relocated superiorly. The procedure may be performed in many different fashions. The resulting scar runs around the areola, vertically down to the inframammary fold, and often within the inframammary fold.

The mammogram will have characteristic skin thickening over the lower portions of the breast in the region of the scars, most evident on the mediolateral oblique or mediolateral view. The breast ducts will appear to terminate lower than the replaced nipple because the nipple has been moved to a higher location. The lower portion of the breast will show architectural distortion, and the overall pattern of the lower portion of the breast will be distorted. Depending on the amount of tissue removed from various areas of the breast, the breast parenchymal pattern can be patchy and much different from the pre-reduction mammogram (Figs. 9-17A-D and 9-18).

Reduction mammaplasty or any breast surgery can result in focal fat necrosis or oil cysts that have a characteristic appearance, or they may be atypical and form a palpable mass (Fig. 9-19). Epidermal inclusion cysts can also form in biopsy scars and produce a dense smooth round or oval mass near the skin surface but not connected to it. These masses represent epidermal cells that are displaced into breast tissue during biopsy, after which they grow and form a benign mass. In the case of fat necrosis, breast ultrasound may be helpful, but biopsy may not be avoided at all times.

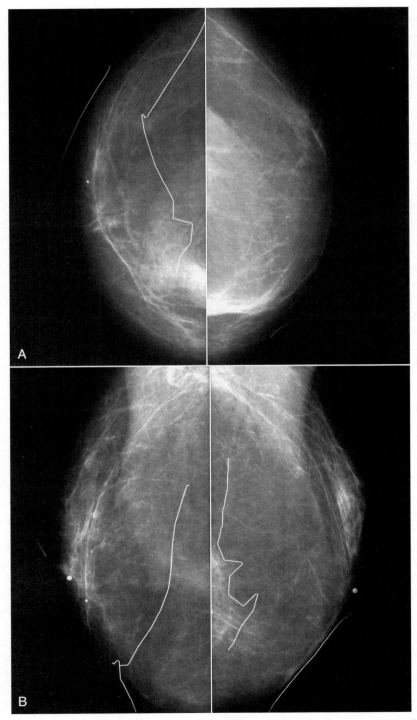

FIGURE 9-16   Transverse Rectus Abdominis Musculocutaneous (TRAM) Flap Reconstruction on Mammography. Craniocaudal (**A**) and mediolateral oblique (**B**) mammograms show fatty tissue and focal density in the breasts reconstructed from abdominal tissue. Note the relative fatty composition of the reconstructed breast and lack of normal glandular elements. Linear metallic scar markers show the location of the scars.

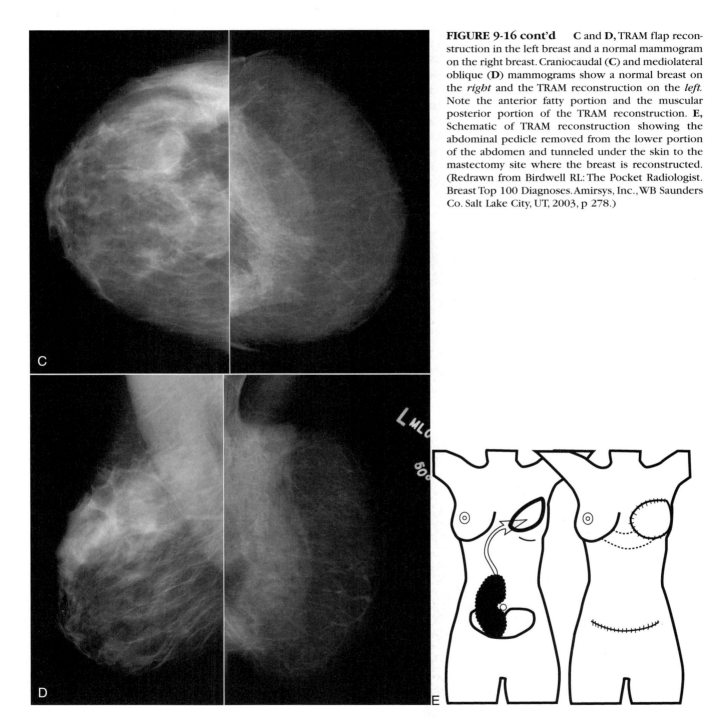

FIGURE 9-16 cont'd   C and **D**, TRAM flap reconstruction in the left breast and a normal mammogram on the right breast. Craniocaudal (**C**) and mediolateral oblique (**D**) mammograms show a normal breast on the *right* and the TRAM reconstruction on the *left*. Note the anterior fatty portion and the muscular posterior portion of the TRAM reconstruction. **E,** Schematic of TRAM reconstruction showing the abdominal pedicle removed from the lower portion of the abdomen and tunneled under the skin to the mastectomy site where the breast is reconstructed. (Redrawn from Birdwell RL: The Pocket Radiologist. Breast Top 100 Diagnoses. Amirsys, Inc., WB Saunders Co. Salt Lake City, UT, 2003, p 278.)

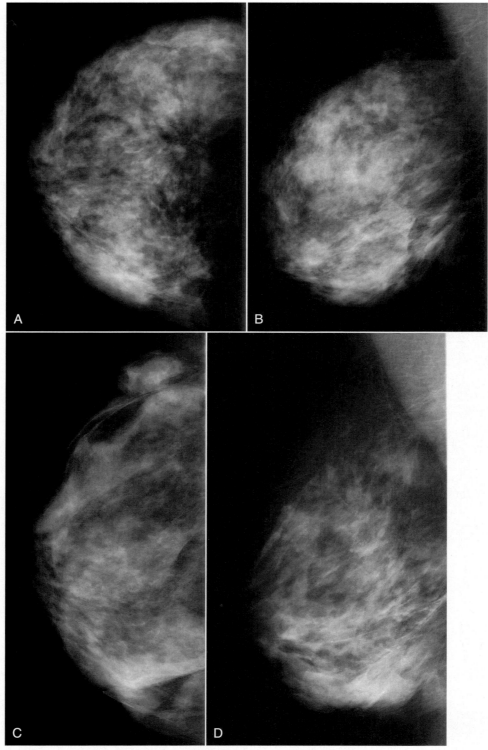

FIGURE 9-17   Reduction Mammaplasty on Mammography. Craniocaudal (**A**) and mediolateral oblique (**B**) mammograms show heterogeneously dense tissue. After reduction mammaplasty, craniocaudal (**C**) and mediolateral oblique (**D**) mammograms show that the breasts are smaller and less dense, with a parenchymal pattern different from that on the previous mammogram. Distortion is apparent in the outer, inner, and lower portions of the breast, and the breast ducts no longer terminate at the reconstructed nipple.

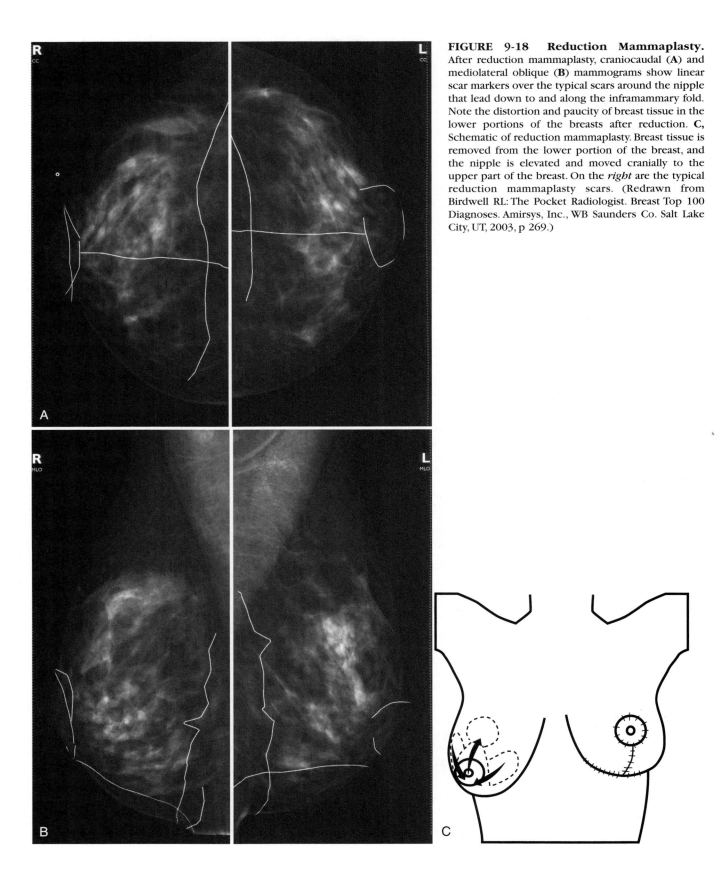

FIGURE 9-18   Reduction Mammaplasty. After reduction mammaplasty, craniocaudal (**A**) and mediolateral oblique (**B**) mammograms show linear scar markers over the typical scars around the nipple that lead down to and along the inframammary fold. Note the distortion and paucity of breast tissue in the lower portions of the breasts after reduction. **C,** Schematic of reduction mammaplasty. Breast tissue is removed from the lower portion of the breast, and the nipple is elevated and moved cranially to the upper part of the breast. On the *right* are the typical reduction mammaplasty scars. (Redrawn from Birdwell RL: The Pocket Radiologist. Breast Top 100 Diagnoses. Amirsys, Inc., WB Saunders Co. Salt Lake City, UT, 2003, p 269.)

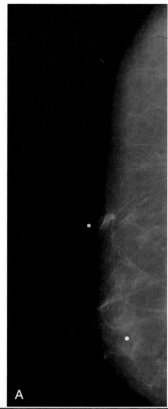

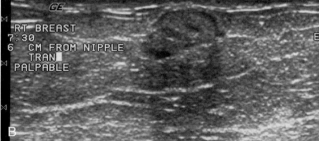

FIGURE 9-19   Fat Necrosis Producing a Mass after Transverse Rectus Abdominis Musculocutaneous (TRAM) Reconstruction. A, A lateral mammogram shows fatty tissue from a TRAM reconstruction with a skin marker over an upper oval equal-density palpable mass. The second skin marker in the lower portion of the breast shows the location of the reconstructed nipple. **B,** Ultrasound shows a hypoechoic mass near the skin surface. The differential diagnosis includes recurrence of cancer, an epidermal inclusion cyst, or fat necrosis. Biopsy showed fat necrosis.

KEY ELEMENTS

No scientific evidence has shown a definite association between silicone breast implants and connective tissue disorders or breast cancer.

In the United States, silicone breast implants are approved for breast reconstruction after mastectomy, and saline implants are approved for breast augmentation.

Breast implants may have single or multiple lumens, each containing silicone or other materials in the different shells.

Implants are placed in subpectoral or subglandular (above the pectoral muscle) locations.

Fibrous capsules form around all implants, sometimes becoming hard or calcified and impairing the implant's look and feel.

Implant complications include rupture, infection, hematoma, and capsular contraction.

Closed capsulotomy, or manual breaking of a hardened fibrous capsule, can result in implant rupture.

Implant rupture is classified as intracapsular (silicone contained in the fibrous capsule) or extracapsular (silicone outside the fibrous capsule).

Symptoms associated with silicone implant rupture are nonspecific and include axillary, breast, or chest wall masses; pain; and changes in breast size, shape, or texture.

Mammography includes standard and implant-displaced craniocaudal and mediolateral or mediolateral oblique views of each breast, for a total of four views of each breast.

About 5% of asymptomatic women have implant ruptures detected on screening mammography.

Extracapsular ruptures appear on mammography as silicone outside the implant in breast tissue, lymph nodes, or ducts or as a deformity in implant contour.

Direct silicone or paraffin injections are used outside the United States for augmentation and cause eggshell-type calcifications or dense masses on mammography, "snowstorm" or "echodense noise" on ultrasound, and hard palpable silicone granuloma masses on physical examination.

Ultrasound of extracapsular rupture shows the "snowstorm" sign or "echodense noise."

Ultrasound of intracapsular rupture shows the "stepladder" sign.

MRI of extracapsular rupture shows blobs of silicone outside the implant and signs of intracapsular rupture.

MRI of intracapsular rupture shows the linguine sign, subcapsular lines, teardrops, or the "keyhole" sign.

Nonspecific findings on MRI are water droplets, reactive fluid, and implant contour abnormalities.

False-positive findings of rupture on ultrasound and MRI are due to intact multiple-lumen implants simulating the stepladder and linguine signs.

False-positive findings of rupture on all imaging methods include previous rupture with implant replacement but without removal of all intraparenchymal silicone.

To avoid false-positive diagnoses of rupture, know the implant type and whether previous rupture and removal of the implant have occurred.

Autologous tissue reconstructions consist of transverse rectus abdominis or latissimus dorsi myocutaneous flaps performed as a pedicle or a free flap.

Mammographic findings of autologous tissue reconstruction include fat and muscle and, commonly, calcifications from fat necrosis and densities from post-surgical changes.

Cancer in reconstructed breasts is often detected by physical examination, with occasional mammographic findings of suspicious masses or calcifications.

Reduction mammaplasty produces a characteristic distortion of the lower portion of the breast and scarring, with relocation of the nipple higher on the breast.

Beware of cancer.

SUGGESTED READINGS

Ahn CY, DeBruhl ND, Gorczyca DP, et al: Comparative silicone breast implant evaluation using mammography, sonography, and magnetic resonance imaging: Experience with 59 implants. Plast Reconstr Surg 94:620-627, 1994.

Ahn CY, Shaw WW, Narayanan K, et al: Residual silicone detection using MRI following previous breast implant removal: Case reports. Aesthetic Plast Surg 19:361-367, 1995.

Baker JL Jr: Augmentation mammaplasty. *In* Owsley JQ Jr, Peterson RA (eds): Symposium on Aesthetic Surgery of the Breast, 1978. St Louis, CV Mosby, 1978.

Beekman WH, Hage JJ, Taets van Amerongen AH, Mulder JW: Accuracy of ultrasonography and magnetic resonance imaging in detecting failure of breast implants filled with silicone gel. Scand J Plast Reconstr Surg Hand Surg 33:415-418, 1999.

Berg WA, Caskey CI, Hamper UM, et al: Diagnosing breast implant rupture with MR imaging, US, and mammography. Radiographics 13:1323-1336, 1993.

Berg WA, Caskey CI, Hamper UM, et al: Single- and double-lumen silicone breast implant integrity: Prospective evaluation of MR and US criteria. Radiology 197:45-52, 1995.

Brown SL, Middleton MS, Berg WA, et al: Prevalence of rupture of silicone gel breast implants revealed on MR imaging in a population of women in Birmingham, Alabama. AJR Am J Roentgenol 175:1057-1064, 2000.

Carlson GW, Moore B, Thornton JF, et al: Breast cancer after augmentation mammaplasty: Treatment by skin-sparing mastectomy and immediate reconstruction. Plast Reconstr Surg 107:687-692, 2001.

Cher DJ, Conwell JA, Mandel JS: MRI for detecting silicone breast implant rupture: Meta-analysis and implications. Ann Plast Surg 47:367-380, 2001.

Chung KC, Wilkins EG, Beil RJ Jr, et al: Diagnosis of silicone gel breast implant rupture by ultrasonography. Plast Reconstr Surg 97:104-109, 1996.

Cicchetti S, Leone MS, Franchelli S, Santi PL: [Evaluation of the tolerability of Hydrogel breast implants: A pilot study.] Minerva Chir 57:53-57, 2002.

Collis N, Coleman D, Foo IT, Sharpe DT: Ten-year review of a prospective randomized controlled trial of textured versus smooth subglandular silicone gel breast implants. Plast Reconstr Surg 106:786-791, 2000.

Collis N, Sharpe DT: Silicone gel-filled breast implant integrity: A retrospective review of 478 consecutively explanted implants. Plast Reconstr Surg 105:1979-1985, discussion 1986-1989, 2000.

Destouet JM, Monsees BS, Oser RF, et al: Screening mammography in 350 women with breast implants: Prevalence and findings of implant complications. AJR Am J Roentgenol 159:973-978, discussion 979-981, 1992.

Eidelman Y, Liebling RW, Buchbinder S, et al: Mammography in the evaluation of masses in breasts reconstructed with TRAM flaps. Ann Plast Surg 41:229-233, 1998.

Eklund GW, Busby RC, Miller SH, Job JS: Improved imaging of the augmented breast. AJR Am J Roentgenol 151:469-473, 1988.

Fajardo LL, Harvey JA, McAleese KA, et al: Breast cancer diagnosis in women with subglandular silicone gel-filled augmentation implants. Radiology 194:859-862, 1995.

Fajardo LL, Roberts CC, Hunt KR: Mammographic surveillance of breast cancer patients: Should the mastectomy site be imaged? AJR Am J Roentgenol 161:953-955, 1993.

Feng LJ, Amini SB: Analysis of risk factors associated with rupture of silicone gel breast implants. Plast Reconstr Surg 104:955-963, 1999.

Ganott MA, Harris KM, Ilkhanipour ZS, Costa-Greco MA: Augmentation mammoplasty: Normal and abnormal findings with mammography and US. Radiographics 12:281-295, 1992.

Gorczyca DP: MR imaging of breast implants. Magn Reson Imaging Clin N Am 2:659-672, 1994.

Gorczyca DP, Schneider E, DeBruhl ND, et al: Silicone breast implant rupture: Comparison between three-point Dixon and fast spin-echo MR imaging. AJR Am J Roentgenol 162:305-310, 1994.

Harris KM, Ganott MA, Shestak KC, et al: Silicone implant rupture: Detection with US. Radiology 187:761-768, 1993.

Hayes MK, Gold RH, Bassett LW: Mammographic findings after the removal of breast implants. AJR Am J Roentgenol 160:487-490, 1993.

Helvie MA, Bailey JE, Roubidoux MA, et al: Mammographic screening of TRAM flap breast reconstructions for detection of nonpalpable recurrent cancer. Radiology 224:211-216, 2002.

Helvie MA, Wilson TE, Roubidoux MA, et al: Mammographic appearance of recurrent breast carcinoma in six patients with TRAM flap breast reconstructions. Radiology 209:711-715, 1998.

Herborn CU, Marincek B, Erfmann D, et al: Breast augmentation and reconstructive surgery: MR imaging of implant rupture and malignancy. Eur Radiol 12:2198-2206, 2002.

Hogge JP, Zuurbier RA, de Paredes ES: Mammography of autologous myocutaneous flaps. Radiographics 19(Spec No):S63-S72, 1999.

Holmich LR, Friis S, Fryzek JP, Vejborg IM, et al: Incidence of silicone breast implant rupture. Arch Surg 138:801-806, 2003.

Hulka BS, Kerkvliet NL, Tugwell P: Experience of a scientific panel formed to advise the federal judiciary on silicone breast implants. N Engl J Med 342:812-815, 2000.

Ikeda DM, Borofsky HB, Herfkens RJ, et al: Silicone breast implant rupture: Pitfalls of magnetic resonance imaging and relative efficacies of magnetic resonance, mammography, and ultrasound. Plast Reconstr Surg 104:2054-2062, 1999.

Janowsky EC, Kupper LL, Hulka BS: Meta-analyses of the relation between silicone breast implants and the risk of connective-tissue diseases. N Engl J Med 342:781-790, 2000.

Kessler DA: The basis of the FDA's decision on breast implants. N Engl J Med 326:1713-1715, 1992.

Kirkpatrick WN, Jones BM: The history of Trilucent implants, and a chemical analysis of the triglyceride filler in 51 consecutively removed Trilucent breast prostheses. Br J Plast Surg 55:479-489, 2002.

Leibman AJ, Kossoff MB, Kruse BD: Intraductal extension of silicone from a ruptured breast implant. Plast Reconstr Surg 89:546-547, 1992.

Marotta JS, Widenhouse CW, Habal MB, Goldberg EP: Silicone gel breast implant failure and frequency of additional surgeries: Analysis of 35 studies reporting examination of more than 8,000 explants. J Biomed Mater Res 48:354-364, 1999.

Mason AC, White CS, McAvoy MA, Goldberg N: MR imaging of slipped stacked breast implants: A potential pitfall in the diagnosis of intracapsular rupture. Magn Reson Imaging 13:339-342, 1995.

Middleton MS: Magnetic resonance evaluation of breast implants and soft-tissue silicone. Top Magn Reson Imaging 9:92-137, 1998.

Mitnick JS, Vazquez MF, Plesser K, Colen SR: "Ductogram" associated with extravasation of silicone from a breast implant. AJR Am J Roentgenol 159:1126-1127, 1992.

Mitnick JS, Vazquez MF, Plesser K, et al: Fine needle aspiration biopsy in patients with augmentation prostheses and a palpable mass. Ann Plast Surg 31:241-244, 1993.

Monticciolo DL, Nelson RC, Dixon WT, et al: MR detection of leakage from silicone breast implants: Value of a silicone-selective pulse sequence. AJR Am J Roentgenol 163:51-56, 1994.

Monticciolo DL, Ross D, Bostwick J 3rd, et al: Autologous breast reconstruction with endoscopic latissimus dorsi musculosub-cutaneous flaps in patients choosing breast-conserving therapy: Mammographic appearance. AJR Am J Roentgenol 167:385-389, 1996.

Mund DF, Wolfson P, Gorczyca DP, et al: Mammographically detected recurrent nonpalpable carcinoma developing in a transverse rectus abdominis myocutaneous flap. A case report. Cancer 74:2804-2807, 1994.

Munker R, Zorner C, McKiernan D, Opitz J: Prospective study of clinical findings and changes in 56 Trilucent implant explantations. Aesthetic Plast Surg 25:421-426, 2001.

Muzaffar AR, Rohrich RJ: The silicone gel–filled breast implant controversy: An update. Plast Reconstr Surg 109:742-747, quiz 748, 2002.

Palmon LU, Foshager MC, Parantainen H, et al: Ruptured or intact: What can linear echoes within silicone breast implants tell us? AJR Am J Roentgenol 168:1595-1598, 1997.

Piza-Katzer H, Pulzl P, Balogh B, Wechselberger G: Long-term results of MISTI gold breast implants: A retrospective study. Plast Reconstr Surg 110:1425-1429, discussion 1460-1465, 2002.

Rieber A, Schramm K, Helms G, et al: Breast-conserving surgery and autogenous tissue reconstruction in patients with breast cancer: Efficacy of MRI of the breast in the detection of recurrent disease. Eur Radiol 13:780-787, 2003.

Rivero MA, Schwartz DS, Mies C: Silicone lymphadenopathy involving intramammary lymph nodes: A new complication of silicone mammaplasty. AJR Am J Roentgenol 162:1089-1090, 1994.

Rizkalla M, Duncan C, Matthews RN: Trilucent breast implants: A 3 year series. Br J Plast Surg 54:125-127, 2001.

Rizkalla M, Webb J, Chuo CB, Matthews RN: Experience of explantation of Trilucent breast implants. Br J Plast Surg 55:117-119, 2002.

Rosculet KA, Ikeda DM, Forrest ME, et al: Ruptured gel-filled silicone breast implants: Sonographic findings in 19 cases. AJR Am J Roentgenol 159:711-716, 1992.

Shaikh N, LaTrenta G, Swistel A, Osborne FM: Detection of recurrent breast cancer after TRAM flap reconstruction. Ann Plast Surg 47:602-607, 2001.

Silverstein MJ, Handel N, Gamagami P: The effect of silicone-gel–filled implants on mammography. Cancer 68(Suppl): 1159-1163, 1991.

Silverstein MJ, Handel N, Gamagami P, et al: Mammographic measurements before and after augmentation mammaplasty. Plast Reconstr Surg 86:1126-1130, 1990.

Soo MS, Kornguth PJ, Walsh R, et al: Intracapsular implant rupture: MR findings of incomplete shell collapse. J Magn Reson Imaging 7:724-730, 1997.

Spear SL, Mardini S: Alternative filler materials and new implant designs: What's available and what's on the horizon? Clin Plast Surg 28:435-443, 2001.

Stewart NR, Monsees BS, Destouet JM, Rudloff MA: Mammographic appearance following implant removal. Radiology 185:83-85, 1992.

Tugwell P, Wells G, Peterson J, et al: Do silicone breast implants cause rheumatologic disorders? A systematic review for a court-appointed national science panel. Arthritis Rheum 44:2477-2484, 2001.

Young VL, Bartell T, Destouet JM, et al: Calcification of breast implant capsule. South Med J 82:1171-1173, 1989.

Young V, Watson M: Breast implant research: Where we have been, where we are, where we need to go. Clin Plast Surg 28:451-483, 2001.

Clinical Breast Problems and Unusual Breast Conditions

Introduction
The Male Breast: Gynecomastia and Breast Cancer
Pregnant Patients and Pregnancy-Associated Breast Cancer
Probably Benign Finding (BI-RADS Category 3)
Nipple Discharge and Galactography
Breast Edema
Hormone Changes
Breast Pain
Axillary Lymphadenopathy
Paget's Disease of the Nipple
Sarcomas
Mondor's Disease
Granulomatous Mastitis
Diabetic Mastopathy
Desmoid Tumor
Trichinosis
Dermatomyositis
Foreign Bodies
Hidradenitis Suppurativa
Neurofibromatosis
Breast Cancer Missed by Mammography
Key Elements

INTRODUCTION

Various breast symptoms and clinical problems are encountered in both benign breast conditions and breast cancer. This chapter will briefly describe these conditions and elucidate how to distinguish them from malignancy.

THE MALE BREAST: GYNECOMASTIA AND MALE BREAST CANCER

The incidence of breast cancer in males is less than 1% of all breast cancers and less than 1% of all male cancers in the United States. Male breast patients seek clinical attention for unilateral or bilateral breast enlargement, breast pain, or a breast lump. Most of these complaints are related to benign gynecomastia and are not due to breast cancer. Gynecomastia is an abnormal proliferation of benign ducts and supporting tissue that causes breast enlargement or a subareolar mass, with or without associated breast pain. It is reversible in its early stages if the cause of the gynecomastia is corrected. Unchecked, the reversible phase of gynecomastia progresses to late periductal edema with irreversible stromal fibrosis.

Broad categories of conditions causing gynecomastia include high estrogen serum levels from endogenous or exogenous sources, low serum testosterone levels, endocrine disorders (hyperthyroidism or hypothyroidism), systemic disorders (cirrhosis, chronic renal failure with maintenance by dialysis, chronic obstructive pulmonary disease), drug induced (cimetidine, spironolactone, ergotamine, marijuana, anabolic steroids, estrogen for prostate cancer), tumors (adrenal carcinoma, testicular tumors, pituitary adenoma), or idiopathic (Box 10-1). Gynecomastia can occur at any age, but it may be seen in particular in neonates as a result of maternal estrogens circulating to the fetus through the placenta, in healthy adolescent boys 1 year after the onset of puberty because of high estradiol levels, or in older men as a result of decreasing serum testosterone levels.

The normal male breast contains major breast ducts only and otherwise has mostly fatty tissue. Under a stimulus producing gynecomastia, breast enlargement occurs as a result of ductal proliferation and stromal hyperplasia, occasionally accompanied by ductal multiplication and elongation, which may be reversible in the active phase if the stimulus is removed. If the stimulus persists, irreversible stromal fibrosis and ductal epithelial atrophy develop, and the breast enlargement may decrease but not completely resolve. Pseudogynecomastia is a fatty proliferation of the breasts without proliferation

Box 10-1 Causes of Gynecomastia			
PHYSIOLOGIC	**DRUG RELATED**	**HORMONAL**	**TUMORS**
Liver disease	Sertraline (Zoloft)	Neonates	Lung
Renal failure	Marijuana	Adolescence	Pituitary
Chronic obstructive pulmonary disease	Tricyclic antidepressants	Older men	Adrenal
Diabetes	Cimetidine	Estrogen therapy	Hepatoma
Hyperthyroidism	Spironolactone	Testicular failure	Testicular
Hypothyroidism	Reserpine	Klinefelter's syndrome	
Starvation/refeeding	Digitalis	Hypogonadism	

of glandular tissue that simulates gynecomastia clinically, but unlike true gynecomastia, proliferation of glandular breast tissue does not occur.

Mammography is performed in men in the same fashion as in women. On the mammogram, the normal male breast consists of fat without obvious fibroglandular tissue, and the pectoralis muscles are usually larger than in women. Both pseudogynecomastia and women with Turner's syndrome have mammograms consisting of mostly fat, similar to the normal male breast.

On the mammogram, gynecomastia is shown as glandular tissue in the subareolar region that is symmetrical or asymmetric, unilateral or bilateral. In a large series by Gunhan-Bilgen et al., gynecomastia was unilateral in 45% and bilateral in 55% of 206 cases on mammograms. In the early phases of gynecomastia, the glandular tissue takes on a flame-like "dendritic" appearance consisting of thin strands of glandular tissue extending from the nipple, similar to fingers extending posteriorly toward the chest wall (Fig. 10-1A-D) (Table 10-1). With continued proliferation of breast ducts, the glandular tissue takes on a triangular "nodular" shape behind the nipple in the subareolar region (Fig. 10-2). If the etiology of the gynecomastia is not eliminated, the proliferation may progress to the appearance of diffuse dense tissue in the later stromal fibrotic phase that is irreversible (Fig. 10-3). On ultrasound, gynecomastia shows hypoechoic flame-like, finger-like, or triangular structures extending posteriorly toward the chest wall from the nipple (Fig. 10-4). Pseudo-gynecomastia shows only fatty tissue on the mammogram and is distinguished from gynecomastia by the absence of glandular tissue.

Male breast cancer accounts for less than 1% of all cancers found in men and is usually diagnosed at or around 60 years of age, older than the mean age for the diagnosis of breast cancer in women (Box 10-2). Male breast cancer has the same prognosis as breast cancer in women, but it is often detected at a higher stage than in women because of delay in diagnosis, and up to 50% of men have axillary adenopathy at initial evaluation. Risk factors include Klinefelter's syndrome, high estrogen

levels such as from prostate cancer treatment, and the development of mumps orchitis at an older age. Male breast cancer is generally manifested as a hard, painless, subareolar mass eccentric to the nipple. When not subareolar, cancers in men are usually found in the upper outer quadrant. Clinical symptoms of nipple discharge or ulceration are not rare in association with male breast cancer.

On mammography, male breast cancers are generally dense noncalcified masses with variable border patterns located in the subareolar region, and they are not usually calcified (Figs. 10-5 and 10-6). On ultrasound, male breast cancers are described as masses with well-circumscribed or irregular borders. Concomitant findings of skin thickening, adenopathy, and skin ulceration are associated with a poor prognosis. Breast cancers in men have the histologic appearance of invasive ductal cancer in 85% of cases, with most of the remaining tumors being medullary, papillary, and intracystic papillary tumors. Invasive lobular carcinoma is rare. Treatment of breast cancer is the same for men as for women and consists of surgery, axillary node dissection, chemotherapy, radiation therapy for invasive tumors, or any combination of these treatments, and the prognosis is identical.

PREGNANT PATIENTS AND PREGNANCY-ASSOCIATED BREAST CANCER

Pregnancy produces a proliferation of glandular breast tissue that results in breast enlargement and nodularity; rarely, the condition progresses to gigantomastia or enlargement of multiple fibroadenomas. Breast masses are difficult to manage in a pregnant patient because the surrounding breast nodularity and size increase over time. Most masses occurring in pregnancy are benign and include benign lactational adenomas, fibroadenomas, galactoceles, or abscesses (Box 10-3), but the diagnosis of exclusion is pregnancy-associated breast cancer.

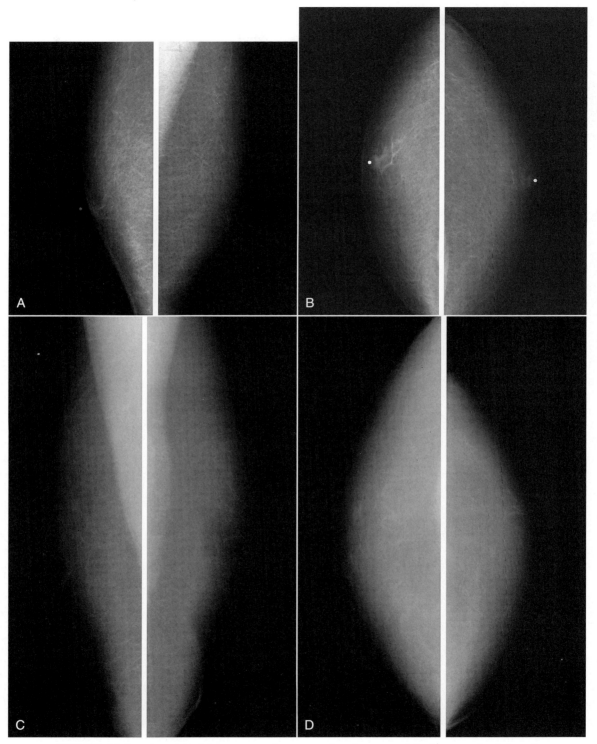

FIGURE 10-1   **A** and **B,** Mammograms in a man showing normal findings on the left and gynecomastia on the right. Craniocaudal (CC) (**A**) and mediolateral oblique (MLO) (**B**) mammograms show flame-like strands of glandular tissue from gynecomastia in the subareolar portion of the right breast and the normal fatty appearance of breast tissue seen in men on the left. **C** and **D,** Turner's syndrome. MLO (**C**) and CC (**D**) views show mostly fatty tissue, similar to the normal male breast in this female patient with Turner's syndrome.

Table 10-1   Mammographic Appearance of Gynecomastia

Type	Mammography	Gynecomastia
Normal	Fatty breast	N/A
Pseudogynecomastia	Fatty breast	N/A
Dendritic	Prominent radiating extensions	Epithelial hyperplasia
Nodular	Fan-shaped triangular density	Later phase
Diffuse	Diffuse density	Dense fibrotic phase

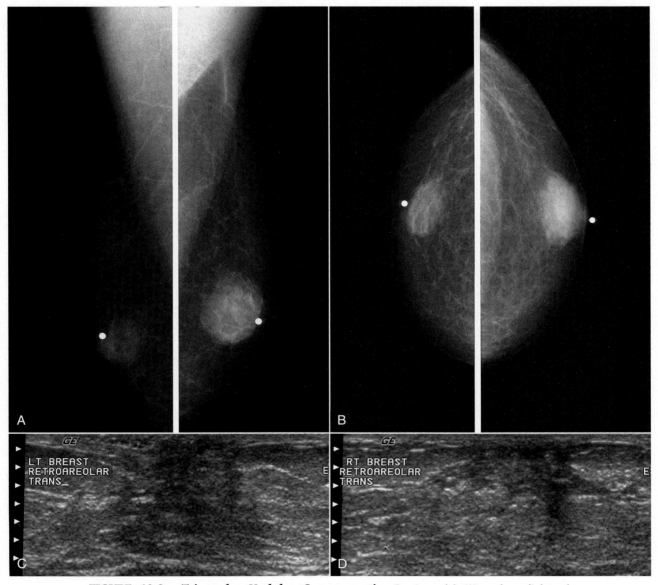

FIGURE 10-2   Triangular Nodular Gynecomastia. Craniocaudal (**A**) and mediolateral oblique (**B**) mammograms show triangular, focally dense breast tissue behind the nipple. Ultrasound of the left (**C**) and right (**D**) breast shows hypoechoic dark strands of tissue extending from the nipple in a finger-like triangular distribution in this male with gynecomastia.

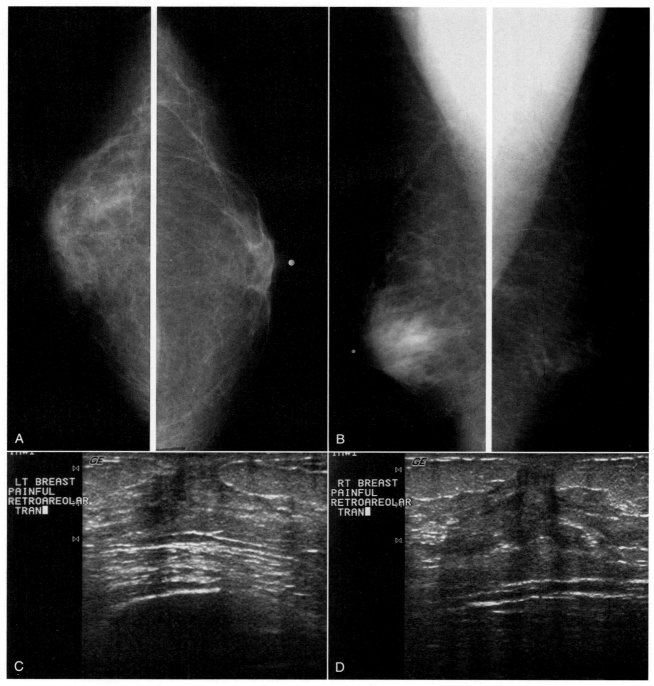

FIGURE 10-3   Diffuse Gynecomastia. Craniocaudal (**A**) and mediolateral oblique (**B**) mammograms show triangular, focally dense breast tissue behind the nipple. Ultrasound of the left (**C**) and right (**D**) breast reveals hypoechoic dark triangular strands of tissue extending down from the nipple.

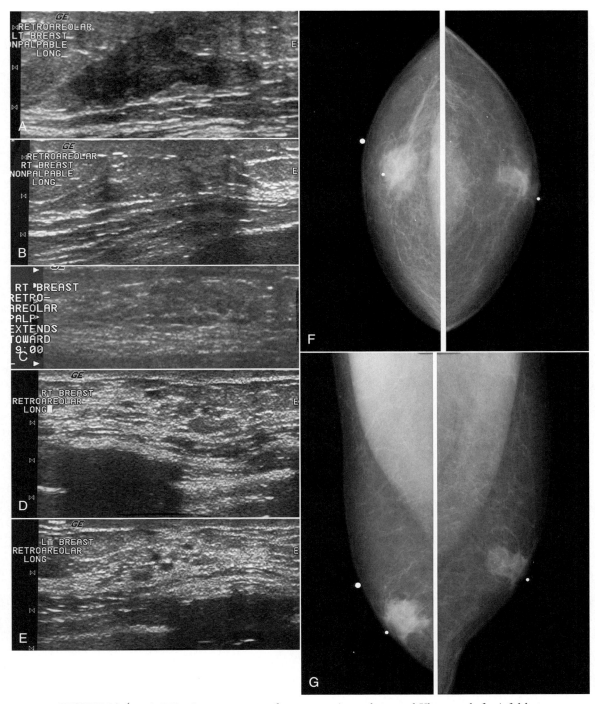

FIGURE 10-4   **A-C,** Varying appearance of gynecomastia on ultrasound. Ultrasound of painful, but nonpalpable left gynecomastia (**A**) shows a triangle of hypoechoic tissue extending to the chest wall from the nipple. The right breast (**B**) is thinner and has a normal appearance. Gynecomastia in another patient has fewer hypoechoic ducts (**C**). **D-G,** Bilateral gynecomastia in another patient with few hypoechoic ducts and echogenic retroareolar glandular tissue in the right (**D**) and left (**E**) subareolar regions. Corresponding craniocaudal (**F**) and mediolateral (**G**) mammograms show dense triangular retroareolar gynecomastia and a marker on an upper right breast lipoma.

Pregnancy-associated cancer is defined as breast cancer discovered during pregnancy or within 1 year of delivery (Box 10-4). The incidence of breast cancer in pregnant women is 0.2% to 3.8% of all breast cancers, or 1 in every 3000 to 10,000 pregnancies. Most pregnancy-associated breast cancers are invasive ductal cancer. These cancers are generally manifested as a hard mass, but they may be associated with bloody nipple discharge or findings of breast edema. The usual initial imaging test in a pregnant patient is breast ultrasound. Many patients are reluctant to undergo mammography because of concern about the effect of radiation on the fetus. However, if cancer is a clinical concern, it is important to perform mammography to make the diagnosis and in particular to detect the presence of suspicious nonpalpable pleomorphic calcifications. The amount of

scattered radiation delivered to the fetus is minimal and can be further reduced with lead shielding. Swinford et al. showed that breast density on mammography ranges from scattered fibroglandular density in pregnant patients to heterogeneously dense or dense breasts in a lactating patient. In their series, mammography was as useful as it is in nonpregnant women with clinical signs and symptoms of breast disease. In lactating patients, breast density can be reduced on the mammogram by pumping milk from the breasts before the study.

Mammographic findings of pregnancy-associated breast cancer were present in 78% of 23 pregnant women reported by Liberman et al. and in 86% of 15 cases reported by Ahn et al. Mammograms showed masses, pleomorphic calcifications (or both masses and calcifications), asymmetric density, or breast edema, but occasionally they were negative because of dense breast tissue. Axillary lymphadenopathy, asymmetric density, and skin or trabecular thickening have been reported as primary or associated findings. In both series, ultrasound was positive in all cases in which it was performed and showed irregular solid masses with irregular margins. In Ahn and colleagues' series, four masses also contained "complex echo patterns" or cystic components, and most showed acoustic enhancement.

Magnetic resonance imaging (MRI) of a normal lactating breast shows dense, enhancing, diffuse glandular tissue and widespread high signal throughout the tissue on T2-weighted images. Breast cancer in a lactating breast on MRI shows higher signal intensity in the initial

Box 10-2	Male Breast Cancer

Average age, 60 years old
Hard painless subareolar mass
Mass eccentric to the nipple or upper outer quadrant
Nipple discharge or ulceration not uncommon
Noncalcified round mass, variable border
Cancer usually ductal in origin
Treatment and prognosis identical to women's cancers

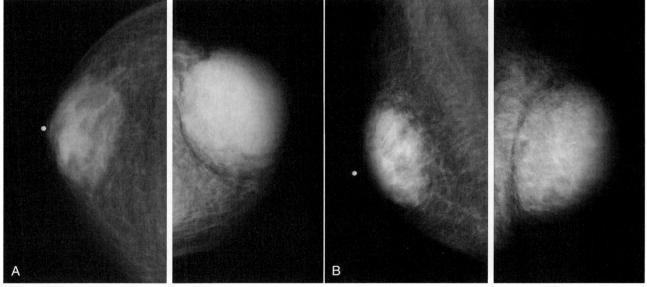

FIGURE 10-5   Male Breast Cancer. In a patient with a palpable mass in the retroareolar region of the left breast, diffuse bilateral gynecomastia with a large oval left retroareolar mass is apparent on craniocaudal (**A**) and mediolateral oblique (**B**) mammograms. Ultrasound-guided fine-needle aspiration of a portion of the mass showed invasive ductal cancer.

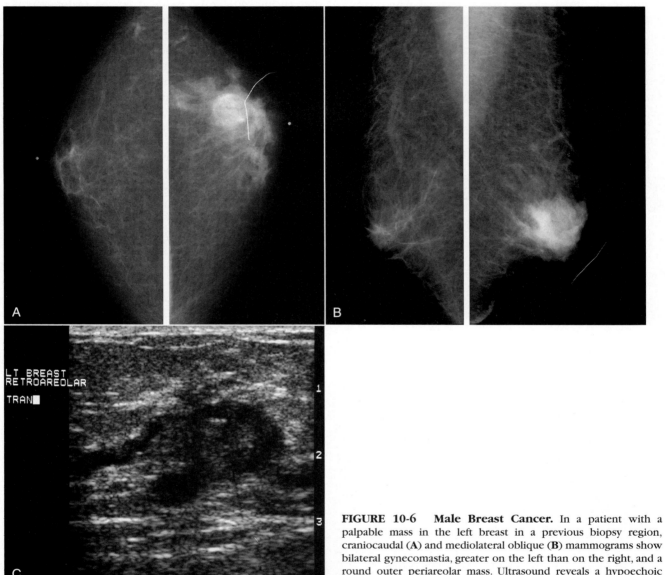

FIGURE 10-6   Male Breast Cancer. In a patient with a palpable mass in the left breast in a previous biopsy region, craniocaudal (**A**) and mediolateral oblique (**B**) mammograms show bilateral gynecomastia, greater on the left than on the right, and a round outer periareolar mass. Ultrasound reveals a hypoechoic mass (**C**) that was diagnosed as invasive ductal cancer.

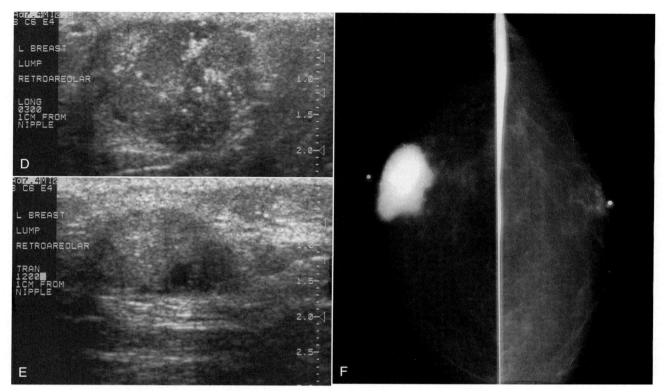

FIGURE 10-6 cont'd Longitudinal (**D**) and transverse (**E**) ultrasound scans in a man with a palpable round mass show a hypoechoic oval mass containing calcifications, with suspicious microcalcifications detected in the left breast on mammography (**F**). Invasive ductal cancer was diagnosed.

Box 10-3	Pregnancy and Lactational Breast Problems

Growing fibroadenoma (rare)
Lactational adenoma (rare)
Cancer (rare)
Mastitis/abscess (common)
Galactocele (uncommon)
Benign bloody nipple discharge (uncommon)

Box 10-4	Pregnancy-Associated Cancer

Cancer diagnosed during pregnancy or within 1 year postpartum
Stage for stage, same prognosis as in nonpregnant patients
Mammography and ultrasound are indicated
Chemotherapy possible after the second trimester
Radiation therapy is an absolute contraindication

enhancement phase than in the surrounding lactational breast tissue, with a washout or plateau in the late phases in the rare reported cases in the radiology literature.

Pregnancy-associated breast cancers have a prognosis similar to that in nonpregnant women when matched for age and stage. In pregnancy, diagnostic delays may cause the diagnosis of breast cancer to be detected at a later stage, thereby leading to a worse prognosis. Modified radical mastectomy was the usual treatment for pregnant women, but more recently, breast-conserving surgery is becoming more common. Chemotherapy has been used

in women after the first trimester. Pregnancy is an absolute contraindication for radiation therapy.

Benign conditions are the most frequent cause of breast masses in pregnant or lactating patients, and cancer is much less common. Both benign fibroadenomas and lactating adenomas are solid tumors diagnosed during pregnancy. Growth of preexisting fibroadenomas may be stimulated by elevated hormone levels, and the fibroadenoma may become clinically apparent. Infarction of fibroadenomas has been reported in the literature during pregnancy as well.

Another benign tumor diagnosed during pregnancy is lactating adenoma, which is a well-circumscribed lobulated mass containing distended tubules with an epithelial lining. Lactating adenoma is a firm painless mass that occurs late in pregnancy or during lactation. The mass can enlarge rapidly and regresses after cessation of lactation. Ultrasound typically shows an oval, well-defined hypoechoic mass that may contain echogenic bands representing the fibrotic bands seen on pathology. Whether lactating adenoma represents change stimulated by hormonal alterations in a fibroadenoma or tubular adenoma or whether the tumors arise de novo has not been resolved.

Sampling of solid masses for histologic examination in a pregnant or lactating patient can be accomplished by either percutaneous core biopsy or surgery. Milk fistula produced by damage to the breast ducts is a known, but uncommon complication of surgery or percutaneous large-core needle biopsy in women in the third trimester of pregnancy or those who are lactating.

Lactational mastitis is a common complication of nursing in which the breast becomes painful, indurated, and tender, usually as a result of *Staphylococcus aureus* infection. A cracked nipple may be the port of entry for the infecting bacteria, but it can be prevented by good nipple hygiene and care, along with frequent nursing to avoid breast engorgement. Treatment is administration of antibiotics and cessation of nursing. On occasion, antibiotic therapy is not sufficient to treat mastitis. If a hot, swollen, painful breast does not respond to antibiotics, ultrasound may identify an abscess that can be treated either by percutaneous drainage if small or by percutaneous palliative drainage until operative methods can be performed. On mammography, an abscess is a developing density or mass seen against a background of breast edema; it does not usually contain gas and is frequently located in the subareolar region (Fig. 10-7A and B). On ultrasound, abscesses are fluid-filled structures with irregular borders in the early phase, but later, well-circumscribed borders develop as the walls of the abscess form. The abscess may contain debris or multiple septations, which may be drained under ultrasound guidance, but some residua may remain because of thick debris (Fig. 10-7C and D). Some authors suggest aspiration, irrigation, and instillation of antibiotics directly into the abscess cavity to aid in resolution of the abscess.

A galactocele produces a fluid-filled breast mass that can mimic benign or malignant solid breast masses. On mammography, a galactocele is a round or oval, well-circumscribed equal- or low-density mass (Fig. 10-8A and B). Because a galactocele is filled with milk, the creamy portions of the milk may rise to the nondependent part of the galactocele and produce a rare, but pathognomonic fluid-fluid or fat-fluid appearance on the horizontal beam image (lateral-medial view) at mammography. Ultrasound shows a fluid-filled mass that can have a wide range of sonographic appearances, depending on the relative amount of fluid and solid milk components within it. Galactoceles that are mostly fluid filled have well-defined borders with thin echogenic walls. Galactoceles containing more solid components of milk show variable findings ranging from homogeneous medium-level echoes to heterogeneous contents with fluid clefts. Both distal acoustic enhancement and acoustic shadowing are seen. The diagnosis is made by an appropriate history of childbirth and lactation, with aspiration yielding milky fluid and leading to resolution of the mass. Aspiration is usually therapeutic.

PROBABLY BENIGN FINDINGS (BI-RADS CATEGORY 3)

Mammography detects small cancers, but it can also uncover nonpalpable benign-appearing lesions indeterminate for malignancy. Fine-detail films and ultrasound in appropriate cases show that some indeterminate findings are typically benign and the patient can therefore resume screening. Other findings have a low probability (<2%) of malignancy after an appropriate work-up that serves as a baseline for follow-up studies (Box 10-5). Sickles, Varas, and Yasmeen and their colleagues have independently provided data that Breast Imaging Reporting and Database System (BI-RADS) category 3, or "probably benign" findings, has a less than 2% chance of malignancy; category 3 was found in 5%, 3%, and 5% of all screening studies after recall in their series, respectively. Probably benign findings in their series included single or multiple clusters of small, round or oval calcifications; single or multiple, bilateral, nonpalpable and noncalcified, round or lobulated, primarily circumscribed solid masses; or nonpalpable focal asymmetries containing interspersed fat and concave scalloped margins that resemble fibroglandular tissue at diagnostic evaluation (Fig. 10-9A-F). Importantly, the asymmetries should contain no masses, distorted architecture, or suspicious calcifications. Probably benign findings are often detected on an initial screening mammogram without comparison films and are managed by short-term mammographic follow-up after recall from screening and a full mammographic and ultrasound work-up.

The 6-month mammographic follow-up serves as an alternative to core or surgical biopsy for probably benign findings, with subsequent yearly follow-up for 2 to 3 years. Because the average breast cancer has a tumor volume doubling time of 100 days, a change should be detected in 2 to 3 years. However, probably benign breast lesions are selected on the basis that they will most likely *not* change in the time interval. Lesions in which change is expected should undergo biopsy.

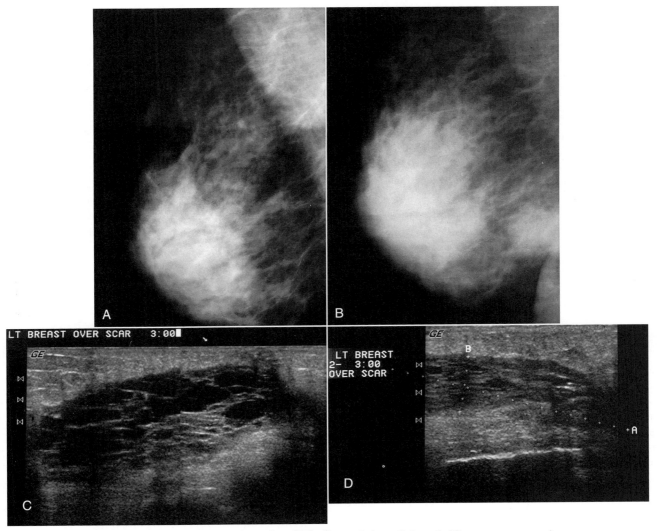

FIGURE 10-7   Pregnancy-Associated Findings. A, A mediolateral oblique mammogram in a lactating patient shows dense tissue. After the development of mastitis and a lump near the chest wall, the mammogram shows a developing density representing an abscess near the chest wall (**B**). **C,** Ultrasound in a patient with a post-surgical abscess shows a 6.5-cm mass with debris and loculated fluid collections. After aspiration of 35 mL of serosanguineous infected fluid through a 14-gauge needle, debris still remains within the abscess along with a few fluid loculations (**D**).

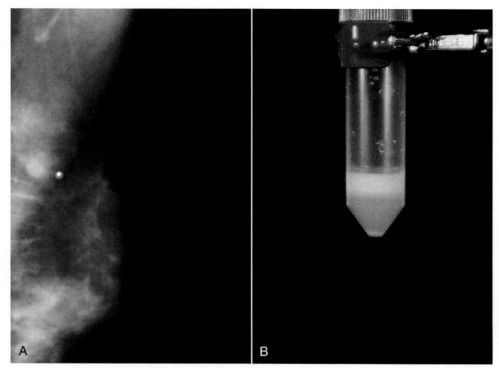

FIGURE 10-8   Galactocele. A mediolateral oblique mammogram in a lactating patient with a marker over a palpable mass shows a low-density mass in the upper portion of the left breast (**A**). Aspiration produced milky fluid with a fat-fluid level (**B**).

Box 10-5   Probably Benign Findings (BI-RADS Category 3)

Nonpalpable findings
<2% chance of malignancy
Found in 5% of all screening cases after recall and diagnostic work-up
Clustered small round or oval calcifications at magnification mammography
Noncalcified oval or lobulated, primarily well-circumscribed solid masses
Asymmetric densities resembling fibroglandular tissue at diagnostic evaluation

From Rosen EL, Baker JA, Soo MS: Malignant lesions initially subjected to short-term mammographic follow-up. Radiology 223:221-228, 2002.

Other criteria for inclusion in the probably benign category include a lesion that is nonpalpable and easy to visualize and classify and a patient who is likely to complete the follow-up regimen. Criteria that may exclude patients from short-term follow-up include extreme anxiety affecting the patient's quality of life, pregnancy or planned pregnancy, or a likelihood of non-compliance with follow-up.

Rosen et al. reviewed the findings of cancers initially subjected to short-term follow-up to identify imaging criteria that should exclude categorization into the "probably benign" classification. Their series of cancers that were mistakenly classified in the "probably benign" category included palpable findings, developing densities,

architectural distortion, irregular spiculated masses, growing masses, pleomorphic calcifications, work-ups showing motion blur on magnification, or lesion progression of any type since the previous mammogram. Their study underscores the reasoning why the "probably benign" classification is reserved only for nonpalpable lesions that fulfill the diagnostic criteria for category 3 after optimal work-up.

Despite the use of these strict criteria, a small number of cancers invariably emerge from category 3 lesions. In Varas and associates' series, 0.4% of cases were initially classified as "probably benign" but were determined to be cancer at subsequent biopsy. These cancers were stage 1 or less, with a favorable prognosis, similar to

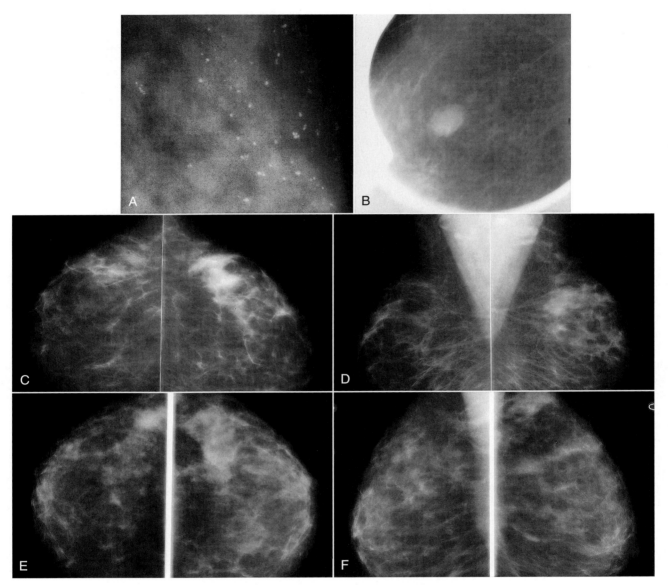

FIGURE 10-9   Probably Benign Findings on Mammography. Findings included scattered and clustered, round punctate, sharply demarcated calcifications (**A**) and a nonpalpable, round, well-circumscribed solid mass (**B**). **C-F,** Asymmetries. Craniocaudal (CC) (**C**) and mediolateral oblique (MLO) (**D**) views show global asymmetry consisting of a nonpalpable greater volume of tissue in the upper outer portion of the left breast than in the right. In another patient, a focal asymmetry resembling fibroglandular tissue is seen in the upper part of the left breast on the CC (**E**) and MLO (**F**) views.

Table 10-2	Nipple Discharge

Color	Cause
Clear or creamy	Duct ectasia
Green, white, blue, black	Cysts, duct ectasia
Milky	Physiologic (neonatal)
	Endocrine (lactation/post-lactation, pregnancy)
	Tumor (prolactinoma or other prolactin-producing tumor)
	Mechanical
	Drugs (dopamine receptor blockers/dopamine-depleting drugs)
Bloody or blood related	Hyperplasia
	Papilloma
	Ductal carcinoma in situ
	Pregnancy

Table 10-3	Imaging of Nipple Discharge

Mammography	Negative (common)
	Dilated duct
	Mass with or without calcifications (papilloma or cancer)
Ultrasound	Negative (common)
	Fluid-filled ducts (normal or pathologic)
	Intraductal mass (papilloma, cancer, debris)
Galactogram	Filling defect (papilloma, cancer, air bubble, debris)
	Duct ectasia or cysts
Magnetic resonance imaging	Fluid in dilated ducts
	Enhancing mass (cancer, papilloma)
	Negative

cancers detected in their mammographic screening series.

The probably benign category was based on imaging features and longitudinal data derived from mammography, which is a well-established imaging modality that has published standards for the acquisition of images, qualifications of personnel, and criteria for interpretation. In clinical practice, the probably benign category has been used with ultrasound and MRI. However, no specific image criteria, definition of lesions, or longitudinal data that are comparable to mammographic studies have been established for ultrasound or MRI.

NIPPLE DISCHARGE AND GALACTOGRAPHY

Nipple discharge is a common reason for women to seek medical advice. Benign nipple discharge usually arises from multiple ducts, whereas nipple discharge from a papilloma or ductal carcinoma in situ usually occurs from a single duct. Nipple discharge is of particular concern if it is spontaneous and from a single duct or if the discharge is bloody. Women may describe intermittent discharge producing tiny stains on their brassiere or nightgown, or they may be able to elicit the discharge themselves. Some women seek imaging after positive findings from ductal lavage in conjunction with an abnormal cytologic evaluation.

The most frequent causes of both nonbloody and bloody nipple discharge are benign conditions. The most common mass producing a bloody nipple discharge is a benign intraductal papilloma, with only approximately 5% of women found to have malignancy at biopsy. The bloody nipple discharge associated with papillomas is due to twisting of the papilloma on its fibrovascular stalk and subsequent infarction and bleeding. Other causes of bloody discharge are cancer, benign findings such as duct hyperplasia/ectasia, and pregnancy as a result of rapidly proliferating breast tissue. Causes of nonbloody nipple discharge are fibrocystic change, medications acting as dopamine receptor blockers or dopamine-depleting drugs, rapid breast growth during adolescence, chronic nipple squeezing, or tumors producing prolactin or prolactin-like substances (Table 10-2).

Papillomas are benign masses that consist of a fibrovascular stalk with an attachment to the wall and breast duct epithelium; they have a variable cellular pattern and can produce nipple discharge. Papillomas may be single or multiple and may extend along the ducts for quite a distance. When large, papillomas can appear to be encysted and multilobulated. Some pathologists support the theory that peripheral papillomas have an increased risk for the subsequent development of carcinoma, whereas solitary or central papillomas do not. Peripheral papillomas are associated with epithelial proliferation, which may have atypical features, thus raising the possibility that atypia within a peripheral papilloma increases the risk of malignancy rather than the location of the papilloma itself.

The mammogram is frequently negative in the setting of nipple discharge (Table 10-3). Mammographic findings described in association with papillomas include a negative mammogram, a single dilated duct in isolation, or a small mass containing calcifications in either papilloma or malignancy (Fig. 10-10A-D). Ultrasound is frequently negative in women with nipple discharge, or fluid-filled dilated ducts without an intraductal mass in

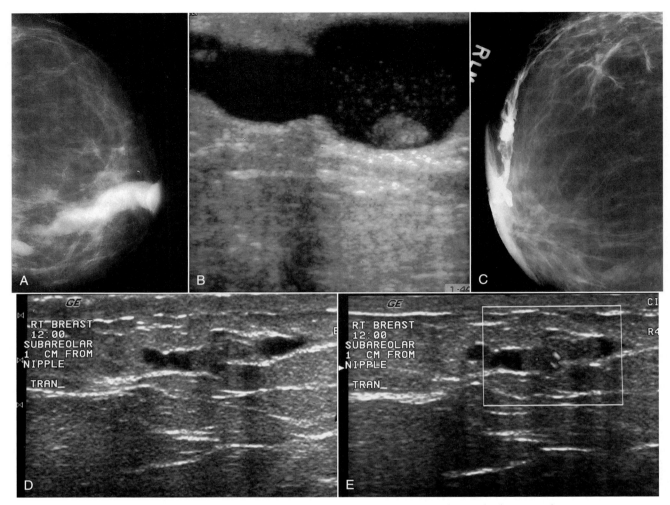

FIGURE 10-10   Papilloma in a Dilated Duct on Mammography and Ultrasound. The mammogram shows a markedly dilated duct (without contrast) extending into the breast from the nipple (**A**). Ultrasound revealed a fluid-filled dilated duct containing a mass that was found to be a papilloma on biopsy (**B**). A papilloma in a contrast-filled duct in another patient has a filling defect (**C**), and ultrasound shows the papilloma as a solid mass surrounded by the distended, contrast-filled duct (**D**). A blood vessel is seen in its fibrovascular component on color Doppler (**E**).

the retroareolar region may be seen (Fig. 10-11A and B). Solid masses in a fluid-filled duct may represent debris, a papilloma, or cancer.

Galactography is used to investigate single-duct nipple discharge, and when positive, it is helpful in subsequent surgical planning by identifying filling defects and their location and distance from the nipple. Galactography may also show normal duct anatomy, duct ectasia, or fibrocystic change. To perform galactography, the radiologist identifies the discharging duct visually by expressing a small amount of the discharge and pinpointing the location of the discharging duct. The radiologist cleans the nipple, may use a topical anesthetic, and with sterile technique, cannulates the discharging duct with a 30-gauge blunt-tipped sialogram needle connected to

tubing and a syringe filled with contrast. Usually, the needle will fall painlessly into the duct, but on occasion, warm compresses are needed to relax the duct opening. A small amount of contrast (0.2 to 1.0 mL) is injected into the duct until resistance is felt or the patient feels "full." Because the ducts are quite fragile, pain or burning may indicate perforation or extravasation of contrast, but neither the cannulation nor the injection should be painful. Either symptom is an indication to stop the procedure and re-evaluate the situation.

After the injection, the needle is withdrawn, and the contrast-filled duct is sealed with collodion or the blunt-tipped catheter is taped in place to the nipple. Standard craniocaudal and mediolateral mammograms are obtained, and some facilities use magnification views to confirm

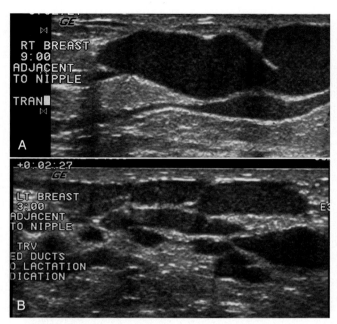

FIGURE 10-11   Ultrasound shows bilateral dilated ducts in the right (**A**) and left (**B**) breasts in a patient taking risperidone. (From Pocket Radiologist. Breast Top 100 Diagnoses. WB Saunders Co. 1st ed. Amirsys Inc, Salt Lake City, UT, 2003, p 36.)

and evaluate the filling defects. After the mammogram, the contrast is expressed from the breast by gentle massage. If duct filling is incomplete, if the contrast is diluted by retained secretions, or if an air bubble is possibly simulating a filling defect, the duct can be reinjected immediately for a second study.

A normal duct arborizes from a single entry point on the nipple into smaller ducts extending over almost an entire quadrant of the breast. Normal ducts are thin and smooth walled and have no filling defects or wall irregularities (Fig. 10-12A). Ductal ectasia is not uncommon, and occasionally, normal cysts or lobules fill from the dilated ducts (Fig. 10-12B). Ducts containing papillomas or cancer may show duct ectasia without a filling defect (false-negative study) (Fig. 10-12C), or they may show a filling defect, an abrupt duct cutoff, or luminal irregularity and distortion from tumors at or outside the duct walls (Fig. 10-13A). Ducts containing malignancy or papillomas are typically dilated between the filling defect and the nipple, and sometimes the papilloma may become encysted (Fig. 10-13D and E). Air bubbles produce filling defects that may mimic papilloma or cancer, but they are usually sharply defined and round and change position inside the duct on repeat injection, unlike fixed intraductal tumors. On the galactogram, extravasation is seen as contrast extending outside the duct lumen into the breast tissue and obscuring the underlying breast tissue and ducts (Fig. 10-13F). In the rare instance of lymphatic or venous uptake of extravasated contrast, a draining

tubular structure leading away from the extravasation site can be seen.

A positive galactogram usually leads to biopsy, either by preoperative needle localization or by ductoscopy. Preoperative needle localization of filling defects after galactography under x-ray guidance may be helpful for surgical planning, especially if the intraductal mass is deep in the breast. Negative galactograms despite the presence of a papilloma on biopsy have been reported, and galactography has a sensitivity ranging from 69% to 78% for tumors.

On MRI, intraductal papillomas can have three patterns. The first pattern is a small smooth enhancing breast mass at the terminus of a dilated breast duct corresponding to the filling defects seen on galactography. The second pattern is an irregular, rapidly enhancing mass with occasional spiculation or rim enhancement in women without nipple discharge; this pattern cannot be distinguished from invasive breast cancer. Finally, despite the presence of a papilloma, MRI may be negative, with the papilloma undetected on both contrast-enhanced and fat-suppressed T1-weighted studies.

In the early 1990s, surgeons reported using a tiny ductoscope to cannulate a discharging duct for identification of papillomas or other intraductal masses while in the operating room as a guide for surgery. Dooley reported that 16% of women undergoing ductoscopy at surgery had lesions detected by ductoscopy that were not seen on either ductograms or mammograms before surgery.

BREAST EDEMA

On clinical examination, breast edema may be evident as *peau d'orange,* a term signifying thickening and elevation of the skin around tethered hair follicles, similar to an orange peel, and the edematous breast may be larger than the contralateral side. The differential diagnosis for breast edema depends on whether the edema is unilateral or bilateral (Box 10-6). Unilateral breast edema is due to mastitis, inflammatory cancer, local obstruction of lymph nodes, trauma, radiation therapy, or *coumarin* necrosis (Fig. 10-14). Bilateral breast edema is due to systemic etiologies such as congestive heart failure, liver disease, anasarca, renal failure, or other conditions that can cause edema elsewhere in the body. Alternatively, bilateral lymphadenopathy or superior vena cava syndrome for any reason may cause bilateral breast edema (Fig. 10-15A and B).

The key to diagnosis is to obtain an accurate clinical history and evaluate the breast for any signs of cancer such as suspicious microcalcifications or masses in appropriate clinical settings. On mammography, breast edema is manifested as skin thickening greater than 2 to

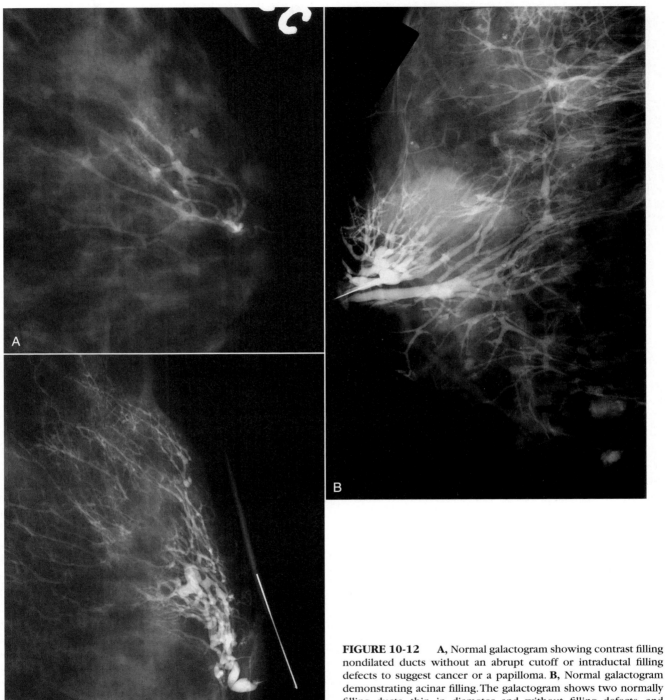

FIGURE 10-12   A, Normal galactogram showing contrast filling nondilated ducts without an abrupt cutoff or intraductal filling defects to suggest cancer or a papilloma. **B,** Normal galactogram demonstrating acinar filling. The galactogram shows two normally filling ducts, thin in diameter and without filling defects, and rounded acini filling in the periphery. **C,** Normal galactogram showing nondilated contrast-filled ducts in a patient with nipple discharge. Ductoscopy revealed two microscopic papillomas.

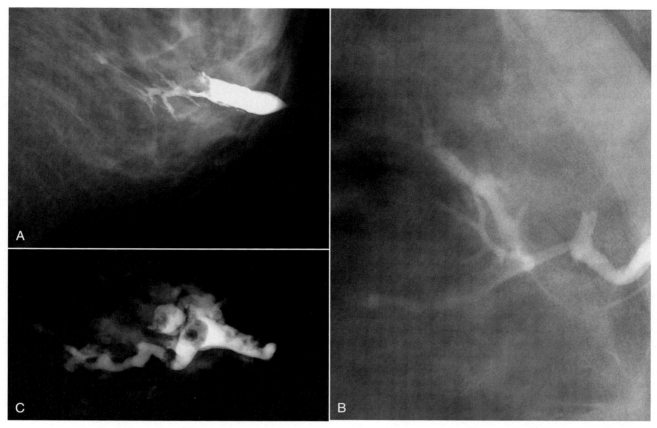

FIGURE 10-13   **A,** Papilloma on galactography. A filling defect on the galactogram corresponded to a retroareolar papilloma at surgery. **B,** Galactogram with an abrupt cutoff in a proximal duct. Biopsy showed papilloma. **C,** Galactogram showing cancer. A magnification view of a galactogram reveals an irregular filling defect in the retroareolar region. Biopsy findings were consistent with ductal carcinoma in situ.

3 mm and coarsening of trabeculae in deep breast tissues and particularly in subcutaneous fat. Fluid within subdermal lymphatics produces thick white lines in subdermal fat just below the skin line that have an appearance similar to Kerley's B lines at the periphery of the lung on chest radiographs in congestive heart failure. An edematous breast will be much denser and more difficult to penetrate and will appear whiter than the contralateral side because of fluid in the breast tissue.

The differential diagnosis for increased bilateral breast density on mammography other than breast edema includes increased breast tissue produced by exogenous hormone therapy or loss of fatty tissue from weight loss. Distinction between breast edema and exogenous hormone therapy or weight loss is made by noting the presence of skin thickening, which is found only with breast edema (Box 10-7). In addition, increased breast density from exogenous hormone therapy is usually bilateral and occurs in regions where breast tissue was previously present (Fig. 10-16A and B). Weight loss

produces increased breast density because of the loss of fat, but the history should lead to the correct diagnosis (Fig. 10-17A and B).

On ultrasound, breast edema is characterized by skin thickening, loss of the normal sharp margins of Cooper's ligaments, increased echogenicity of surrounding tissues, and in severe cases, fluid in dilated subdermal lymphatics, which are seen as tubular fluid-filled structures just under the skin line. In inflammatory cancer, breast ultrasound may detect a hypoechoic shadowing mass that may represent an invasive ductal cancer hidden on the mammogram by overlying breast edema.

On MRI, breast edema is manifested as skin thickening and coarsening of breast trabeculae and Cooper's ligaments. With locally advanced cancer, the cancer is usually seen as an irregular mass with rapid initial enhancement, a late plateau or washout phase, and enhancement within the skin if skin invasion has occurred.

Inflammatory cancer, a rare (1% of all cancers) aggressive breast cancer with a poor prognosis, is the

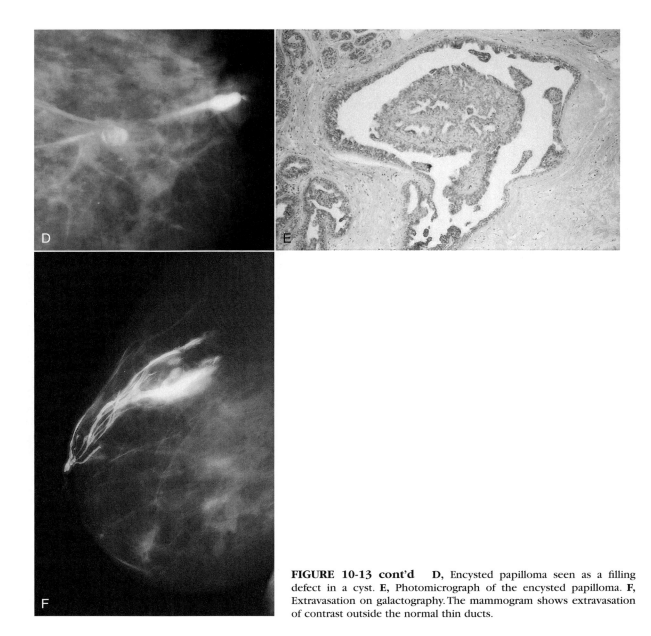

FIGURE 10-13 cont'd **D,** Encysted papilloma seen as a filling defect in a cyst. **E,** Photomicrograph of the encysted papilloma. **F,** Extravasation on galactography. The mammogram shows extravasation of contrast outside the normal thin ducts.

Box 10-6   Causes of Breast Edema

UNILATERAL

Mastitis
   Staphylococcus aureus (common)
   Tuberculosis (rare)
   Syphilis (rare)
   Hydatid disease (rare)
   Molluscum contagiosum
Abscess complicating mastitis
Recurrent subareolar abscess
Inflammatory cancer
Trauma
Coumarin necrosis
Unilateral lymph node obstruction
Radiation therapy

BILATERAL

Congestive heart failure
Anasarca
Renal failure
Lymphadenopathy
Superior vena cava syndrome
Liver disease

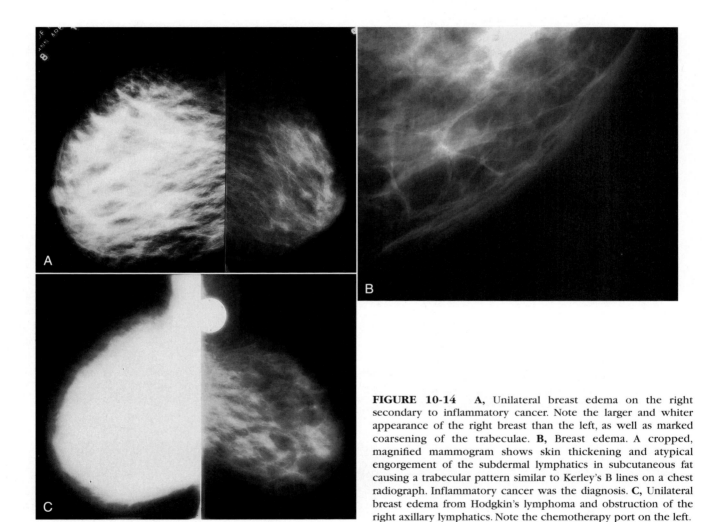

FIGURE 10-14   A, Unilateral breast edema on the right secondary to inflammatory cancer. Note the larger and whiter appearance of the right breast than the left, as well as marked coarsening of the trabeculae. **B,** Breast edema. A cropped, magnified mammogram shows skin thickening and atypical engorgement of the subdermal lymphatics in subcutaneous fat causing a trabecular pattern similar to Kerley's B lines on a chest radiograph. Inflammatory cancer was the diagnosis. **C,** Unilateral breast edema from Hodgkin's lymphoma and obstruction of the right axillary lymphatics. Note the chemotherapy port on the left.

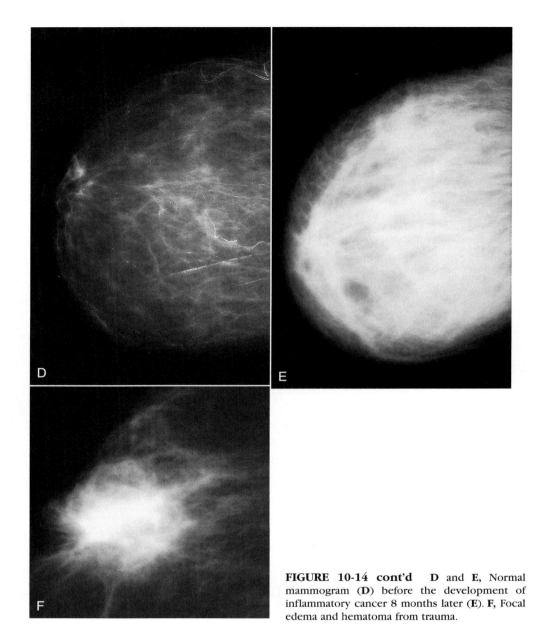

FIGURE 10-14 cont'd **D** and **E,** Normal mammogram (**D**) before the development of inflammatory cancer 8 months later (**E**). **F,** Focal edema and hematoma from trauma.

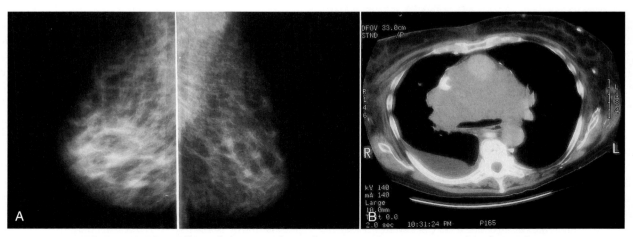

FIGURE 10-15 **Bilateral Breast Edema from Superior Vena Cava (SVC) Syndrome Secondary to Granulomatous Disease.** A bilateral mammogram shows bilateral breast edema, worse on the right (**A**) because the patient was used to lying on her right side. Contrast-enhanced computed tomography shows SVC syndrome from mediastinal adenopathy along with right pleural effusion (**B**).

Box 10-7 Hormone Changes versus Breast Edema on Mammography	
HORMONE CHANGES	**BREAST EDEMA**
Increased breast density	Increased breast density
Breast density increases at sites with glandular tissue	Diffuse or focal; may develop where no glandular tissue occurred previously
Normal skin	Skin thickening
Normal subcutaneous fat	Subcutaneous trabecular thickening
Normal skin on physical examination	Peau d'orange on physical examination

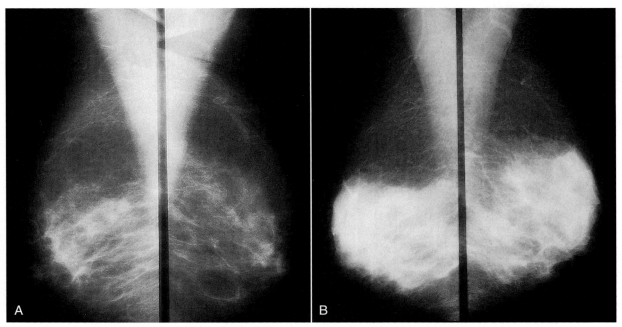

FIGURE 10-16   Exogenous Hormone Replacement Therapy. Bilateral mediolateral oblique mammograms before (**A**) and after (**B**) hormone replacement therapy show increased glandular tissue bilaterally in locations where glandular tissue previously existed. Unlike breast edema, there is no skin thickening or coarsening of trabeculae in subcutaneous fat.

most important differential diagnosis for unilateral breast edema. The definition of inflammatory cancer varies, but it usually has the clinical signs of an enlarging erythematous breast with peau d'orange, and it should be distinguished from locally advanced breast cancer, producing a focal, red, raised skin metastasis. Inflammatory cancer is often mistaken for mastitis because of its clinical features, but it does not respond to antibiotics. Mammography of inflammatory cancer reveals findings of breast edema (skin thickening, diffuse increased breast density, trabecular thickening), but it may also demonstrate findings of cancer, including a breast mass, asymmetric focal density, microcalcifications, nipple retraction, or axillary adenopathy. Ultrasound may show findings of breast edema in 96% of cases, masses in 80%, and dilated lymphatic channels in 68%. On MRI, one report of inflammatory cancer described a "patch enhancement" pattern with some "areas of focal enhancement" and washout on the late phase of the dynamic curve. The enhancement rate on MRI for inflammatory cancer is reported to be quite rapid in the initial post-contrast phase and slightly less rapid in mastitis. On biopsy, breast cancer is present in the dermal lymphatics in 80% of cases. The usual management is biopsy to make the diagnosis of inflammatory cancer, neoadjuvant chemotherapy with or without subsequent surgery, and radiation therapy,

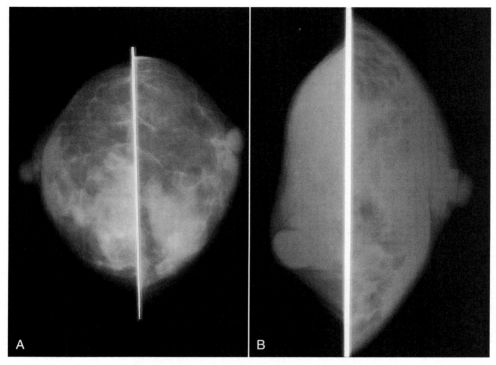

FIGURE 10-17   Weight Loss. Bilateral craniocaudal mammograms before (**A**) and after (**B**) weight loss show increased breast density on the mammogram because of loss of fat.

depending on tumor response, or any combination of these modalities.

Mastitis and abscesses are common causes of unilateral breast edema, and clinical findings of pain, erythema, and peau d'orange are typically noted. The most common cause of mastitis is *S. aureus*. Rare causes of breast infection include tuberculosis, syphilis, hydatid disease, and molluscum contagiosum. Clinically, mastitis produces breast cellulitis, which if untreated, may progress to small focal microabscesses or a larger abscess collection that may become walled off. On mammography, an abscess is an ill-defined or irregular mass without calcifications that is generally located in the subareolar region. Usually, no gas is seen in the abscess on the mammogram. On ultrasound, abscesses are tender, irregular, ill-defined hypoechoic masses, sometimes containing septations or debris, that become enhanced though transmission of sound. Rarely, an abscess contains gas, which is most commonly seen if previous aspiration has been attempted. Because antibiotics cannot cross abscess walls, larger abscesses require either percutaneous or operative drainage. For this reason, ultrasound is particularly helpful in the setting of mastitis to detect and define abscesses requiring drainage.

A recurrent subareolar abscess is a special entity caused by plugging of the major breast ducts and subsequent infection; it is commonly associated with a

---

Box 10-8   Coumarin Necrosis

Rare cause of breast edema
Exact mechanism unknown
Associated protein C or S deficiency
Painful swelling and petechiae
Hemorrhagic bullae
Full-thickness skin necrosis
Discontinue or change anticoagulants

---

fistulous tract that forms from the abscess inside the breast and drains to the skin. The resulting abscess is chronic and may be drained percutaneously or operatively many times without resolution or with frequent recurrence. A recurrent subareolar abscess is treated by surgically removing both the abscess and the fistulous tract.

An extremely rare cause of unilateral breast edema is necrosis of the breast from coumarin (warfarin [Coumadin]) therapy. Necrosis occurs more commonly in the abdomen, buttocks, and thighs, rather than in breast, and it occurs in 0.01% to 1% of coumarin-treated patients (Box 10-8). Although it has been associated with protein C or protein S deficiency, the exact mechanism

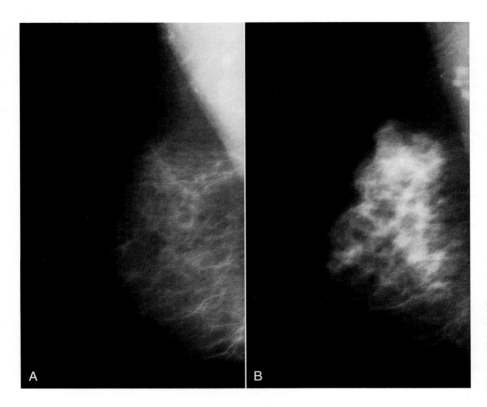

FIGURE 10-18   Exogenous Hormone Replacement Therapy. Mediolateral oblique mammograms before (**A**) and after (**B**) hormone replacement therapy show a denser breast where breast tissue previously existed.

of coumarin-induced necrosis is unknown. Painful lesions, swelling, and petechiae from thrombosis of small vessels and inflammation occur after the initiation of coumarin treatment; large hemorrhagic bullae result and develop to full-thickness fat and skin necrosis. Discontinuing the use of coumarin is recommended. Heparin or other anticoagulants may be necessary in patients who require sustained anticoagulation in the short term. Heparin-induced skin necrosis has also been reported in association with type II heparin-induced thrombocytopenia, but heparin is often used in the setting of coumarin necrosis. In some cases, the skin lesions heal spontaneously after shallow tissue sloughing. In other cases, skin grafts are required, whereas in extreme cases, mastectomy is required.

HORMONE CHANGES

Normal women have extremely dense breast tissue when young that is replaced by fat during the aging process. On mammography, the breasts usually appear very white in younger patients and become darker and darker as glandular tissue is replaced by fatty tissue with age. The overall breast density at any time in the patient's life depends on the patient's age, her genetic predisposition for glandular tissue, and her hormonal status.

Exogenous hormone replacement therapy, pregnancy, or lactation reverses the trend toward fatty breast tissue by causing a proliferation of the glandular elements and periductal stroma of the breast and thereby resulting in a denser mammogram. Unlike breast edema, only the breast tissue becomes denser, and the skin does not become thickened more than 2 to 3 mm as it does with breast edema (Fig. 10-18A and B)

Some women report breast tenderness, pain, fullness, and lumpiness with exogenous hormone replacement therapy. The frequency of increased breast density on mammography in women undergoing exogenous hormone therapy varies from 23% to 34%. The highest percentage of women with increased density were receiving continuous-combined hormone therapy consisting of conjugated equine estrogen, 0.625 mg/day, plus medroxyprogesterone acetate, 2.5 mg/day, or other combinations, with the progestin component most affecting the increase in breast density. In another report, continuous-combined hormone therapy produced increased breast density on mammography, but estrogen-only therapy did not.

Other medications also have effects on breast density. Raloxifene hydrochloride, a drug used for bone mineral density, has been reported to produce increased breast density on mammography in a very small number of women. Case studies of two women undergoing injections of medroxyprogesterone (Depo-Provera) for contraception reported a decrease in breast density on mammograms during the injections and an increase in breast density when the injections were discontinued. Tamoxifen used for adjuvant or prophylactic treatment of breast cancer has been reported to decrease mammographic tissue density in some women, with one case report describing a return to baseline breast density after termination of drug therapy. Isoflavones are phytoestrogens contained in soy foods and have been reported to have both estrogenic and antiestrogenic effects. A double-blind randomized trial of women undergoing mammography after isoflavone supplements showed no significant decrease in breast density or change in dense tissue over a 12-month period.

Because breast density changes with hormone therapy, new or focal densities on mammograms are correlated with older films and the clinical history, in addition to being evaluated for a new mass or a developing density as a result of cancer. In questionable cases, spot compression, fine-detail views, and ultrasound may be helpful to exclude the presence of a mass. If questions still remain after additional work-up, discontinuing exogenous hormone therapy for 3 months and re-imaging may exclude a mass. Similarly, the increased breast enhancement noted on contrast-enhanced breast MRI in women receiving exogenous hormone replacement therapy is reversible when the therapy is discontinued.

BREAST PAIN

Patients with focal breast pain should be evaluated with mammography and breast physical examination. Although focal breast pain is worrisome to the patient, studies have shown that it is most often *not* caused by cancer. However, because both breast pain and cancer are common, mammography is reasonable to exclude cancer and reassure the patient. Consideration should be given to ultrasound in women with focal pain to exclude a breast cyst that may be causing the pain.

Cyclic mastalgia has many causes, including cyclic enlargement as a result of menses or multiple cysts. Relief from breast pain may be achieved in some cases by aspiration of the cyst, decrease in caffeine intake, or analgesics. Home remedies for breast pain have included 400 U of vitamin E per day, vitamin B_6, analgesics, decrease in fat and salt intake, use of sports brassieres, or evening primrose oil. In extreme cases, progestins, danazol, tamoxifen, or bromocriptine is used to relieve mastodynia.

Breast pain is a common complaint. Although it is not often a symptom of breast cancer, both breast pain and breast cancer are common, so the purpose of the work-up is to reassure the patient and exclude a coexistent cancer.

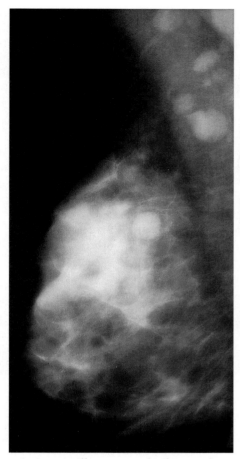

FIGURE 10-19   Axillary Lymphadenopathy. Abnormal dense round lymph nodes in the axilla have lost their fatty hila and are rounder and bigger than normal lymph nodes as a result of lupus and rheumatoid arthritis.

AXILLARY LYMPHADENOPATHY

Axillary lymphadenopathy is visualized on mammography as replacement of the fatty hilum of lymph nodes by dense tissue, a rounded shape of the lymph nodes, and an overall generalized increased density with or without lymph node enlargement (Fig. 10-19). Abnormal lymph nodes may also contain calcifications, gold deposits mimicking calcifications from treatment of rheumatoid arthritis, or silicone from a previously ruptured breast implant. The differential diagnosis for axillary adenopathy without a definite breast mass varies for unilateral versus bilateral findings (Box 10-9). Causes of unilateral axillary adenopathy include metastatic breast cancer or mastitis. Bilateral axillary adenopathy is usually due to systemic etiologies such as infection, collagen vascular diseases such as rheumatoid arthritis, lymphoma, leukemia, or metastatic tumor.

"Calcific" particles in abnormal axillary lymph nodes may represent calcified metastasis from breast cancer or calcifying infections such as tuberculosis (Box 10-10). In the case of tuberculous mastitis, patients have axillary swelling and breast enlargement without a breast mass, as well as enlarged dense or matted axillary lymph nodes or breast edema with or without findings of pulmonary tuberculosis. The finding of macrocalcifications rather than pleomorphic microcalcifications in the lymph nodes may suggest tuberculous mastitis, but biopsy is necessary to exclude metastatic breast cancer. Migration of silicone into axillary lymph nodes from ruptured silicone breast implants or migration of gold particles from therapy for rheumatoid arthritis may mimic calcifications in lymph nodes, but the clinical history should provide clues to the correct diagnosis.

Detection of lymphadenopathy on mammography in women with no underlying palpable breast mass or clinical reason for the abnormal lymph nodes should prompt a critical review of the breast for pleomorphic calcifications or other signs of breast cancer. In one clinical series of 21 women with lymphadenopathy detected at screening mammography, 50% was due to malignancy (lymphoma, metastatic carcinoma, leukemia), and the other 50% was due to benign causes (reactive changes, healed granulomatous disease, rheumatoid arthritis, amyloid, infection).

Primary breast cancer manifested as isolated lymph node metastasis in women with normal mammographic and physical examination findings is an uncommon clinical problem that accounts for less than 1% of all breast cancers (Fig. 10-20A and B). Both breast ultrasound

Box 10-9	Axillary Lymphadenopathy	
UNILATERAL	**BILATERAL**	
Mastitis	Widespread infection	
Cancer	Rheumatoid arthritis	
	Collagen vascular disease	
	Lymphoma	
	Leukemia	
	Metastatic cancer	

Box 10-10	Lymphadenopathy with "Calcifications"
Metastatic calcifying cancer	
Granulomatous disease	
Gold particles from rheumatoid arthritis therapy	
Migrated silicone from implant rupture	

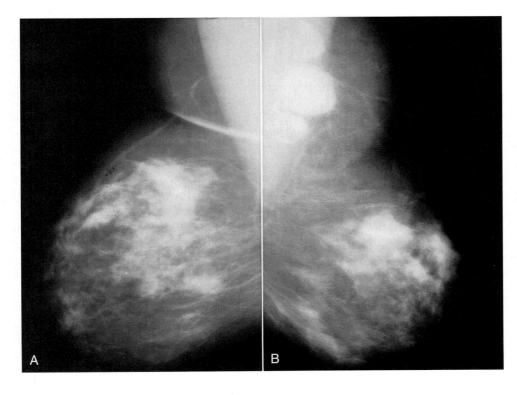

FIGURE 10-20   Breast Cancer Manifested As Axillary Lymphadenopathy. Normal right (A) and abnormal left (B) mammograms show adenopathy in the left axilla, which was consistent with the diagnosis of breast cancer. Additional views of the left breast by mammography and ultrasound did not demonstrate any masses. Examination after mastectomy showed no primary breast cancer. The patient was treated for breast cancer empirically. No breast cancer in the opposite breast and no additional tumors were found elsewhere in 5 years of follow-up.

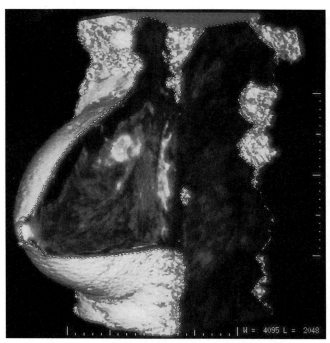

FIGURE 10-21 A shaded, cut-surface display of contrast-enhanced magnetic resonance imaging of the breast shows an irregular-enhancing suspicious mass in the upper part of the breast representing an occult malignancy not seen on mammography. (Image courtesy of Bruce L. Daniel, M.D., Stanford University, Stanford, CA.)

and contrast-enhanced breast MRI have been used to detect the primary breast cancer in this scenario, with improved results in comparison to mammography, and breast conservation rather than mastectomy was a potential option in these patients (Fig. 10-21). In some cases the primary breast cancer is never identified. In a pathology series by Haupt et al. in which 43 women with this clinical dilemma were reviewed, the primary tumor was found in 31 (72%) specimens but never identified in the remaining 12. Survival rates between the two groups were similar, and the 12 women in whom a tumor was never discovered did have another primary malignancy detected in the follow-up period.

PAGET'S DISEASE OF THE NIPPLE

Paget's disease of the nipple is a distinct clinical entity that heralds an underlying breast cancer. Ductal carcinoma almost always coexists with Paget's disease, either in the ducts beneath the nipple or elsewhere in the breast, and it has a high rate of overexpression of the c-*erb*-B2 oncogene. Affected women have a bright, reddened nipple and eczematous nipple changes that may extend to the areola, with subsequent ulceration and nipple destruction if the process is unchecked. A delay of

Box 10-11 Paget's Disease of the Nipple
Heralds underlying ductal cancer
Bright red nipple
Eczematous nipple/areolar changes
Ulceration
Cancer location often subareolar, but may be anywhere in the breast
Normal mammogram in 50%
Nipple change, skin/areolar thickening in 30%
Subareolar mass/calcifications suspicious

several months often occurs before women seek advice, unless associated nipple discharge is present.

The nipple and mammogram are normal in almost 50% of cases despite clinical signs of Paget's disease and the presence of an underlying breast cancer (Box 10-11). On abnormal mammograms, the underlying malignancy has the appearance of suspicious microcalcifications or a spiculated mass, or both. The cancer is often located in the subareolar region or deep in the breast and does not necessarily lie directly adjacent to the nipple or areola (Fig. 10-22A). In women with Paget's disease, skin or areolar thickening, nipple retraction, subareolar masses, or calcifications leading to the nipple should be viewed with suspicion on mammography (Fig. 10-22B). Conversely, nipple/areolar abnormalities or thickening detected at mammography should be correlated with the physical examination to exclude clinical findings of Paget's disease.

SARCOMAS

Sarcomas are rare tumors of the breast or the underlying chest wall, and their classification depends on the cell type involved (Fig. 10-23A and B). Ultrasound shows a hypoechoic mass and may be helpful in determining whether the origin of the sarcoma is from the breast or chest wall (Fig. 10-24A and B). Mammography shows high-density masses without calcifications or spiculation, unless the tumor has osseous elements (Fig. 10-25).

MRI of angiosarcoma shows low signal intensity on T1-weighted images, higher signal intensity on T2-weighted images, and enhancement of the mass with a low-intensity central region.

MONDOR'S DISEASE

Mondor's disease is acute thrombophlebitis of the superficial veins of the breast (Box 10-12). It is rare, is

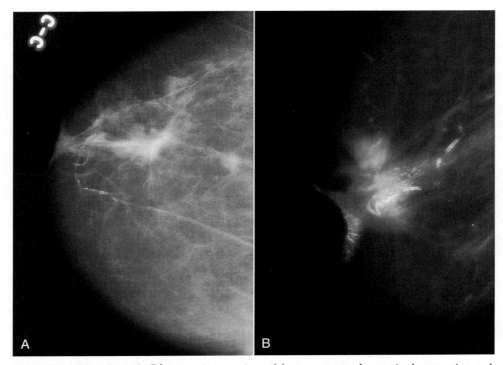

FIGURE 10-22   Paget's Disease. A, A craniocaudal mammogram shows nipple retraction and a second invasive ductal cancer deep in the breast in a patient with Paget's disease. **B,** A mediolateral oblique mammogram in a patient with Paget's disease shows destruction of the nipple covered with a radiopaque salve and a retroareolar dense mass producing retraction.

often associated with trauma or recent surgery, has been reported to occur after sonography-guided or stereotactic core biopsy, but may also be idiopathic in origin. Patients report acute pain, discomfort, and tenderness along the lateral aspect of the breast, the chest wall, or the region of the thrombosed vein; they may also report a cord-like painful elongated mass just below the skin. Extension of the arm may produce a long narrow furrow in the skin as a result of retraction from the thrombosed vein, similar to skin dimpling from breast cancer.

Physical examination shows a tender palpable cord extending toward the outer portion of the breast that is produced by fibrosis and obliteration of the superficial vein and occasionally accompanied by discoloration of the overlying skin in the acute phase. Thereafter, the vein diminishes in painfulness over a period of 3 to 4 weeks as a result of either recanalization or complete obliteration of the vein by phlebosclerosis and hyalinization. Because Mondor's disease is self-limited and the palpable finding resolves over a 2- to 12-week period, supportive care is the appropriate treatment.

Case reports describe negative mammographic findings in women with Mondor's disease or, rarely, a long linear or tubular density on the mammogram corresponding to the thrombosed vein (Fig. 10-26A-C). Case reports of ultrasound in Mondor's disease show a noncompressible hypoechoic tubular cord in the subcutaneous tissue, with or without flow on color Doppler imaging, depending on the degree of recanalization.

GRANULOMATOUS MASTITIS

Granulomatous mastitis is a rare disease that occurs in young premenopausal women after their last childbirth. It has been correlated with breast-feeding and oral contraceptive use, and a possible autoimmune component has been implicated in its etiology. Affected patients may have galactorrhea, inflammation, a breast mass, induration, and skin ulcerations.

Women undergoing mammography are found to have asymmetric density, focal asymmetric or ill-defined breast masses, or negative results. Calcifications are not a feature. On ultrasound, findings include irregular masses, focal regions of inhomogeneous patterns associated with hypoechoic "tubular/nodular structures," or decreased parenchymal echogenicity with acoustic shadowing, all suggestive of malignancy.

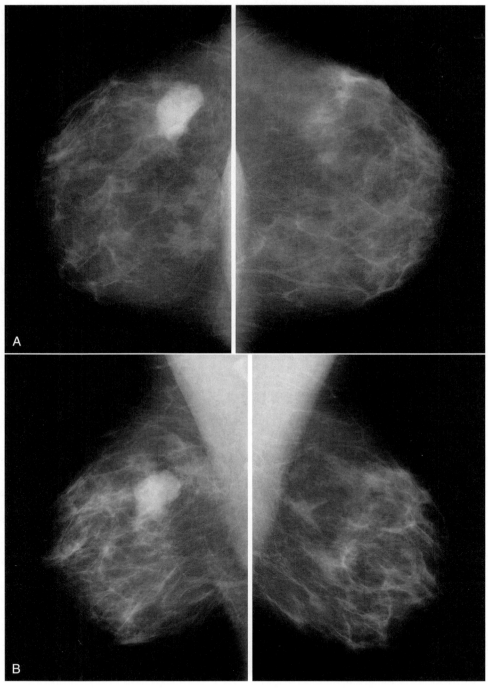

FIGURE 10-23   Carcinosarcoma. Craniocaudal (**A**) and mediolateral oblique (**B**) mammograms in a 37-year-old woman with a palpable mass show a dense lobulated mass in the right breast with an obscured lower border. Pathologic examination demonstrated the epithelial and mesenchymal differentiation required to make the diagnosis. (From Smathers RL: Mammography: Diagnosis and Intervention, Medical Interactive (MedInter.com). Copyright Mammography Specialists Medical Group, Inc. Contribution from Mahendra Ranchod, M.D., San Jose, CA.)

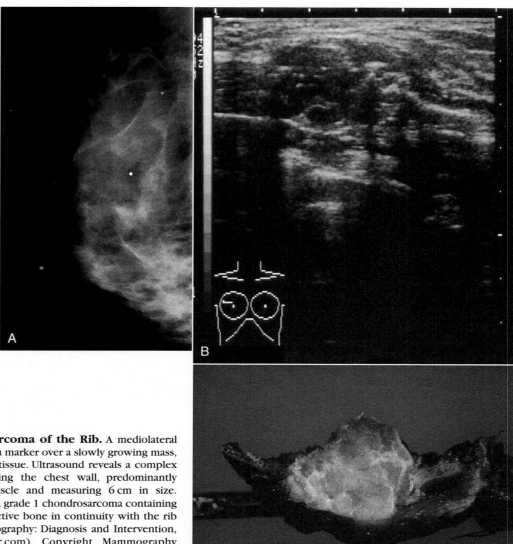

FIGURE 10-24   Chondrosarcoma of the Rib. A mediolateral oblique mammogram (**A**) shows a marker over a slowly growing mass, which proved to be only dense tissue. Ultrasound reveals a complex heterogeneous mass (**B**) invading the chest wall, predominantly posterior to the pectoralis muscle and measuring 6 cm in size. Pathologic examination showed a grade 1 chondrosarcoma containing mature hyaline cartilage and reactive bone in continuity with the rib (**C**). (From Smathers RL: Mammography: Diagnosis and Intervention, Medical Interactive (MedInter.com). Copyright Mammography Specialists Medical Group, Inc. Contribution from Suzanne Dintiz, M.D., Stanford, CA.)

Because the mammographic and sonographic features suggest breast cancer, biopsy is frequently performed on women with this condition. Biopsy shows a chronic granulomatous inflammation composed of giant cells, leukocytes, epithelioid cells, macrophages, and abscesses. Treatment consists of surgical excision, oral steroid therapy, anti-inflammatory drugs or colchicines, or methotrexate, as well as antibiotic treatment of any associated abscesses. Recurrence rates of up to 50% have been reported, but they can be reduced by immunosuppressive treatment until complete remission.

DIABETIC MASTOPATHY

Diabetic mastopathy produces hard, irregular, sometimes painful mobile breast masses that may be recurrent or bilateral in patients with a history of long-term insulin-dependent diabetes, in younger premenopausal diabetic women, or in rare patients with thyroid disease (Box 10-13). Diabetic mastopathy is due to an autoimmune reaction to the accumulation of abnormal matrix proteins caused by hyperglycemia. It leads to atrophy and

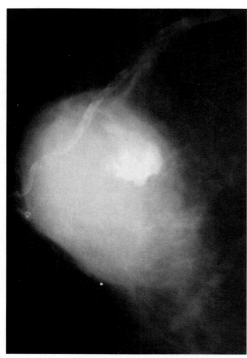

FIGURE 10-25   Fibrosarcoma of the Breast with Osseous Trabeculae. A craniocaudal mammogram shows a dense mass containing dense calcification resembling bone. (From Elson BC, Ikeda DM, Andersson I, Wattsgard C: Fibrosarcoma of the breast: Mammographic findings in 5 cases. AJR 158:994, 1992.)

obliteration of glandular breast tissue and the production of fibrosis, which forms a hard mass simulating breast cancer. Because of the hardness of the mass, needle biopsy is often performed, but it may be insufficient for diagnosis and therefore necessitate histologic sampling. Pathologic examination reveals fibrosis with a dense lymphocytic infiltration around breast lobules and ducts.

Mammography shows a regional asymmetric density with ill-defined margins but no microcalcifications or dense glandular tissue. Ultrasound demonstrates a hypoechoic mass or region displaying marked acoustic shadowing in most cases, findings suggestive of scirrhous breast cancer. On color Doppler imaging of the breast, no flow is seen in the mass.

Case reports of diabetic mastopathy on MRI describe a decreased area of signal intensity with "poor" or "heterogeneous" enhancement or "nonspecific" enhancement in the initial post-contrast phase. Heterogeneous "spotting enhancement" or a "benign gradual-type dynamic curve" is reported in the late enhancement phase.

On biopsy, fibrosis with perivascular, periductal, or perilobular lymphocytic infiltrates is seen. Frequently, patients will undergo surgical excisional biopsy. Unfortunately, surgery may exacerbate the disease, with recurrences developing in the same location.

Box 10-12   Mondor's Disease

Thrombophlebitis of the superficial veins of the breast
Painful, rope-like, palpable cord
Thrombosed vein causes a furrow/dimpling
Self-limited
Related to trauma or surgery
Mammography is negative, or a long tubular density is noted
Ultrasound: hypoechoic tube or cord with or without flow

DESMOID TUMOR

Desmoid tumor, or extra-abdominal desmoid, is also known as fibromatosis. Desmoid tumor is an infiltrative, locally aggressive fibroblastic/myofibroblastic process that may recur locally, may be multicentric, has been associated with previous trauma or surgery, and has been reported in women with breast implants. In the breast, desmoid tumor is manifested as a solitary, hard painless mass, occasionally fixed to the skin or pectoral fascia. Because treatment involves wide surgical excision, the primary tumor is evaluated for its origin within either the breast or the underlying musculo-aponeurotic structures. The extent of invasion into surrounding structures is also evaluated to facilitate surgical planning.

On mammography, desmoid tumors are spiculated masses. Ultrasound shows a hypoechoic shadowing mass. Because these masses simulate spiculated breast cancer, biopsy is required (Fig. 10-27).

Treatment of desmoid tumors is complete local surgical excision. Recurrence of desmoid tumor is less likely with wide excision and clear histologic margins. Tumor recurrence usually occurs within 3 years of excision, and for this reason breast reconstruction is generally delayed for 3 years. Because surgical trauma has been associated with recurrence, informed consent is necessary before breast reconstruction. Recurrences are treated by radical excision, just as the primary tumor. Radiation therapy is used as an alternative to surgery for tumors in which complete excision would result in a poor functional outcome or for some tumors with positive margins (Box 10-14).

TRICHINOSIS

Trichinosis is caused by the ingestion of raw or undercooked meat containing encysted larvae of the *Trichinella* genus. Diarrhea is produced during the

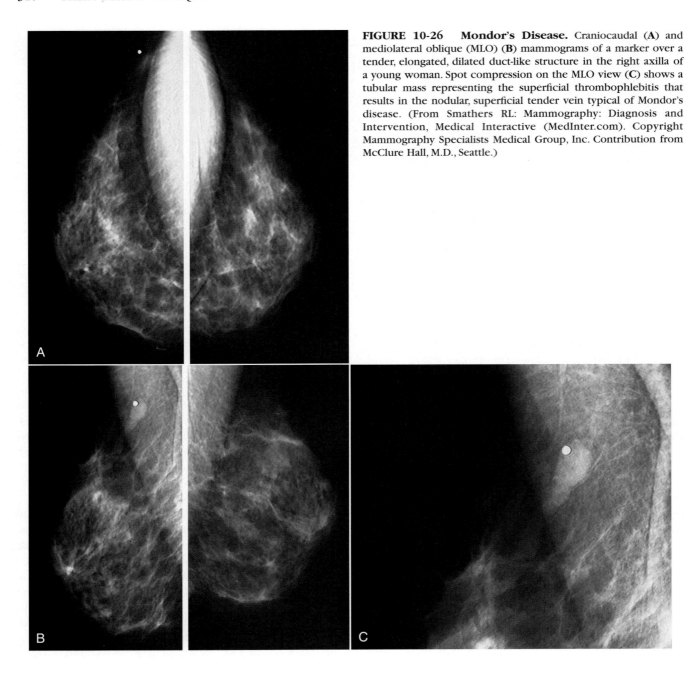

FIGURE 10-26   Mondor's Disease. Craniocaudal (**A**) and mediolateral oblique (MLO) (**B**) mammograms of a marker over a tender, elongated, dilated duct-like structure in the right axilla of a young woman. Spot compression on the MLO view (**C**) shows a tubular mass representing the superficial thrombophlebitis that results in the nodular, superficial tender vein typical of Mondor's disease. (From Smathers RL: Mammography: Diagnosis and Intervention, Medical Interactive (MedInter.com). Copyright Mammography Specialists Medical Group, Inc. Contribution from McClure Hall, M.D., Seattle.)

Box 10-13   Diabetic Mastopathy

Long-term insulin-dependent diabetics
Thyroid disease (rare)
Autoimmune reaction causing fibrosis
Periductal and perilobular lymphocytic infiltration
May result in a hard mass
Surgery can result in recurrent masses

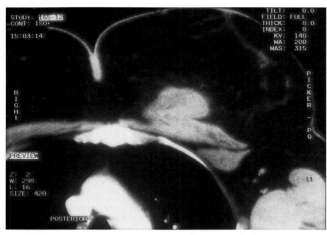

FIGURE 10-27 Computed tomography shows a soft tissue mass adjacent to the pectoralis muscle in the left breast. Biopsy revealed a desmoid tumor.

Box 10-14   Desmoid Tumor

Synonyms: extra-abdominal desmoid/fibromatosis
Recurrent unless widely resected
Associated with previous trauma or surgery, implants
Solitary spiculated hard painless mass, occasionally fixed
If recurrent, occurs within 3 years

Box 10-15   Trichinosis

Ingestion of encysted worm larvae in undercooked meat
Tiny linear calcified encysted larvae in the pectoralis
    muscle
No calcifications in breast tissue

---

intestinal phase of adult development, and then myositis, fever, and periorbital edema develop during larval migration (Box 10-15). After gastric digestion releases the encysted larvae, the larvae migrate into the intestinal mucosa, mature, and mate. The adult female releases new larvae into mucosal blood vessels, and the larvae are distributed throughout the body over a period of 4 to 6 weeks. The larvae enter skeletal muscles, most commonly the diaphragm, tongue, periorbital muscles, deltoid, pectoralis, gastrocnemius, and intercostal muscles, where the larvae encyst and calcify in 6 to 18 months, with a further life span of 5 to 10 years in the encysted form. During migration, larvae may also produce myocarditis, pneumonitis, or central nervous system symptoms from vasculitis of small arteries or capillaries,

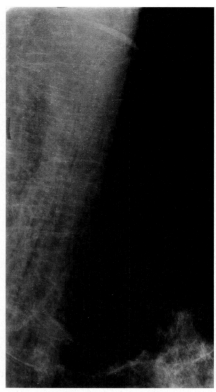

FIGURE 10-28   Trichinosis. A magnified mediolateral oblique view of the upper part of the breast shows innumerable tiny calcifications aligned along the pectoralis muscle that represent the calcified encysted larvae of *Trichinella.*

but encystment does not usually occur in these locations. Ingestion of the encysted larvae by a new host perpetuates the life cycle of the organism. In the United States, most *Trichinella* infections are asymptomatic and are acquired by ingesting undercooked pork, feral meat, wild boar, bear, or walrus.

On mammography, the calcified encysted larvae are seen as tiny linear calcifications smaller than 1 mm that are aligned along the long axis of the pectoralis muscle, parallel to the muscular fibers (Fig. 10-28). Because the calcifications are within the muscle, they should not be mistaken for breast cancer. At this point patients are asymptomatic.

Parasitic diseases that have been reported to calcify in breast tissue include hydatid disease, paragonimiasis, *Dirofilaria repens* infection, schistosomiasis, myiasis, and loiasis.

DERMATOMYOSITIS

Dermatomyositis and some collagen vascular diseases can rarely produce calcifications within the soft tissues

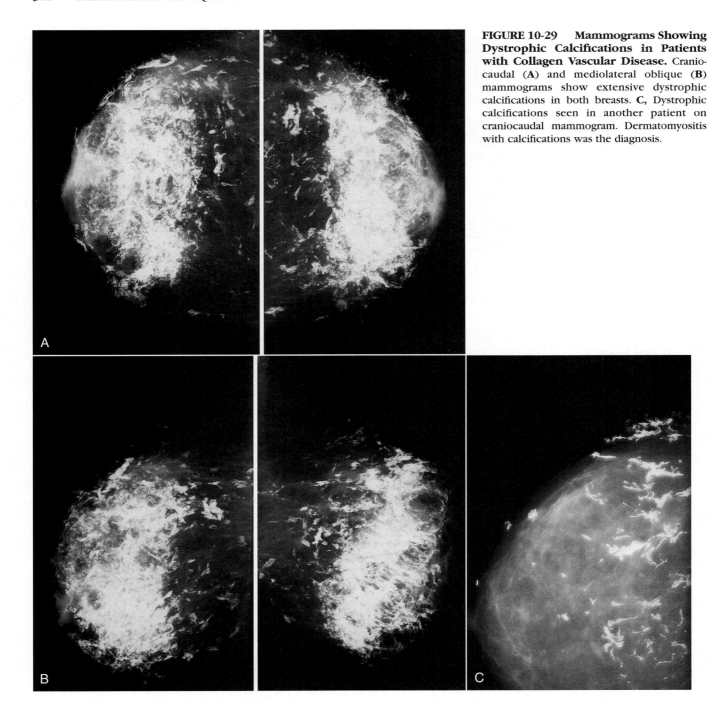

FIGURE 10-29 **Mammograms Showing Dystrophic Calcifications in Patients with Collagen Vascular Disease.** Cranio-caudal (**A**) and mediolateral oblique (**B**) mammograms show extensive dystrophic calcifications in both breasts. **C,** Dystrophic calcifications seen in another patient on craniocaudal mammogram. Dermatomyositis with calcifications was the diagnosis.

of the arms and legs. In the breast, bizarre sheet-like calcifications form in a configuration similar to that of fat necrosis; the calcifications align along the breast tissues and generally point at the nipple (Fig. 10-29A and B). Dermatomyositis is not a specific indicator of breast cancer. However, mammography is often performed because of an association of dermatomyositis with malignancies.

FOREIGN BODIES

Foreign bodies can be seen within the breast on mammography. Some acupuncture practitioners break acupuncture needle tips off in the breast tissue after placement, and the tiny sheared-off metallic needle tip fragments can be seen inside the breast tissue (Fig. 10-30A and B).

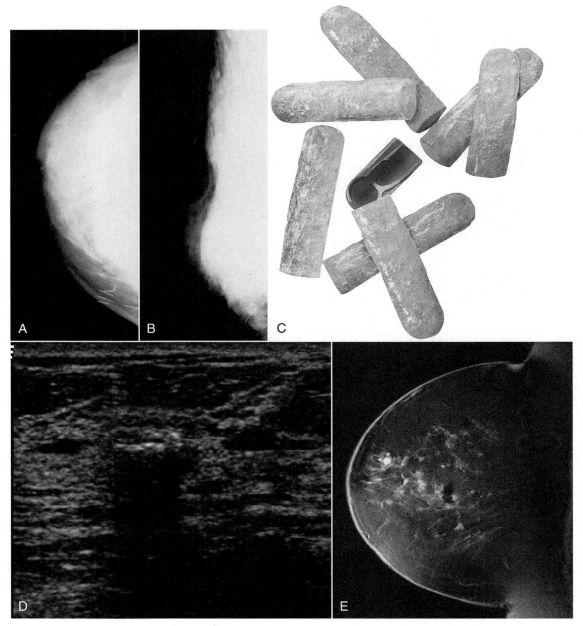

FIGURE 10-30   Foreign Bodies. Mediolateral oblique (**A**) and craniocaudal (**B**) mammograms show dense small masses throughout the breast tissue representing silicone injections, as well as thin metallic slivers in the peripheral breast parenchyma representing retained acupuncture needles. **C-J,** Metallic clip and ultrasound-visible pellets for marking the biopsy site after percutaneous needle biopsy. **C,** Pellets and a metallic marker. **D,** Echogenic ultrasound appearance after a gel marker is placed. **E,** Magnetic resonance imaging signal void from a metallic marker.   *Continued*

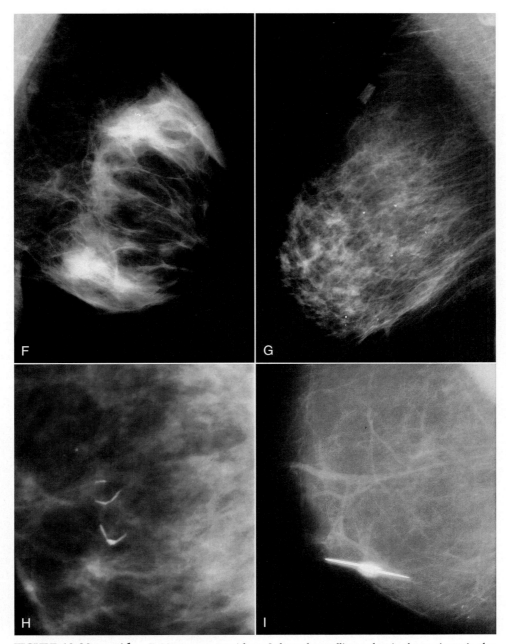

FIGURE 10-30 cont'd   **F,** Mammogram with an S-shaped metallic marker in dense tissue in the upper part of the breast. **(C-F** From SenoRx Inc., 11 Columbia, Suite A, Alisa Viejo, CA 92656.) **G,** A retained Dacron Hickman catheter cuff in the upper part of the right breast is seen as a radiopaque tube. **H,** Mammography shows sutures containing knots and a small calcified suture fragment. **I,** A needle was iatrogenically placed by this patient into her own breast, and it subsequently broke and calcified.

The most common foreign bodies seen in the breast on mammography are metallic markers placed percutaneously after core needle biopsy guided by stereotaxis, ultrasound, or MRI (Fig. 10-30C-F). The markers have different shapes, depending on the manufacturer, and may contain a pellet or pellets that are visible by ultrasound. For patients who desire removal of the markers, case reports describe the use of an 11-gauge stereotactic vacuum-assisted probe technique that can remove the markers percutaneously. Percutaneous breast biopsy devices may produce tiny residual metallic shavings or fragments from the biopsy probe or needle itself and are usually not seen on the mammogram. These fragments are ferromagnetic and can occasionally cause signal voids on MRI.

Fragments of preoperatively placed hookwires have been reported in the breast after preoperative needle localization; these fragments may have been transected at surgery or may be due to breakage of the wire at the hooked end. Specimen radiography is used to determine whether the lesion prompting biopsy has been removed, as well as whether the hookwire and hookwire tip are included in the specimen. Information regarding the lesion, hookwire, and hookwire tip should be conveyed to the surgeon in the operating room to ensure complete removal of both the lesion and the hookwire tip. Although some hookwire fragments have been reported to be stable within the breast 1.5 to 11 years after surgery, other fragments become symptomatic as a result of migration within and through the breast into the soft tissues of other parts of the body.

Round Dacron Hickman catheter cuffs may be left inside the breast after removal of a Hickman catheter. The rounded, short tube-like structure made of Dacron has a characteristic appearance in the upper part of the breast on mammography (Fig. 10-30G).

Sutures used to close breast cancer biopsy sites may calcify after lumpectomy and radiation therapy, thereby delaying absorption of the suture material and promoting calcification. The result is linear or curvilinear calcification of the suture, and the diagnosis can be made if the suture still contains a knot (Fig. 10-30H).

Surgeons occasionally place metallic surgical clips in breast cancer biopsy cavities to delineate the extent of the tumor site for radiation oncologists to plan electron beam boosts. This practice is becoming less common because of the increasing use of MRI for follow-up and the use of ultrasound to delineate the breast biopsy cavity to guide planning for electron beam boost therapy.

Other materials may lodge in the breast, and the clinical history may help in the diagnosis (Fig. 10-30I).

HIDRADENITIS SUPPURATIVA

This condition involves hidradenitis of the apocrine sweat glands, which are usually located in the axilla and the inguinal region. In the breast, these glands are also found in the inframammary folds, between the breasts, and around the areola. Hidradenitis suppurativa has been reported in obese patients in regions where the skin surfaces of the breasts or chest wall rub together. Severe hidradenitis causes masses with local inflammation. Severe cases are treated by excision of local disease, but local recurrence is common after treatment.

NEUROFIBROMATOSIS

This autosomal dominant disease is composed of two main types, the most common of which is also known as von Recklinghausen's disease (type I) and is found in 90% of patients. Affected patients may have café au lait skin lesions, neurofibromas of the neural plexus or peripheral nerve sheaths, and neurilemomas.

The skin lesions of neurofibroma can mimic a deep breast tissue mass and limit evaluation of the breast. However, like any skin lesion, neurofibromas may be outlined with air, and correlation with the breast history form is advisable. Furthermore, the description of cutaneous findings on the technologist's sheet should enable the radiologist to distinguish neurofibromas on the skin from masses of ductal origin inside the breast (Fig. 10-31A and B).

BREAST CANCER MISSED BY MAMMOGRAPHY

Non-detection of breast cancer on mammography is of concern to the patient, the referring physician, and the radiologist. Detection of cancer on mammography is the result of a variety of factors, including the mammographic technique, experience of the radiologist, morphology of the breast tumor, and the background on which it is displayed. Cancers can best be displayed by good mammographic technique, optimal positioning, and a tumor location that can be displayed on the film. About 10% to 15% of breast cancers are mammographically occult, even on good images, and will not be detected on mammography in the best of hands.

Cancer may not be detected on previous mammograms for several reasons (Box 10-16). First, the tumor may have a morphology that is undetectable on the mammographic background on which it is displayed and is therefore mammographically occult.

Second, the tumor may display findings that are visible, but below the threshold of any radiologist for consideration as cancer. Such findings have been termed "nonspecific," examples of which include mammographic findings suggesting normal islands of fibroglandular tissue, a few benign-appearing calcifications, or a benign-appearing mass among many other benign-appearing masses that do not represent cancer.

Third, the tumor may show subtle findings representing cancer but are atypical, such as a single dilated duct, a developing density, or other less common features of breast cancer that are perceptible but may have been unrecognized.

Fourth, signs that are classic for breast cancer may have been present on the mammogram but either were

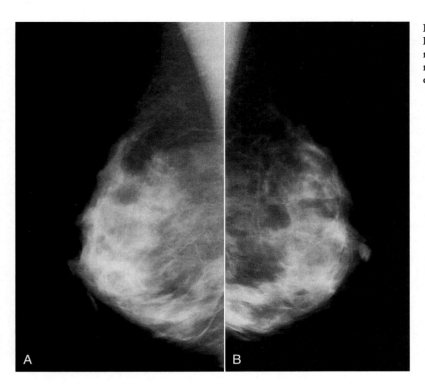

FIGURE 10-31 Neurofibromatosis Simulating Breast Masses. Right lateral (**A**) and left lateral (**B**) mammograms show a neurofibroma simulating a retroareolar mass on the left and a long neurofibroma extending from inferior to the nipple on the right.

Box 10-16	Types of Findings on Previous Mammograms in Patients with Missed Breast Cancer

Occult on mammography (negative)
Nonspecific findings (normal or benign findings)
Atypical findings (subtle)
Classic cancer findings overlooked or misinterpreted

Box 10-17	Factors Contributing to Missed Cancers on Mammography

Suboptimal technique
Cancer not included on the image
Seen on one view
Distracting lesions
Radiolucent lines of fat through the lesion
Overlooked calcifications or small masses
Calcifications look like calcifying blood vessel
Dense breast tissue
Lesion at the edge of glandular tissue
Lesion at the edge of the film
Lesion in the axilla that looks like a lymph node
Benign-appearing lesion
Large breast
Obscured by a blood vessel

not perceived or were misinterpreted at the time of diagnosis.

Box 10-17 shows factors that may contribute to cancer being missed on previous mammograms. Birdwell et al. reviewed possible reasons why tumors were not identified on previous mammograms. They postulated that findings were hidden among many other findings ("busy breasts") or that distracting findings other than the cancer were present on the film. Other contributing factors included dense breast tissue, small calcifications or masses that may have been overlooked, cancers hiding in the axilla and simulating lymph nodes, linear microcalcifications simulating vascular calcifications, findings seen on only one mammographic view, and findings at the edge of the film or at the edge of the glandular tissue producing either a tent sign or concavity that was missed at the time of screening. Of note, most of these cancers were located in the upper outer quadrant, where 50% of all cancers occur. Also of note, not all the cancers that were missed were small inasmuch as at least half the tumors were 1 cm or larger at the time that they were missed.

To decrease the number of missed breast cancers, the radiologist should use a systematic approach to reviewing the mammogram that minimizes distractions, paper shuffling, or other busy work in the reading room at the time of interpretation. Next, comparison to older films may reveal subtle changes not apparent on only the current examination. Finally, the radiologist should be aware of subtle or nonspecific findings of breast cancer.

KEY ELEMENTS

The normal male breast shows only fat on mammography.

Gynecomastia is unilateral or bilateral, symmetrical or asymmetric, and is shown as glandular tissue in a retroareolar flame-like dendritic, triangular nodular, or diffuse appearance on mammography.

Gynecomastia causes breast lumps and pain and has physiologic, drug-related, and medical-related etiologies.

Breast cancer in men is rare, is manifested as a mass eccentric to the nipple or in the upper outer quadrant, and has the same prognosis as breast cancer in women.

Breast cancer in men develops at 1% the rate in women, occurs in older men, and on mammography is usually a noncalcified spiculated or circumscribed retroareolar or periareolar mass.

Pregnancy-related conditions include mastitis, lactational adenoma, enlarging fibroadenoma, galactocele, and pregnancy-associated breast cancer.

Pregnancy-associated breast cancer is defined as cancer diagnosed during pregnancy or within 1 year of delivery.

Stage for stage, the prognosis for pregnancy-associated breast cancer is the same as for nonpregnant women.

On mammography, pregnancy-associated breast cancer is detected as masses or pleomorphic calcifications.

Probably benign findings (BI-RADS category 3) include non-palpable single or multiple clusters of small, round or oval calcifications; single, unilateral or multiple, nonpalpable, non-calcified, round or lobulated, primarily circumscribed solid masses; and nonpalpable focal or global asymmetries that resembles fibroglandular tissue at diagnostic evaluation.

Nipple discharge characteristics that should be investigated are new, bloody, or spontaneously occurring copious serous discharge.

Mammograms and ultrasound are frequently negative in the setting of nipple discharge.

A positive galactogram shows a filling defect, an abrupt duct cutoff, or luminal irregularity.

The differential diagnosis of intraductal masses on galactography includes papilloma, cancer, debris, and an air bubble.

Unilateral breast edema may be caused by mastitis, inflammatory cancer, local obstruction of lymph nodes, trauma, radiation therapy, or coumarin necrosis.

Bilateral breast edema is due to systemic etiologies such as congestive heart failure, liver disease, anasarca, renal failure, bilateral lymphadenopathy, or superior vena cava syndrome.

Although breast edema, exogenous hormone therapy, and weight loss all result in increased breast density, distinction between these causes is made by the presence of skin thickening, which is seen only with breast edema.

Inflammatory cancer is the most important differential diagnosis for unilateral breast edema and is a rare (1% of all cancers) aggressive breast cancer with a poor prognosis.

The most common cause of mastitis is *S. aureus;* rare causes include tuberculosis, syphilis, hydatid disease, and molluscum contagiosum.

An extremely rare cause of unilateral breast edema is coumarin (warfarin [Coumadin]) therapy producing necrosis of the breast.

Axillary lymphadenopathy on mammography is shown as replacement of the fatty hilum of lymph nodes by dense tissue, a rounded lymph node shape, and overall generalized increased density with or without lymph node enlargement.

The differential for abnormal lymph nodes containing "calcifications" includes calcifying metastatic disease, granulomatous disease, gold deposits from therapy for rheumatoid arthritis mimicking calcifications, or silicone from a previously ruptured breast implant.

The differential for unilateral axillary adenopathy includes metastatic breast cancer or mastitis.

The differential for bilateral axillary adenopathy is systemic conditions such as infection, collagen vascular diseases such as rheumatoid arthritis, lymphoma, leukemia, and metastatic tumor.

Primary breast cancer manifested as isolated lymph node metastasis in women with normal mammographic findings and normal physical examinations is uncommon and accounts for less than 1% of all breast cancers.

Paget's disease of the nipple heralds an underlying breast cancer with a high rate of overexpression of the c-*erb*-B2 oncogene.

Women with Paget's disease of the nipple have a bright red nipple, eczematous nipple changes that may extend to the areola, and subsequent ulceration or nipple destruction.

Sarcomas are rare malignant tumors of the breast or underlying chest wall, and their classification depends on the cell type; mammography shows high-density masses without calcifications or spiculation.

Mondor's disease is a rare benign and self-limited acute thrombophlebitis of the superficial veins of the breast. It is often associated with trauma or recent surgery and produces a tender palpable cord extending toward the outer portion of the breast.

Mammography is usually negative in women with Mondor's disease or rarely shows a long linear or tubular density corresponding to the thrombosed vein.

Granulomatous mastitis is a rare benign cause of a breast mass in young premenopausal women after their last childbirth; it has been correlated with breast-feeding and oral contraceptive use, and a possible autoimmune component has been implicated in its etiology.

Patients with granulomatous mastitis may have galactorrhea, inflammation, a breast mass, induration, and skin ulcerations. Treatment is surgery, but the recurrence rate is high.

Diabetic mastopathy is a benign cause of hard, irregular, sometimes painful mobile breast masses in long-term insulin-dependent diabetes, younger premenopausal diabetic women, or rare patients with thyroid disease.

Diabetic mastopathy is due to an autoimmune reaction to the accumulation of abnormal matrix proteins caused by hyperglycemia. It produces a hard fibrotic mass with a lymphocytic reaction; treatment is surgery, but the recurrence rate is high.

Desmoid tumor is also known as an extra-abdominal desmoid or fibromatosis.

Desmoid tumor is an infiltrative, locally aggressive fibroblastic/myofibroblastic process that is treated by surgery, may recur locally, may be multicentric, is associated with previous trauma or surgery, and has been reported in women with breast implants.

Trichinosis is caused by ingesting raw or undercooked meat containing encysted larvae of the *Trichinella* genus. The larvae give rise to tiny linear calcifications in the pectoralis muscles and not in the breast.

Dermatomyositis and some collagen vascular diseases can rarely produce bizarre sheet-like calcifications that are found to align along the breast tissues on mammography.

Foreign bodies in the breast seen on mammography include percutaneous metallic markers, acupuncture needle tips, hookwire fragments, calcifying sutures, vascular clips to mark breast cancer cavities for planning radiation therapy, Dacron Hickman catheter cuffs, and other foreign objects.

Hidradenitis suppurativa is a benign condition that produces breast lumps representing hidradenitis of the apocrine sweat glands in the axilla, between the breasts, and in the inframammary folds.

Neurofibromatosis is an autosomal dominant disease also known as von Recklinghausen's disease (type I); affected patients may have café au lait skin lesions and neurofibromas of the neural plexus or peripheral nerve sheaths. The skin lesions can cause apparent breast masses on mammography.

Missed breast cancers may be due to cancers that are occult on the mammogram, nonspecific findings, atypical findings, or misinterpretation of the classic features of cancer.

Factors influencing why cancers were missed on previous mammograms include findings hidden among many other findings, distracting findings, dense breast tissue, overlooked small calcifications or masses, location simulating lymph nodes, simulation of vascular calcifications, visualization on only one mammographic view, and findings at the edge of the film or at the edge of glandular tissue.

SUGGESTED READINGS

Ad-El DD, Meirovitz A, Weinberg A, et al: Warfarin skin necrosis: Local and systemic factors. Br J Plast Surg 53:624-626, 2000.

Ahn BY, Kim HH, Moon WK, et al: Pregnancy- and lactation-associated breast cancer: Mammographic and sonographic findings. J Ultrasound Med 22:491-497, quiz 498-499, 2003.

American College of Radiology: ACR Breast Imaging Reporting and Data System, Breast Imaging Atlas. Reston, VA, American College of Radiology, 2003.

Bayer U, Horn LC, Schulz HG: Bilateral, tumorlike diabetic mastopathy—progression and regression of the disease during 5-year follow up. Eur J Radiol 26:248-253, 1998.

Bejanga BI: Mondor's disease: Analysis of 30 cases. J R Coll Surg Edinb 37:322-324, 1992.

Bergkvist L, Frodis E, Hedborg-Mellander C, Hansen J: Management of accidentally found pathological lymph nodes on routine screening mammography. Eur J Surg Oncol 22:250-253, 1996.

Berkowitz JE, Gatewood OM, Goldblum LE, Gayler BW: Hormonal replacement therapy: Mammographic manifestations. Radiology 174:199-201, 1990.

Birdwell RL, Ikeda DM, O'Shaughnessy KF, Sickles EA: Mammographic characteristics of 115 missed cancers later detected with screening mammography and the potential utility of computer-aided detection. Radiology 219:192-202, 2001.

Brenner RJ: Follow-up as an alternative to biopsy for probably benign mammographically detected abnormalities. Curr Opin Radiol 3:588-592, 1991.

Brenner RJ: Percutaneous removal of postbiopsy marking clip in the breast using stereotactic technique. AJR Am J Roentgenol 176:417-419, 2001.

Bruwer A, Nelson GW, Spark RP: Punctate intranodal gold deposits simulating microcalcifications on mammograms. Radiology 163:87-88, 1987.

Camuto PM, Zetrenne E, Ponn T: Diabetic mastopathy: A report of 5 cases and a review of the literature. Arch Surg 135:1190-1193, 2000.

Chow JS, Smith DN, Kaelin CM, Meyer JE: Case report: Galactography-guided wire localization of an intraductal papilloma. Clin Radiol 56:72-73, 2001.

Crowe DJ, Helvie MA, Wilson TE: Breast infection. Mammographic and sonographic findings with clinical correlation. Invest Radiol 30:582-587, 1995.

Dale PS, Wardlaw JC, Wootton DG, et al: Desmoid tumor occurring after reconstruction mammaplasty for breast carcinoma. Ann Plast Surg 35:515-518, 1995.

Daniel BL, Gardner RW, Birdwell RL, et al: Magnetic resonance imaging of intraductal papilloma of the breast. Magn Reson Imaging 21:887-892, 2003.

Dershaw DD, Moore MP, Liberman L, Deutch BM: Inflammatory breast carcinoma: Mammographic findings. Radiology 190:831-834, 1994.

Diesing D, Axt-Fliedner R, Hornung D, et al: Granulomatous mastitis. Arch Gynecol Obstet 2003 (in press).

Doberl A, Tobiassen T, Rasmussen T: Treatment of recurrent cyclical mastodynia in patients with fibrocystic breast disease. A double-blind placebo-controlled study—the Hjorring project. Acta Obstet Gynecol Scand Suppl 123:177-184, 1984.

Dooley WC: Ductal lavage, nipple aspiration, and ductoscopy for breast cancer diagnosis. Curr Oncol Rep 5:63-65, 2003.

Duijm LE, Guit GL, Hendriks JH, et al: Value of breast imaging in women with painful breasts: Observational follow up study. BMJ 317:1492-1495, 1998.

Elson BC, Ikeda DM, Andersson I, Wattsgard C: Fibrosarcoma of the breast: Mammographic findings in five cases. AJR Am J Roentgenol 158:993-995, 1992.

Evans GF, Anthony T, Turnage RH, et al: The diagnostic accuracy of mammography in the evaluation of male breast disease. Am J Surg 181:96-100, 2001.

Finder CA, Kisielewski RW, Kedas AM: Residual metal shavings and fragments associated with large-core biopsy needles: A follow-up. Radiology 208:833-834, 1998.

Garstin WI, Kaufman Z, Michell MJ, Baum M: Fibrous mastopathy in insulin dependent diabetics. Clin Radiol 44:89-91, 1991.

Godwin Y, McCulloch TA, Sully L: Extra-abdominal desmoid tumour of the breast: Review of the primary management and the implications for breast reconstruction. Br J Plast Surg 54:268-271, 2001.

Gunhan-Bilgen I, Bozkaya H, Ustun EE, Memis A: Male breast disease: Clinical, mammographic, and ultrasonographic features. Eur J Radiol 43:246-255, 2002.

Gunhan-Bilgen I, Ustun EE, Memis A: Inflammatory breast carcinoma: Mammographic, ultrasonographic, clinical, and pathologic findings in 142 cases. Radiology 223:829-838, 2002.

Harenberg J, Hoffmann U, Huhle G, et al: Cutaneous reactions to anticoagulants. Recognition and management. Am J Clin Dermatol 2(2):69-75, 2001.

Haupt HM, Rosen PP, Kinne DW: Breast carcinoma presenting with axillary lymph node metastases. An analysis of specific histopathologic features. Am J Surg Pathol 9:165-175, 1985.

Homer MJ, Smith TJ: Asymmetric breast tissue. Radiology 173:577-578, 1989.

Hook GW, Ikeda DM: Treatment of breast abscesses with US-guided percutaneous needle drainage without indwelling catheter placement. Radiology 213:579-582, 1999.

Ikeda DM, Birdwell RL, O'Shaughnessy KF, et al: Analysis of 172 subtle findings on prior normal mammograms in women with breast cancer detected at follow-up screening. Radiology 226:494-503, 2003.

Ikeda DM, Helvie MA, Frank TS, et al: Paget disease of the nipple: Radiologic-pathologic correlation. Radiology 189:89-94, 1993.

Ikeda DM, Sickles EA: Mammographic demonstration of pectoral muscle microcalcifications. AJR Am J Roentgenol 151:475-476, 1988.

Kedas AM, Byrd LJ, Kisielewski RW: Residual metal shavings and fragments associated with large-core breast biopsy. Radiology 200:585, 1996.

Kushwaha AC, Whitman GJ, Stelling CB, et al: Primary inflammatory carcinoma of the breast: Retrospective review of mammographic findings. AJR Am J Roentgenol 174:535-538, 2000.

Leibman AJ, Kossoff MB: Mammography in women with axillary lymphadenopathy and normal breasts on physical examination: Value in detecting occult breast carcinoma. AJR Am J Roentgenol 159:493-495, 1992.

Liberman L, Giess CS, Dershaw DD, et al: Imaging of pregnancy-associated breast cancer. Radiology 191:245-248, 1994.

Liberman L, Morris EA, Benton CL, et al: Probably benign lesions at breast magnetic resonance imaging: Preliminary experience in high-risk women. Cancer 98:377-388, 2003.

Liu GJ, Chen WG, Duan G, et al: Mammographic findings of gynecomastia. Di Yi Jun Yi Da Xue Xue Bao 22:839-840, 2002.

Matsuoka K, Ohsumi S, Takashima S, et al: Occult breast carcinoma presenting with axillary lymph node metastases: Follow-up of eleven patients. Breast Cancer 10:330-334, 2003.

Memis A, Bilgen I, Ustun EE, et al: Granulomatous mastitis: Imaging findings with histopathologic correlation. Clin Radiol 57:1001-1006, 2002.

Montrey JS, Levy JA, Brenner RJ: Wire fragments after needle localization. AJR Am J Roentgenol 167:1267-1269, 1996.

Murray ME, Given-Wilson RM: The clinical importance of axillary lymphadenopathy detected on screening mammography. Clin Radiol 52:458-461, 1997.

Orel SG, Dougherty CS, Reynolds C, et al: MR imaging in patients with nipple discharge: Initial experience. Radiology 216:248-254, 2000.

Parsi K, Younger I, Gallo J: Warfarin-induced skin necrosis associated with acquired protein C deficiency. Australas J Dermatol 44:57-61, 2003.

Rieber A, Tomczak RJ, Mergo PJ, et al: MRI of the breast in the differential diagnosis of mastitis versus inflammatory carcinoma and follow-up. J Comput Assist Tomogr 21:128-132, 1997.

Rosen EL, Baker JA, Soo MS: Malignant lesions initially subjected to short-term mammographic follow-up. Radiology 223:221-228, 2002.

Sachs DD, Gordon AT: Hidradenitis suppurativa of glands of Moll. Arch Ophthalmol 77:635-636, 1967.

Sawhney S, Petkovska L, Ramadan S, et al: Sonographic appearances of galactoceles. J Clin Ultrasound 30:18-22, 2002.

Schnarkowski P, Kessler M, Arnholdt H, Helmberger T: Angiosarcoma of the breast: Mammographic, sonographic, and pathological findings. Eur J Radiol 24:54-56, 1997.

Serels S, Melman A: Tamoxifen as treatment for gynecomastia and mastodynia resulting from hormonal deprivation. J Urol 159:1309, 1998.

Sickles EA: Periodic mammographic follow-up of probably benign lesions: Results in 3,184 consecutive cases. Radiology 179:463-468, 1991.

Sickles EA: Nonpalpable, circumscribed, noncalcified solid breast masses: Likelihood of malignancy based on lesion size and age of patient. Radiology 192:439-442, 1994.

Sickles EA: Probably benign breast lesions: When should follow-up be recommended and what is the optimal follow-up protocol? Radiology 213:11-14, 1999.

Stomper PC, Waddell BE, Edge SB, Klippenstein DL: Breast MRI in the evaluation of patients with occult primary breast carcinoma. Breast J 5:230-234, 1999.

Swinford AE, Adler DD, Garver KA: Mammographic appearance of the breasts during pregnancy and lactation: False assumptions. Acad Radiol 5:467-472, 1998.

Talele AC, Slanetz PJ, Edmister WB, et al: The lactating breast: MRI findings and literature review. Breast J 9:237-240, 2003.

Tilanus-Linthorst MM, Obdeijn AI, Bontenbal M, Oudkerk M: MRI in patients with axillary metastases of occult breast carcinoma. Breast Cancer Res Treat 44:179-182, 1997.

Varas X, Leborgne JH, Leborgne F, et al: Revisiting the mammographic follow-up of BI-RADS category 3 lesions. AJR Am J Roentgenol 179:691-695, 2002.

Woo JC, Yu T, Hurd TC: Breast cancer in pregnancy: A literature review. Arch Surg 138:91-98, discussion 99, 2003.

Yasmeen S, Romano PS, Pettinger M, et al: Frequency and predictive value of a mammographic recommendation for short-interval follow-up. J Natl Cancer Inst 95:429-436, 2003.

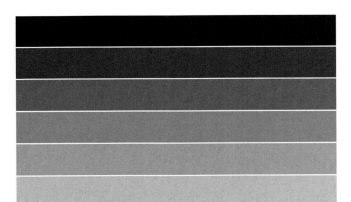

Index

Note: Page numbers followed by the letter f refer to figures, those followed by the letter t refer to tables, and those followed by b refer to boxed material.

A

Abscess, 126, 128, 128f. See also Infection; Mastitis.
  after percutaneous biopsy, 185
  during lactation, 288, 289f
  during pregnancy, 280
  edema associated with, 126, 152, 153f, 288, 301
  in granulomatous mastitis, 308
  mammographic appearance of, 126, 288, 289f, 301
  post-surgical, 289f
  recurrent subareolar, 301
  ultrasound imaging of, 126, 128f, 152–153, 153f, 288, 289f, 301
  vs. mucinous carcinoma, on MRI, 206
Accreditation of facilities, 1–2, 1b, 12
  for digital mammography, 18
  labeling of mammograms and, 8
  mammographic views and, 5–6
Acini, 26, 27f
  calcifications in, 62, 63f, 71
  galactography of, 295f
Acoustic enhancement
  as BI-RADS descriptor, 134f, 135
  by cyst, 136–137, 138, 138f
  by fibroadenoma, 110
  by galactocele, 288
  by medullary cancer, 106, 108f, 146f
  by mucinous carcinoma, 106, 147
  by necrotic tumor, 147
  by phyllodes tumor, 113
  by pregnancy-associated breast cancer, 285
  variations of, 145f
Acoustic shadowing, 92, 95f
  as BI-RADS descriptor, 134t, 135
  by biopsy scar, 153
  by desmoid tumor, 309
  by diabetic mastopathy, 309
  by fibroadenoma, 110
    as suspicious finding, 141
  by galactocele, 128, 288
  by granulomatous mastitis, 306

Acoustic shadowing—cont'd
  by invasive ductal cancer, 95, 96f, 97, 144f
    recurrent, 248f
  by nipple, 136, 137f
  by spiculated masses, 144
    inflammatory cancer as, 148f, 149
    invasive ductal cancer as, 95, 96f, 97
    post-biopsy scar as, 100
    radial scar as, 103
  technique and, 133–134
  vs. edge shadowing, 144, 145f
Acoustic spiculation, 92
  of invasive ductal cancer, 95, 97
  of post-biopsy scar, 100
ACR. See American College of Radiology (ACR).
ACR BI-RADS. See BI-RADS lexicon.
Activated charcoal marking, after biopsy, 178, 180
Acupuncture needle tips, retained, 312, 313f
Adenoid cystic carcinoma, 116
Adenoma. See also Fibroadenoma(s).
  lactating, 116, 116f, 280, 287, 288
Adenopathy. See Lymphadenopathy.
Adenosis
  of fibroadenoma, 110
  of radial scar, 103
  sclerosing, 103
    calcifications in, 62, 85f–86f, 103
ADH. See Atypical ductal hyperplasia (ADH).
Adjuvant chemotherapy. See also Chemotherapy.
  mortality decrease due to, 24
  tamoxifen as, 303
AEC (automatic exposure control)
  for digital mammography, 17
  for screen-film mammography, 2, 4, 4f, 5
Age
  breast cancer risk and, 24, 25
  density of breast and, 26, 28, 136, 302
Alcohol use, breast cancer and, 24
ALH (atypical lobular hyperplasia), on core biopsy, 184
ALND. See Lymph nodes, axillary, dissection of.
American College of Radiology (ACR)
  accreditation by, 1, 8, 12, 18
  screening trials of

American College of Radiology (ACR)—cont'd
  of digital vs. film, 17
  of ultrasound, 160–161
  terminology of. See BI-RADS lexicon.
Amorphous calcifications, 62, 64f, 67, 67f
  indeterminate for malignancy, 85f–86f
  new, 87f
Analgesics, 180, 185, 303
Analog-to-digital converter, 15, 17
Anechoic pattern, 134, 134t
Anesthesia. See Local anesthesia.
Angiogenesis, tumor, MRI of, 189, 199
Angiosarcoma
  MRI of, 305
  vs. pseudoangiomatous stromal hyperplasia, 120, 184
Anode-filter combinations, 3, 3b
Antiperspirant, 70, 71f
Architectural distortion. See also Scar.
  asymmetry associated with, 288
  differential diagnosis of, 32t
  exclusion from "probably benign" category, 290
  implant removal and, 262, 264f
  in breast cancer, 28, 32t, 34, 36f, 149
    as ductal carcinoma, 148f
    as lobular carcinoma, 98, 98f
  in fibrocystic change, proliferative, 103f
  mass associated with, 92
  on ultrasound report, 135
  post-biopsy scar with, 100, 101f, 225, 226b, 227f–228f, 245f
  radial scar with, 105f
  reduction mammaplasty causing, 271
Areola. See also "Retroareolar" entries; "Subareolar" entries.
  apocrine sweat glands and, 315
  mammographic appearance of, 34
  Paget's disease of nipple and, 305
  post-radiation swelling of, 239
  subcutaneous mastectomy and, 249
Arterial calcification, 81, 81f, 316
Artifacts
  mammographic, 6, 9f–11f
    simulating calcifications, 70–71, 71f–72f
  MRI, 197–198, 197f, 197t

Artifacts—*cont'd*
    core biopsy needles and, 221
    metal biopsy markers and, 181
    ultrasound. *See* Ultrasound, artifacts in.
Aspiration. *See* Fine-needle aspiration;
    Vacuum-assisted biopsy.
Asymmetry. *See* Density of breast,
    asymmetric.
Ataxia-telangiectasia syndrome, 25
Atherosclerosis, calcification in, 81, 81f
Atlas, breast, for MRI, 201, 203f-212f,
    205-206, 208
Atypical ductal hyperplasia (ADH)
    breast cancer risk and, 25
    core biopsy of, 183, 184
    excisional biopsy of, 183
    radial scar associated with, 103, 184
    vacuum-assisted biopsy of, 183
Atypical hyperplasia, vacuum-assisted biopsy
    of, 177
Atypical lobular hyperplasia (ALH), on core
    biopsy, 184
Automatic exposure control (AEC)
    for digital mammography, 17
    for screen-film mammography, 2, 4, 4f, 5
Axilla
    deodorant in, 70, 71f
    hidradenitis suppurativa in, 315
    mammographic appearance of, 34, 37,
        38f-39f
    MRI of, 193
    silicone extruded into, 268, 269f
    skin calcifications in, 73
Axillary breast tissue, 37, 38f
Axillary lymph nodes. *See* Lymph nodes,
    axillary.
Axillary lymphadenopathy, 303-305, 304b,
    304f-305f. *See also* Lymph nodes,
    axillary.

B
Baker classification, 254, 254t
BBs, on skin above lesion, 169, 176f
Benign calcifying entities, 70, 70b, 82b. *See*
    also Calcifications, benign; *specific*
    entity.
Benign mammographic findings, probable,
    37, 39b, 84, 288, 290, 290b, 291f, 292
Benign mass(es). *See also* Cyst(s); *specific*
    diagnosis.
    borders of, 90, 91
    MRI of, 199, 199b, 200f-202f, 201, 201b,
        201t
    rounded or expansile, 106b, 110,
        111f-116f
    that should be left alone, 126b
    ultrasound of, 92, 140-143, 141b,
        142f-143f
Bilateral breast cancer, MRI of, 214, 218f
Biopsy
    complications of. *See also* Core needle
        biopsy, complications of; Hematoma;
        Postoperative appearance.
        breast edema as, 151
        epidermal inclusion cyst as, 128
    core needle. *See* Core needle biopsy.
    Doppler imaging prior to, 155, 160f
    excisional. *See* Excisional biopsy.
    fine-needle. *See* Fine-needle aspiration.
    galactogram as indication for, 294
    history of, 32, 33f, 34
    in pregnancy, 288
    key elements of, 186

Biopsy—*cont'd*
    mammographic follow-up instead of, 288
    markers in site of. *See* Markers, metallic.
    MRI enhancement in site of, 190
    MRI-guided, 217, 219, 219b, 221, 221f
    of calcifications, 60, 70, 82, 84, 85f-87f
        with mass, 92, 93f
    of desmoid tumor, 309
    of diabetic mastopathy, 309
    of fibroadenoma, 110, 111f-112f, 142, 183
    of granulomatous mastitis, 308
    of inflammatory cancer, 300
    of intracystic tumors, 140, 171
    of palpable mass, with normal
        mammogram and ultrasound, 150, 213
    of spiculated mass, 103, 105b
    percutaneous. *See also* Core needle
        biopsy; Fine-needle aspiration.
        advantages of, 163
        cancellation of, 164
        follow-up to, 186
        informed consent for, 164, 164b, 186
        local anesthesia for, 164, 171, 173
        metal fragments left by, 314-315
        neoadjuvant chemotherapy and, 155,
            156f
        noncompliance of patient after, 186
        patient work-up for, 163-164, 164b
        risks of, 164
        role of, 229
    rate of
        true-positive rate and, 84
        with digital screening, 17
    sentinel lymph node, 82, 233-235, 233t,
        234b, 235f
BI-RADS lexicon, 5
    for breast density, 28, 28b
    for calcifications, 61, 61b, 62, 65f, 67, 70,
        70b
    for mammography reporting, 37, 39b
        "probably benign" category in, 37, 39b,
            84, 288, 290, 290b, 291f, 292
    for masses, 90, 91, 91f, 91t
        associated findings and, 92b
        reporting and, 94, 95b
        ultrasound findings and, 92, 94t,
            134-135, 134t, 144-145
    for MRI reporting, 198, 198t, 199
    for ultrasound labeling, 134, 134b
Blackhead, 128
Bleed, silicone gel, 254, 255, 255t, 264, 270
Bleeding. *See also* Hematoma; Nipple
    discharge, bloody.
    from core biopsy, 177, 185
Blue dye, for sentinel node biopsy, 233, 234,
    235
Blurring
    in mammography, 4, 10f
    in MRI, 197t, 198
Bracket localization, of calcifications, 168,
    170f
Branching calcifications, 67, 68f, 70
    malignant, 82
    of secretory disease vs. DCIS, 79
BRCA1 gene, 25
    screening MRI and, 210-211, 214f
BRCA2 gene, 25
    screening MRI and, 210-211
Breast
    apocrine sweat glands of, 315
    axillary tissue of, 37, 38f
    lactating. *See* Lactating breast.
    metastasis to, 109-110, 110f

Breast—*cont'd*
    normal anatomy of, 26, 27f
    asymmetric glandular tissue in, 28,
        29f-30f
        sonographic, 135-136, 135f-137f, 136b
    normal MRI findings in, 194-197,
        195f-196f
    painful. *See* Pain, breast.
    positions in
        describing, 32, 34f
        on label of ultrasound, 92, 94b
    veins of, thrombophlebitis of, 305-306,
        309b, 310f
Breast atlas, for MRI, 201, 203f-212f,
    205-206, 208
Breast augmentation. *See* Implants; Silicone
    injections.
Breast bud, 136, 137f
Breast cancer. *See also* Ductal carcinoma in
    situ (DCIS); Invasive ductal cancer;
    Invasive lobular carcinoma; Mass(es);
    Occult breast cancer.
    bilateral, MRI of, 214, 218f
    computer-aided diagnosis of, 18-20,
        19f-21f
    dermatomyositis associated with, 312
    doubling time of, 288
    family history of, 25
    galactography of, 294, 296f
    implants and, 252, 255, 256f
    in lactating breast, 285, 287
    incidence of
        in men, 279
        in 90-year life span, 25
        increased, in United States, 24
    locally advanced. *See also* Inflammatory
        breast cancer.
        edema in, 296, 300
        treatment of, 155
    male, 279, 280, 285, 285b, 285f-287f
        inflammatory, ultrasound imaging of,
            148f
        sentinel node biopsy in, 235
    mammography of, 28, 32t
        inflammatory, 298f-299f, 300
        male, 280, 285f-287f
        missed, 315-317, 316b
        pregnancy-associated, 285
        recurrent, 246-247, 246b, 247f-248f
        sarcoma as, 305, 307f-309f
    metastatic. *See* Metastasis(es).
    missed by mammography, 315-317, 316b.
        See also Occult breast cancer.
    lobular carcinoma as, 150, 236
    mortality of, screening mammography and,
        1, 2, 24
    MRI of, 199, 199b, 200f-202f, 201, 201b,
        201t
        inflammatory, 300
        invasive ductal, 97
        invasive lobular, 98
        mammographically occult, 189, 190f,
            210, 213
        multicentric or bilateral, 214, 218f
        multifocal, 214, 217f, 238f
        recurrent, 240, 246, 246f
    multicentric
        breast conservation precluded by, 236,
            237f
        MRI of, 214, 218f
        radiation therapy and, 233
        sentinel node biopsy of, 235
    multifocal, MRI of, 214, 217f, 238f

Breast cancer.—*cont'd*
nipple discharge in, 292-293, 292t, 294, 296f
occult. *See* Occult breast cancer.
pregnancy-associated, 285, 287, 287b
prior history of, 25
"probably benign" category and, 290, 292
radiation-induced, 2, 25, 247
recurrent. *See* Recurrent breast cancer, local.
risk factors for, 24-25, 24b, 25b
on history sheet, 32, 33f
peripheral papillomas as, 114
radiation exposure as, 2, 25, 247
screening mammography and, 1, 2, 28
signs and symptoms of, 25-26, 26b
bloody nipple discharge as, 292
silicone injections and, 262
staging of
MRI in, 213-214, 213b, 216f-218f
sentinel node biopsy in, 82, 233-235, 233f, 234b, 235f
TNM classification for, 229, 232t
treatment of, 229, 231, 233. *See also* Breast-conserving therapy; Chemotherapy; Mastectomy; Radiation therapy.
MRI in, 213b, 214, 219f
ultrasound of, 92, 94b, 144-147, 144b, 144f-148f, 146b, 149
inflammatory, 148f, 149, 296, 300
male, 280, 286f-287f
pregnancy-associated, 285
recurrent, 246-247, 247f-248f
secondary signs in, 148f, 149, 149b
vs. radial scar, 103, 104f-105f
Breast coil, dedicated, in MRI, 193, 193b, 193f
for imaging implants, 264
for needle localization, 217
Breast examination, clinical. *See also* Palpable mass.
American Cancer Society guidelines for, 1, 1b
implants and, 255
recurrence found at, 246
Breast history
for mammography, 28, 32, 33f, 37
for MRI, 190
previous biopsies on, 229
Breast Imaging Reporting and Data System. *See* BI-RADS lexicon.
Breast lift, 271
Breast-conserving therapy, 231, 233, 236t, 271. *See also* Lumpectomy; Radiation therapy; Surgical excision.
contralateral reduction following, 271
in pregnancy, 287
key elements of, 249
MRI and, 214
perioperative imaging for, 236, 236t, 239, 240f
post-radiation imaging with, 236t, 239-240, 241f-246f, 243b, 246
preoperative imaging for, 236, 236t, 237f-239f
recurrence after, 233, 233b
calcifications in, 80f, 81
risk of breast cancer and, 25
specimen radiography for, 236
treatment failure with, 246-247, 246b, 247f-248f, 248b
Breast-feeding. *See* Lactating breast.
Brightness, in digital mammography, 17

Bromocriptine, for breast pain, 303
Bucky factor, 5

C

CAD (computer-aided diagnosis), 18-20, 19f-21f, 32, 37
Caffeine, 303
Calcifications, 60-88. *See also* Microcalcifications.
anatomy of, 61-70
duct structure and, 61-62, 61f-62f
group shape, 65b, 67, 68f-69f, 70, 70b
individual forms, 62, 63f-67f, 65b, 67
size of cluster, 62
benign, 60
follow-up hindered by, 236
forms of, 62, 63f, 65f, 70, 70b
group shape, 67, 68f, 70, 70b
locations of, 61
on core biopsy, 183
probably benign, 37, 39b, 84, 288, 290b, 291f
specific entities with, 70, 70b. *See also* *specific entity.*
biopsy of, 60, 70, 82, 84, 85f-87f
core biopsy as, 177-178, 178f-179f, 181, 182f, 183
displacement by, 181, 183
follow-up of, 184
pathologic-radiologic correlation and, 168, 168t, 169f-170f
BI-RADS terminology for, 61, 61b, 62, 65f, 67, 70, 70b
computer-aided detection of, 18, 19, 20, 21f
dermal, 61, 73, 74f-75f, 75b, 82, 164
in autologous flap, 271
foreign-body, 81, 82f, 314f, 315
implant-associated, 254, 255, 256f-257f, 259, 262
after subcutaneous mastectomy, 271
in autologous flap, 271
in collagen vascular disease, 311-312, 312f
in dermatomyositis, 311-312, 312f
in fat necrosis, 143, 240, 244f
in autologous flap, 271
in lymph nodes, 303, 304, 304b
in Paget's disease of nipple, 61, 88f, 305
in parasitic diseases, 311, 311b, 311f
in recurrent breast cancer, 246, 246b
indeterminate, 60, 62, 64f, 84, 85f-87f
key elements of, 84
locations of, 61
magnification views of, 50, 60-61, 240
malignant, 81-82, 82b, 83f, 84b. *See also* *specific diagnosis.*
causes of formation of, 60, 62
cluster size of, 62, 82
forms of, 62, 64f-67f, 65b, 67
group shapes of, 65b, 67, 68f-69f, 70
in male breast cancer, 287f
locations of, 61-62
significance of, 60
mammogram interpretation and, 32, 34
mammographic technique for, 60-61, 61b
mass with, 92, 92b, 93f
MRI and, 208, 219
new, 84, 87f
nipple discharge and, 292
osteogenic sarcoma with, 82, 305, 309f
pleomorphic. *See* Pleomorphic calcifications.

Calcifications—*cont'd*
post-biopsy, 239, 240, 240f, 244f
radiolucent centers in, 73, 74f, 77, 164, 225, 229f, 240
report on, 61, 61b
specimen radiography of, 168, 168t, 169f-170f, 177-178, 179f
implant-associated, 257f
ultrasound imaging of, 84, 88f, 92, 142, 144-145, 147, 147f, 149
BI-RADS terminology for, 135
in DCIS, 149, 149f
not seen on, 145f, 147
vascular, 81, 81f, 316
Calcium oxalate, 168
Calcium phosphate, 168
Cancer. *See* Breast cancer; Ovarian cancer.
Cancerization of lobules, 62f, 67
Carbon marking, after stereotactic biopsy, 180
Carcinoma. *See* Adenoid cystic carcinoma; Ductal carcinoma in situ (DCIS); Intracystic carcinoma; Invasive ductal cancer; Invasive lobular carcinoma; Lobular carcinoma in situ (LCIS); Mucinous carcinoma; Papillary carcinoma; Squamous cell carcinoma; Tubular carcinoma.
Carcinosarcoma, 307f. *See also* Sarcoma.
Casting calcifications, 62, 65f-66f, 67
Catheter cuff, retained, 314f, 315
Caudal-cranial view. *See* From below (FB) view.
CC (craniocaudal) view, 5, 6, 6f-7f
in digital mammography, 16f
normal, 26, 27f, 29f-31f
rolled, 40-41, 42f, 50f-51f
Cellulitis, 126, 128f, 301
Chemotherapy
adjuvant
mortality decrease due to, 24
tamoxifen for, 303
contrast-enhanced MRI and, 208, 214, 240, 246
in pregnancy, 287
neoadjuvant, 155
false-negative axilla caused by, 235
for inflammatory breast cancer, 300
marker placement and, 155, 156f-158f
MRI of response to, 214, 219f
percutaneous biopsy and, 155, 156f
Chest wall. *See also* Pectoralis muscle; Pneumothorax, risk of.
lesions close to
cyst as, ultrasound of, 138
mammographic views of, 47, 54f
MRI of, 215f, 236
MRI of, 193
with invasion, 213, 217f
with lesions close to wall, 215f, 236
pain along, in Mondor's disease, 306
sarcoma in, 305, 308f
ultrasound image of, 134, 136f
with cyst, 138
Child, breast bud in, 136, 137f
Chondrosarcoma, 308f. *See also* Sarcoma.
Circumscribed mass, 91, 91f, 92
Cleavage view (CV), 40t, 41t, 47, 52f
of sternalis muscle, 26
Cleopatra view, 40t, 47, 53f
Clips, 313f, 315. *See also* Markers, metallic.
for electron beam boost, 239-240, 243f, 315
MRI-guided biopsy with, 221

Clips—*cont'd*
 stereotactic core biopsy with, 177,
  178f–179f, 180t, 181, 182f, 183
 ultrasound-guided placement of, 94, 95f,
  313f
 with core biopsy, 175f–176f
Clustered calcifications, 60, 61, 62, 63f, 65f,
 68f–69f, 70
 BI-RADS terminology for, 67
 dermal, 73
Collagen vascular disease
 axillary adenopathy in, 303, 303f, 304
 calcifications in, 311–312, 312f
 radiation therapy and, 233
Collimators
 in digital mammography, 18
 in screen-film mammography, 4, 5
Colloid carcinoma. *See* Mucinous carcinoma.
Color Doppler ultrasound, 155, 160, 160f. *See
 also* Doppler ultrasound.
 in Mondor's disease, 306
 of cyst, 138, 139f, 140
 of diabetic mastopathy, 309
 of lymph nodes, 120, 121f
 of papilloma, intraductal, 293f
 of round cancer, 138, 139f
 retroareolar vascularity on, 136
Comedo-type DCIS, calcifications in, 62, 67,
 82
Comedo-type intraductal carcinoma,
 recurrence of, 246
Complex fibroadenomas, 110, 141
Complex sclerosing lesions, 103
Compression of breast, 4, 4f. *See also* Spot
 compression.
 for MRI, 193
 image quality and, 6, 8f
 implants and, 255
 importance of, 2
 pain caused by, 2
 thickness produced by, 3
Compression plate, 2, 4, 4b, 4f, 15
 fenestrated
  for fine-needle aspiration, 173
  for needle localization, 164–166, 165f
  for stereotactic biopsy, 177
Computer-aided diagnosis (CAD), 18–20,
 19f–21f, 32, 37
Conservation. *See* Breast-conserving
 therapy.
Contraceptives
 injected, breast density and, 303
 oral
  granulomatous mastitis and, 306
  MRI enhancement and, 201, 204f
Contralateral breast cancer,
 mammographically occult, 214, 218f
Contrast
 in digital mammography, 17, 18
 in screen-film mammography, 3, 5, 6, 17
Contrast agents
 in galactography, 293–294, 295f–297f
 in MRI. *See* Magnetic resonance imaging
  (MRI), contrast enhancement in.
 in ultrasound imaging, 160
Cooper's ligaments, 26
 distortion of, 34, 36f
  by post-biopsy scar, 100
  in breast cancer, 149
  in lobular carcinoma, 98
  invasion through, 106
 on MRI image, 199
  edema and, 296

Cooper's ligaments,—*cont'd*
 on ultrasound image, 135, 135f–136f, 136,
  136b
  edema and, 151, 152f, 296
  technique and, 133–134
Core needle biopsy, 177–186. *See also* Biopsy,
 percutaneous.
 air at site of, 180–181
 auditing the practice of, 186
 calcifications displaced by, 181, 183
 calcifications in, 177–178, 178f–179f, 181,
  182f, 183
  follow-up of, 184
 complete lesion removal by, 180–181
  with benign lesions, 177
 complications of, 177, 185–186, 185b
  informed consent and, 164, 186
  pneumothorax as, 164, 171, 173, 175f,
   185–186
 excision based on, 180–181, 182f, 183,
  183b
  controversial, 183–184, 184b
 follow-up to benign findings of, 184–185
 freehand, of palpable mass, 171, 173
  MRI-guided, 221
 hemostasis after, 180
 in pregnancy, 288
 mammographic follow-up instead of, 288
 mammography before and after, 177,
  178f–179f, 180, 180t, 181, 182f
  as follow-up, 186
  pathology report and, 183, 184
 markers in site of. *See* Markers, metallic.
 MRI-guided, 219, 221, 221f
 noncompliance of patient after, 186
 of diabetic mastopathy, 309
 patient comfort after, 180
 repeated
  findings on, 184–185
  indications for, 183, 183b, 184
 specimen radiography of core from,
  177–178, 179f
 stereotactic. *See* Stereotactic core needle
  biopsy.
 ultrasound-guided, 173, 175f–176f, 177
  Mondor's disease following, 306
  of MRI-detected lesion, 217
  pneumothorax caused by, 164, 171, 173,
   175f, 185–186
  with implant, 259, 259f
 vacuum-assisted. *See* Vacuum-assisted
  biopsy.
 vs. diagnostic MRI, 211
 wound care after, 180
Coumarin necrosis, 294, 301–302, 301b
Cowden syndrome, 25
Craniocaudal (CC) view, 5, 6, 6f–7f
 in digital mammography, 16f
 normal, 26, 27f, 29f–31f
 rolled, 40–41, 42f, 50f–51f
Cribriform DCIS, calcifications in, 62, 67,
 82
CV (cleavage view), 40t, 41t, 47, 52f
 of sternalis muscle, 26
Cyst(s)
 apocrine-lined, 136
 aspiration of, 136, 137, 140, 140f, 169, 171,
  173f–174f
  for pain relief, 303
 carcinoma in, 109, 109f, 124, 140
  in male, 280
  ultrasound imaging of, 137, 140, 141f
  vs. intracystic papilloma, 109, 109f, 140

Cyst(s)—*cont'd*
 complex, 126f
  ultrasound imaging of, 134, 138, 139f,
   140, 140b, 140f–141f
  vs. mucinous cancer, 146f, 147
  vs. necrotic cancer, 124, 147
 debris in, 138, 139f–141f, 140
 epidermal inclusion, 128, 271, 276f
 in fibroadenoma, 110
 in juvenile papillomatosis, 114
 in lactating adenoma, 116
 in squamous cell carcinoma, 120
 incidence of, in breast, 136
 milk of calcium in, 73, 75, 76f–77f, 77, 77t
 MRI of, 201, 202f–203f
  vs. mucinous carcinoma, 206
 multiple, painful, 303
 oil cyst(s), 73, 74f, 122, 124f
  intradermal, in steatocystoma multiplex,
   122
  post-biopsy, 225, 229f
  post-surgical, 271
 papilloma in, 124, 126, 294, 297f
  ultrasound imaging of, 140, 141f
  vs. cyst, 140
  vs. intracystic carcinoma, 109, 109f,
   140
 pneumocystography of. *See*
  Pneumocystography.
 recurrence after aspiration of, 136
 sebaceous, 128, 129f
 septated, 137, 138f, 140
  vs. mucinous cancer, 146f
 simple, 122, 124, 126f
  MRI of, 201
  ultrasound criteria for, 136–137, 137b,
   138, 138f, 140, 140f
  vs. necrotic cancer, 124
 ultrasound characterization of, 133, 134,
  136–138, 137b, 138f–141f, 140b
  vs. cystic mass, 140, 140b
  vs. medullary cancer, 106
  vs. mucinous carcinoma, 106, 147
  vs. necrotic tumor, 147
  vs. solid mass, 136–138, 138f–139f, 140
Cystic mass(es), 140, 140b. *See also* Mass(es),
 fluid-containing.
 in pregnancy-associated breast cancer,
  285
Cystosarcoma phyllodes. *See* Phyllodes
 tumor.
Cytokeratins, in sentinel lymph node, 234
Cytologic examination, 171, 173
 ductal lavage for, 292
 fine-needle aspiration for, 171, 173
 of sentinel lymph node, 234

D

Dacron Hickman catheter cuff, retained, 314f,
 315
Danazol, for breast pain, 303
Dazzle glare, 8
DCG (depth-compensated gain) curve, 134,
 137
DCIS. *See* Ductal carcinoma in situ (DCIS).
Dense breast
 category of, 28, 28b, 29f
 missed breast cancer and, 316
 MRI of, 189, 213
 palpable mass in, ultrasound evaluation of,
  150
 ultrasound screening of, 160
Dense mass, 91t, 92

Density
  focal, postoperative, 225, 226b
  vs. mass, 34, 90
Density of breast, 28, 28b, 29f, 302. *See also*
  Dense breast.
  asymmetric
    differential diagnosis of, 32t
    in breast cancer, 28, 32t, 34, 36f
      inflammatory, 300
      pregnancy-associated, 285
    in diabetic mastopathy, 309
    in granulomatous mastitis, 306
    medial, 37
    normal, 28, 29f–30f, 32, 34
    probably benign, 288, 290b, 291f
  breast cancer obscured by, 28
  developing over time, 28, 31f, 32t, 37, 290,
    315
  edematous. *See* Edema, breast.
  hormone therapy and, 296, 300b, 300f,
    302–303, 302f
  in lactating patient, 28, 285
  in pregnancy, 285
  post-radiation, 239
  weight loss and, 296, 301f
Deodorant, 70, 71f
Depth-compensated gain (DCG) curve, 134,
  137
Dermal calcifications, 61, 73, 74f–75f, 75b
Dermatomyositis, 311–312, 312f
Desmoid tumor, 309, 311b, 311f
Diabetes mellitus
  abscess of breast in, 126
  mastopathy in, 308–309, 310b
Diagnostic mammography
  CAD systems for, 20
  views in. *See* Views, in diagnostic
    mammography.
  vs. screening mammography, 37, 40, 40t
Diet, breast pain and, 303
Diffuse calcifications, 70
Digital mammography, 15, 15f–16f, 17–18
  calcifications in, 60
  computer-aided diagnosis with, 15, 19,
    19f
  magnifier for viewing of, 32, 37
  quality assurance in, 18, 18b
  viewing conditions for, 28
Digitized screen-film mammograms, 19,
  19f–20f, 20
Discharge. *See* Nipple discharge.
Dixon technique, modified three-point, 264
Dopamine-related drugs, nipple discharge
  and, 292
Doppler ultrasound. *See also* Color Doppler
  ultrasound; Power Doppler ultrasound.
  of lymph nodes, 120, 121f
  of lymphatics, in breast edema, 151, 152f
Dose. *See* Radiation dose.
Double reading, 18–19
Duct(s), breast. *See also* Galactography.
  anatomy of, 26, 27f, 61f–62f
    on galactography, 294, 295f
  calcifications in, 61–62
  dilated. *See* Duct ectasia.
  fistula of, traumatic, 288
  of male breast, in gynecomastia, 279, 280
  plugged, recurrent subareolar abscess and,
    301
  vs. lymphatics, on ultrasound, 151
Duct ectasia
  as single dilated duct
    missed breast cancer in, 315

Duct ectasia—*cont'd*
  with breast cancer, 28, 292
  with papilloma, 292, 293f
  galactography of, 293, 294
  in secretory disease, 77
  MRI of, 199, 201, 203f, 294
  ultrasound imaging of, 293f–294f
  with nipple discharge, 292–293, 293f–294f
Ductal cancer. *See* Ductal carcinoma in situ
  (DCIS); Invasive ductal cancer.
Ductal carcinoma in situ (DCIS)
  ADH associated with, 183
  as extensive intraductal component (EIC),
    92
  bloody nipple discharge from, 114
  calcifications in, 62, 62f, 64f–69f, 67, 82,
    82b, 83f, 84
    absent, MRI and, 213
    at site of recurrence, 80f
    mass associated with, 92, 93f, 95, 149
    new, 87f
    on mammography vs. ultrasound, 149
    stability of, 82, 84
    ultrasound imaging of, 88f, 149, 149f, 160
    vs. fibrocystic dysplasia, 83f
    vs. fingerprint artifact, 71, 72f
    vs. milk of calcium, 76f, 77, 77t
    vs. sclerosing adenosis, 103
    vs. secretory disease, 62, 65f, 68f, 77, 79, 79t
    vs. vascular calcifications, 81
  core needle biopsy of, 177, 180, 183, 184,
    185
  cribriform, 62, 67, 82
  galactography of, 296f
  histologic types of, 82
  in fibroadenoma, 110
  LCIS associated with, 184
  management of, 82
  micropapillary, 62, 67, 82
  MRI of, 199, 206, 208, 212f, 213
    for screening, 214f
    preoperative, 236
  nipple discharge from, 292
  papillary, on core biopsy, 1843
  papillary carcinoma associated with, 106
  radial scar associated with, 103, 105f, 184
  recurrence in form of, 233, 240
  sentinel node biopsy with, 235
  surgical excision of, 183
    needle localization for, 165f, 170f
    residual tumor left by, 239
  ultrasound imaging of, 149, 149f
Ductal hyperplasia. *See also* Atypical ductal
  hyperplasia (ADH).
  bloody nipple discharge caused by, 292
Ductal lavage, 292
Ductoscopy, 211, 294
Dust artifacts, 6, 10f
Dynamic scanning MRI, 193–194, 194b, 198,
  199, 201b, 201f
Dystrophic calcifications, 80–81, 80f, 80t
  in collagen vascular disease, 312f
  on implant capsule, 255, 256f–257f, 262
  post-biopsy, 240

E

Echo pattern, 134, 134t
Echodense noise, on silicone image, 261f,
  262, 262t, 264, 265f–266f
Edema, breast, 294, 296, 298f–299f
  abscess with, 126, 152, 153f, 288, 301
  differential diagnosis of, 32t, 151, 151b,
    239, 294, 296, 297b

Edema—*cont'd*
  focal, post-biopsy, 225, 226b, 227f
  in breast cancer, 28, 32t, 149
    inflammatory, 151, 294, 298f–299f
    pregnancy-associated, 285
  in male, 279
  mass associated with, 92
  MRI of, 296
  peau d'orange in, 26, 151, 232t, 294
    infection with, 301
    inflammatory cancer with, 300
    post-radiation, 239
  physical signs of, 151
  post-radiation, 239, 241f–242f
  tuberculous mastitis with, 304
  ultrasound imaging of, 135, 136, 151, 152f,
    296
    with abscess, 152, 153f
    with post-biopsy scar, 154f
  vs. hormone therapy, 296, 300b, 300f, 302
  vs. weight loss, 296, 301f
Edge shadowing, 144, 145f
  by implant, 253f
  vs. "snowstorm," 264
Eggshell-type calcifications, 73, 74f
  of foreign-body granulomas, 81, 82f, 259
  of oil cysts, 225, 229f
  on injected silicone or paraffin, 259, 263f
EIC (extensive intraductal component), 92
Electron beam boost, 239–240, 243f, 315
Electron beam current (mA), 3
Enhancement. *See* Acoustic enhancement;
  Magnetic resonance imaging (MRI),
  contrast enhancement in.
Epidermal inclusion cyst(s), 128, 271, 276f
Epinephrine, lidocaine with, 164
Equipment
  for digital mammography, 15, 15f, 17, 18
  for MRI, 190, 193, 193b, 193f
  for screen-film mammography, 2–5, 2f, 3b,
    4b, 4f
  quality assurance for, 2, 12, 13b
  for ultrasound, 133
c-*erb*-B2 oncogene, in Paget's disease of
  nipple, 305
Erythema, in breast infection, 301
Estrogen. *See also* Hormone therapy.
  breast cancer risk and, 25
    in males, 280
  density of breasts and, 302, 303
  gynecomastia caused by, 279
  phytoestrogens, 303
Evening primrose oil, 303
Examination. *See* Breast examination,
  clinical.
Excisional biopsy. *See also* Biopsy; Needle
  localization; Surgical excision.
  carbon marking for, 180
  in pregnancy, 288
  indications for, 183, 183b, 184
  key elements of, 186
  mammographic follow-up instead of, 288
  metallic marker of site for, 155, 159f
  of DCIS, 82, 92, 177
  of diabetic mastopathy, 309
  of mass with calcifications, 92, 93f
  of papillomas, 116, 184
  of PASH, 120
  post-biopsy imaging findings
    calcifications in, 80–81, 80f, 80t
    key elements of, 249
    mammographic, 225, 226b, 226f–230f,
      229

Excisional biopsy.—*cont'd*
  MRI, 214, 229, 231, 231b
  ultrasound, 229, 230f–231f
  role of, 229
Excretory ducts, 26, 27f
Expander, tissue, 233, 247, 270, 271
Exposure. *See also* Automatic exposure
    control (AEC).
  electron beam current and, 3
  image quality and
    in digital mammography, 17
    in screen-film mammography, 6, 8f
Extensive intraductal component (EIC), 92

F

False negative mammogram, 28, 32t. *See also*
    Occult breast cancer.
Fast spin echo (FSE) MRI, 193, 194b, 201,
    202f
  of silicone implants, 264, 269
Fat
  age of woman and, 136
  dietary, 303
  in lymph nodes, 120, 121f
    ultrasound image of, 135f, 136
  mammographic appearance of, 37, 91
  masses containing, 92, 120, 120b,
    121f–125f, 122. *See also* Oil cyst(s).
    galactocele as, 288, 290f
  MRI of, 195–196, 195f
  post-radiation thickening of, 239
  retroglandular, 26, 27f, 37
  ultrasound image of, 135, 135f–136f, 136,
    136b
    as pseudolesion, 143
    edematous, 151, 152f
    gain adjustment and, 134
    in lymph node, 135f, 136
    screening and, 160
Fat necrosis
  calcifications in, 143, 240, 244f
    in autologous flap, 271
  foreign-body granuloma with, 81
  in surgical bed, 80, 81, 100, 103
  MRI of, 206, 208
  oil cyst caused by, 73, 74f, 122, 124
  post-biopsy, 225, 229f
  post-surgical, 271, 276f
  simulating treatment failure, 247
  spiculated appearance of, 100, 103
Fat suppression, in MRI, 193, 194, 194b
  for imaging silicone, 264, 269
  interpretation and, 199
  poor, 197, 197f, 197t
Fatty breast, 28, 28b, 29f
Fatty pseudolesions, 143
FB (from below) view, 41t, 47, 54f
FDA (Food and Drug Administration)
  breast implants and, 252
  regulation of mammography by, 1, 2, 3, 12,
    18
FFDM (full-field digital mammography). *See*
    Digital mammography.
Fibroadenolipoma, 120, 122, 122f–123f
Fibroadenoma(s), 110, 111f–112f
  biopsy of, 110, 111f–112f, 142, 183
  calcifying, 79–80, 79f, 110, 142, 142f–143f,
    143
  complex, 110, 141
  giant, 110, 141
  in pregnancy, 280, 287
  infarction of, in pregnancy, 287
  juvenile, 110

Fibroadenoma(s)—*cont'd*
  lactating adenoma and, 288
  MRI of, 198, 199, 201, 202f, 205, 207f
    incidental enhancing lesions and, 210
    vs. DCIS or invasion, 208
  triangulation of, 49f
  ultrasound imaging of, 56f, 140–143, 141b,
    142f–143f
  vs. malignant tumor, 142, 144b, 146, 147
    invasive ductal cancer as, 107f
    medullary cancer as, 106
    papillary cancer as, 143f
    phyllodes tumor as, 113
Fibrocystic change
  calcifications in, 62, 63f–64f, 67f, 70,
    85f–86f
    on core biopsy, 183
    round, 71
    vs. DCIS, 83f
    with spiculated image, 103, 103f
  in excised mass, diagnosed as ADH, 183
  juvenile papillomatosis with, 114
  MRI of, 198, 199, 201, 205, 205f
    vs. DCIS, 208
  nipple discharge in, 292
  on core biopsy, 183, 184
  on galactography, 293
  spiculated appearance in, 103, 103f
Fibrofatty nodules, benign, 150
Fibromatosis, 309, 311b, 311f
Fibrosarcoma, 117
Fibrosis
  focal
    on post-biopsy mammogram, 225, 226f
    vs. DCIS, on MRI, 208
    gynecomastia progressing to, 279, 280,
      283f
    in diabetic mastopathy, 309
    post-radiation, 239
Film. *See also* Screen-film cassettes; Screen-
    film mammography (SFM).
  labeling of, 8, 12b
  optical density (OD) of, 5, 6, 17
  processing of, 5, 5t
    artifacts caused by, 6, 10f–11f
    quality assurance for, 13–14, 14t
  viewing conditions for, 8, 12f, 28, 37,
    316–317
Fine-needle aspiration. *See also* Biopsy,
    percutaneous.
  complications of, 185–186
    informed consent and, 164, 186
  freehand, of palpable masses, 173
  mammographic follow-up to, 186
  noncompliance of patient after, 186
  of cyst, 136, 137, 140, 140f, 171,
    173f–174f
    for pain relief, 303
  of galactocele, 288
  ultrasound-guided, 173, 175f–176f, 177
    of abscess, 288, 289f
  x-ray–guided, 173
Fingerprints, on film, 6, 10f–11f, 71, 72f
Fistula
  milk, 288
  recurrent subareolar abscess and, 301
Flake-like calcifications, 62, 64f
Flap, tissue, autologous, 233, 247, 270–271,
    272f–273f
Fluid-containing mass(es), 122, 124, 126,
    126b, 126f–130f, 128. *See also* Cyst(s).
  galactocele as, 128, 130f, 280, 288, 290f
  ultrasound imaging of, 140, 140b

Focal spot
  in contact mammography, 3, 3t, 4f
  in magnification mammography, 3–4, 3t, 4f,
    60
Focal zone, ultrasound, 133, 134
Food and Drug Administration (FDA)
  breast implants and, 252
  regulation of mammography by, 1, 2, 3, 12, 18
Foreign body(ies), 312, 313f–314f, 314–315.
    See also Markers, metallic.
  calcifications caused by, 81, 82f, 259, 314f,
    315
  granuloma(s) associated with
    calcifications in, 81, 82f, 259
    silicone-induced, 81, 82f, 254, 255, 259
From below (FB) view, 41t, 47, 54f
Frozen section, of sentinel lymph node, 234
FSE (fast spin echo) MRI, 193, 194b, 201, 202f
  of silicone implants, 264, 269
Full-field digital mammography (FFDM). *See*
    Digital mammography.

G

Gadolinium contrast. *See* Magnetic resonance
    imaging (MRI), contrast enhancement in.
Gain. *See* Depth-compensated gain (DCG)
    curve; Time-compensated gain (TCG)
    curve.
Galactocele, 128, 130f, 280, 288, 290f
Galactography, 293–294
  extravasation of contrast in, 293, 294, 297f
  normal findings in, 294, 295f
  of papilloma, 115f, 116, 205, 294, 295f–297f
  unrevealing, MRI in case of, 211
Galactorrhea, in granulomatous mastitis, 306
Gamma probe, of sentinel node, 234, 235
Gel bleed, 254, 255, 255t, 264, 270
Gel marker, 313f
Genetic testing, 25
Ghosting, in MRI, 197, 197t
Giant fibroadenoma, 110, 141
Gigantomastia, in pregnancy, 280
Gold deposits, in lymph nodes, 303, 304
Gradient echo imaging, of implants, 264
Granular calcifications, 62, 66f–67f, 67
  in DCIS, 83f, 87f
Granuloma
  foreign-body
    calcifications in, 81, 82f, 259
    silicone-induced, 81, 82f, 254, 255, 259
  in TRAM flap, vs. recurrent cancer, 271
  simulating treatment failure, 247
Granulomatous mastitis, 306, 308
Grid, antiscatter, 2, 4, 5
  artifacts associated with, 6, 9f
  eliminated in slot scanning, 17
Gynecomastia, 279–280, 280b, 281f–284f, 282t
  breast cancer with, 286f
    inflammatory, 148f

H

Hair artifacts, 71, 72f
Half-value layer (HVL), 3, 3b
Halo, echogenic, 134, 134t, 144, 144f, 145
  of invasive ductal cancer, 117, 117f, 145f, 148f
Hamartoma, 120, 122, 122f–123f
Hematoma, 124, 127f
  after biopsy
    excisional, 127f, 225, 228f
    percutaneous, 164, 170f, 177, 180, 185
  calcified, in autologous flap, 271
  implant-associated, 254
  MRI of, 206

Hematoxylin and eosin (H&E) staining
  micrometastases not identified by, 235
  of calcifications, 168
Heparin-induced skin necrosis, 302
Heterogeneously dense breast, 28, 28b
Hickman catheter cuff, retained, 314f, 315
Hidradenitis suppurativa, 315
History, breast
  for mammography, 28, 32, 33f, 37
  for MRI, 190
  previous biopsies on, 229
Hodgkin's lymphoma, breast edema in, 298f
Hookwire. See also Needle localization.
  retractable, 94
Hormone therapy, 302–303, 302f. See also
    Estrogen.
  breast cancer and, 24
  breast density and, 28
    vs. edema, 296, 300b, 300f, 302
  MRI and, 190
  pseudoangiomatous stromal hyperplasia
    and, 118
  simple cyst and, 122
Hormone-related enhancement, on MRI, 201,
    204f
  vs. DCIS, 208
HVL (half-value layer), 3, 3b
Hydatid disease, 301, 311
Hydrogel implants, 254
Hyperechoic pattern, 134, 134t
Hyperplasia
  atypical. See also Atypical ductal
    hyperplasia (ADH).
    lobular, 184
    vacuum-assisted biopsy of, 177
  bloody nipple discharge caused by, 292
  lobular
    atypical, 184
    sclerosing adenosis caused by, 103
  of fibroadenoma, 110
  of radial scar, 103
  pseudoangiomatous stromal, 118, 120,
    120f, 184
Hypoechoic pattern, 134, 134t

I

IBTRs (in-breast tumor recurrences). See
    Recurrent breast cancer, local.
IELs (incidental enhancing lesions), 208, 210
IHC (immunohistochemistry), of sentinel
    lymph node, 234, 235
Image quality. See also Quality assurance.
  computer-aided detection and, 20
  in digital mammography, 17
    quality assurance for, 18, 18b
  in screen-film mammography
    breast cancer detection and, 1
    quality assurance for, 14, 14b, 14t, 15b
    variables affecting, 5–6, 5t, 6f–11f
Image receptor, in screen-film mammography,
    2, 4–5, 4b, 4f
Image-guided procedures. See MRI-guided
    procedures; Ultrasound-guided
    procedures; X-ray–guided procedures.
Immunocompromised patient, abscess in,
    126
Immunohistochemistry (IHC), of sentinel
    lymph node, 234, 235
Implants, 252–270. See also Reconstruction,
    breast; Silicone injections.
  after mastectomy, 247, 249, 252
    latissimus dorsi flap for, 271
    tissue expander for, 270

Implants—cont'd
  axillary lymphadenopathy caused by, 235
  complications of, 252–254, 254b, 254f
    desmoid tumor as, 309
    rupture as, 252, 254f, 255, 255t
      asymptomatic, 255, 259
      mammography of, 255, 259,
        260f–261f, 262t
      MRI of, 262, 262t, 264, 268–270,
        268f–270f, 270b
      silicone in lymph nodes from, 259,
        261f, 262t, 303, 304
      ultrasound of, 256f, 259, 262, 262t,
        264, 265f–267f
    fibrous capsule on, 254, 254f, 254t, 255
      after implant removal, 262
      calcifications in, 81, 82f, 254, 255,
        256f–257f, 262
      intracapsular rupture in, 255, 255t, 262t,
        264, 267f, 268f
      MRI of, 268–269, 269f–270f
      polyurethane-coated implants and,
        252
  key elements of, 276
  normal image of
    mammographic, 253f, 255, 256b,
      256f–258f
    MRI, 213, 268, 268b, 270b
    ultrasound, 253f, 255
  placement of, 254, 254f
  polyurethane-covered, 252, 255, 257f,
    262
  regulatory status of, 252, 253
  removal of, 257f, 260f–261f, 262, 264f
  saline, 252
    mammography of, 255, 257f
      with residual silicone, 261f
      with rupture, 255, 256f
    saline outer/silicone inner, 253b, 255
    stacked, 252, 253b
      mammography of, 256f
      MRI of, 270
    technologist's marks indicating, 32
    Trilucent, 252–253
    types of, 252–254, 253b
      MRI interpretation and, 270, 270f
In situ breast cancer. See also Ductal
    carcinoma in situ (DCIS); Lobular
    carcinoma in situ (LCIS).
  incidence of, 24
Incidental enhancing lesions (IELs), 208,
    210
Indistinct mass, 91
  invasive ductal carcinoma as, 106
  ultrasound image of, 134, 134t, 144
Infection. See also Abscess; Mastitis.
  axillary adenopathy in, 303, 304
  cellulitis in, 126, 128f, 301
  core biopsy as cause of, 177, 185
  implant-associated, 254, 268
Infiltrating lobular carcinoma. See Invasive
    lobular carcinoma.
Inflammatory breast cancer, 151, 294, 296,
    298f–299f, 300–301
  ultrasound imaging of, 148f, 149, 296
Informed consent, for percutaneous biopsy,
    164, 164b, 186
Infraclavicular lymph nodes
  as sentinel nodes, 234, 235f
  TNM staging and, 232t
Intercostal muscles, on ultrasound image,
    136, 137f
Interlobular ducts, 26, 27f

Intracystic carcinoma, 109, 109f, 124, 140
  in male, 280
  ultrasound imaging of, 137, 140, 141f
  vs. intracystic papilloma, 109, 109f, 140
Intracystic mass, aspiration and, 171
Intracystic papilloma, 124, 126, 294, 297f
  ultrasound imaging of, 140, 141f
  vs. cyst, 140
  vs. intracystic carcinoma, 109, 109f, 140
Intraoperative ultrasound, 169, 181
Invasive ductal cancer
  bilateral, MRI of, 214, 218f
  calcifications in, 62, 67, 67f, 82, 83f, 84, 93f,
    95, 96f
    in round mass, 107f
    ultrasound imaging of, 84, 88f, 147f,
      149
  core needle biopsy of, 159f, 180, 183, 184,
    185
  extensive intraductal component (EIC) in,
    92
  in males, 280, 285f–287f
  indistinct margins in, 116–117, 117f
  inflammatory cancer coexisting with, 296
  LCIS and risk of, 25
  management of, 82
  medullary variant of, 106, 108f
  MRI of, 206, 209f
    as incidental enhancing lesion, 210
    vs. DCIS, 208, 212f
    with needle localization, 220f
  needle localization of, preoperative, 165f,
    170f
  neoadjuvant chemotherapy for, 156f–158f
  not otherwise specified (NOS), 94, 106,
    107f
  on implant capsule, 256f
  Paget's disease of nipple in, 305, 306f
  papillary DCIS with, 184
  pregnancy-associated, 285
  recurrence of, 233, 245f–246f, 246,
    247f–248f
  round forms of, 105–106, 107f, 108b
    ultrasound imaging of, 145–146, 146b,
      146f
  spiculated, 94–95, 96f–97f, 97
  ultrasound imaging of, 144f–148f,
    145–146
    with coexisting inflammatory cancer,
      296
    with implant, 259f
  views of
    magnification view, 57f
    spot view, 45f–46f
    triangulation with, 48f, 51f
    XCCM view, 54f
  vs. axillary breast tissue, 39f
  vs. lymphoma, 117, 118f
  vs. radial scar, 103
Invasive lobular carcinoma, 97–98, 98b, 98f
  calcifications in, 88f, 97
  in men, 280
  indistinct margins in, 117
  LCIS and risk of, 25
  missed by mammography, 150, 236
  missed by ultrasound, 150, 236
  MRI of, 206, 208, 210f, 213, 236
Inversion recovery fast spin echo (IRFSE)
    pulse sequences, 264
Isoechoic pattern, 134, 134t
Isoflavones, 303
Isosulfan blue dye, for sentinel node biopsy,
    233, 234, 235

J

Jewish women, breast cancer in, 25
Juvenile fibroadenoma, 110
Juvenile papillomatosis, 113, 114

K

Kerley's B lines, breast edema similar to, 296, 298f
Keyhole sign, 262t, 268f, 269, 269f
Klinefelter's syndrome, 280
kVp (peak kilovoltage), 2-3, 3b

L

Labeling
    of films, 8, 12b
    of ultrasound images, 92, 94b, 134, 134b
Lactating adenoma, 116, 116f, 280, 287, 288
Lactating breast
    biopsy in, 288
    breast cancer in, 285, 287
    density of, 28, 285, 289f, 302
    galactocele in, 128, 130f, 280, 288, 290f
    granulomatous mastitis and, 306, 308
    infection in, 152, 288, 289f
    MRI of, 285, 287
Lactational mastitis, 288, 289f
Laser printer, 17, 18
Laterally exaggerated craniocaudal (XCCL) view, 40t, 41t, 47, 52f-53f
Lateral-medial (LM) view, 41t
    triangulation with, 41, 47f, 49f, 51f, 91
Latissimus dorsi flap, 247, 271
Lavage, ductal, 292
LCIS. See Lobular carcinoma in situ (LCIS).
Leukemia, 303, 304
Lexicon. See BI-RADS lexicon.
Lidocaine anesthesia, for percutaneous biopsy, 164
Li-Fraumeni syndrome, 25
Linear calcifications, 62, 65f-66f, 67, 68f, 70
    malignant, 82
    vs. fingerprint artifact, 71, 72f
Line-pair resolution (lp/mm). See Spatial resolution.
Linguine sign, 262t, 268-269, 268f-270f
Lipid cyst(s). See Oil cyst(s).
Lipid implants, 252-253
Lipoma, 122, 125f
Liposarcoma, 122
LM (lateral-medial) view, 41t
    triangulation with, 41, 47f, 49f, 51f, 91
Lobes, 26
Lobular carcinoma. See Invasive lobular carcinoma.
Lobular carcinoma in situ (LCIS)
    breast cancer risk and, 25
    calcifications in, 82, 87f
    in fibroadenoma, 110
    management of, 25
    on core biopsy, excision of, 184
Lobular hyperplasia, sclerosing adenosis caused by, 103
Lobules
    calcifications in, 61, 62, 62f, 63f, 71
    cancerization of, 62f, 67
    galactography of, 294, 295f
Local anesthesia
    for galactography, 293
    for needle localization
        ultrasound-guided, 168
        x-ray-guided, 166

Local anesthesia—cont'd
    for percutaneous biopsy, 164
        core biopsy, 173
        fine-needle, of palpable mass, 171
Local control, 231. See also Recurrent breast cancer, local.
Local recurrence. See Recurrent breast cancer, local.
Locally advanced breast cancer. See also Inflammatory breast cancer.
    edema in, 296, 300
    treatment of, 155
lp/mm (line-pair resolution). See Spatial resolution.
Lump. See Palpable mass.
Lumpectomy, 231, 233. See also Breast-conserving therapy; Excisional biopsy; Surgical excision.
    MRI in planning of, 214
    site of
        mammography of, 236, 239, 240f
        ultrasound imaging of, 153, 154f
Lump-o-gram, 47, 56f
Lupus erythematosus, axillary adenopathy in, 303f
Lymph nodes. See also Lymphadenopathy.
    axillary
        adenopathy in, 303-305, 304b, 304f-305f
        calcifications in, 303, 304, 304b
        cancer mistaken for, 316
        dissection of, 82
            complications of, 234
            DCIS and, 183
            in men, 280
            mastectomy with, 233
            sentinel node biopsy and, 233-234
        levels of, 233, 233t
        lymphoma in, 117, 118f, 303, 304
        metastases to, 92, 109, 110f, 303, 304-305, 304b, 304f-305f
            as micrometastases, 235
            from occult primary, 213, 216f
            in men, 280
            in pregnancy, 285
            inflammatory cancer with, 300
            MRI of, 210f
            palpable, 233, 235
            radiation therapy and, 233
            staging and, 232t, 233-235
            treatment options with, 231
            ultrasound imaging of, 147f-148f, 149
        normal, 120, 121f
        sentinel node biopsy of, 82, 233-235, 233t, 234b, 235f
        silicone in, 259, 261f, 262t, 303, 304
    benign reactive, 149, 235, 304
    intramammary
        as sentinel nodes, 234-235
        metastasis to, 109, 232t
        MRI of, 202f, 205, 206f, 208
        normal, 120, 121f
    mediastinal
        breast edema and, 299f
        MRI of, 193
    MRI technique and, 193
    normal, 26, 29f, 34, 37, 38f, 120, 121f
        MRI of, 120, 201, 202f
        on core biopsy, 183
        ultrasound imaging of, 135f, 136
    obstruction of, edema and, 294, 298f
    staging of breast cancer and, 232t, 233-235

Lymphadenopathy. See also Lymph nodes.
    axillary, 303-305, 304b, 304f-305f
    breast edema caused by, 294, 299f
    differential diagnosis of, 32t, 303, 304b
    in breast cancer, 28, 32t
        male, 280
        neoadjuvant chemotherapy and, 155
    in lymphoma, 117, 118f, 303, 304
    mammographic appearance of, 37, 38f
    ultrasound appearance of, 147f, 149
Lymphatic vessels
    breast edema and, 151, 294, 296, 298f
        in inflammatory cancer, 300
    sentinel node biopsy and, 234, 235
    tumor invasion of, recurrence and, 233
Lymphoma, 117-118, 118f-119f, 303, 304
    Hodgkin's, breast edema in, 298f
    ultrasound imaging of, 148f, 149
Lymphoscintigraphy, of sentinel nodes, 234-235, 235f

M

Macrocalcifications, BI-RADS definition of, 135
Macromastia, reduction mammaplasty for, 271
Magnetic resonance imaging (MRI), 189-221
    advantages of, for breast cancer, 189-190, 190b
    artifacts in, 197-198, 197f, 197t
        core biopsy needles and, 221
        metal biopsy markers and, 181
    basic principles of, 189
    benign features in, 199, 199b, 200f-202f, 201, 201b, 201t
    biopsy guided by, 217, 219, 219b, 221, 221f
    calcifications and, 208, 219
    contraindications to, 190, 192f
    contrast enhancement in
        advantages of, 189-190, 190b
        catheter and injector for, 190, 193b, 193f
        compression of breast and, 193
        dynamic studies of, 190b, 193-194, 194b, 198, 199, 201b, 201f
        hormonal therapy and, 303
        image processing with, 194, 199
        indications for, 210, 213b
        menstrual cycle and, 190
        poor, 197t, 198
        protocols for, 193-194, 194b
    equipment for, 190, 193, 193b, 193f
    fat suppression in, 193, 194, 194b
        for imaging silicone, 264, 269
        interpretation and, 199
        poor, 197, 197f, 197t
    in breast-conserving therapy, 236, 238f-239f, 240, 246, 246f
    indications for, 210-211, 213-214, 213b, 214f-219f
    interpretation of, 194-210
        approach to lesions in, 198-199, 199b, 200f-202f, 201b, 201t
        artifacts in, 181, 197-198, 197f, 197t, 221
        atlas for, 201, 203f-212f, 205-206, 208
        diagnostic limitations in, 208, 210, 213b
        lexicon for, 198, 198t
        normal findings in, 194-197, 195f-196f
    key elements of, 221
    malignant features in, 199, 199b, 200f-202f, 201, 201b, 201t
    metallic materials and, 181, 190, 192f, 313f, 315
    needle localization guided by, 217, 219, 219b, 220f, 221

Magnetic resonance imaging (MRI)—*cont'd*
  of breast cancer. *See* Breast cancer, MRI of.
  of breast edema, 296
  of cyst(s), 201, 202f–203f
    vs. mucinous carcinoma, 206
  of diabetic mastopathy, 309
  of duct ectasia, 199, 201, 203f, 294
  of fibroadenoma, 110
  of implants, 213, 268, 268b, 270b
    ruptured, 262, 262t, 264, 268–270,
      268f–270f, 270b
  of lactating breast, 285, 287
  of lymph nodes, 120, 201, 202f
  of papilloma, 198, 199, 205, 208, 208f, 210,
    294
  patient selection for, 190, 191b, 191f–192f
  pharmacokinetic scans with, 199
  physiologic scans with, 199
  postoperative findings on, 229, 231, 231b
    as scar, 206, 208, 214
  protocols for, 193–194, 194b
  reporting of breast findings with, 198, 198t
  safety form for, 190, 191f–192f
  screening with, 210–211, 213b, 214f
  staging with, 213–214, 213b, 216f–218f, 229
  three-dimensional, 193–194, 199, 305f
  views in, 194
Magnification mammography, 3–4, 3t, 4f
  in galactography, 293–294
  of calcifications, 50, 60–61
    post-biopsy, 240
  of lumpectomy site, 236, 239
  of lymph nodes, 26
  of mass, 91
  scatter reduction in, 5
  spot compression with, 40b, 40t, 41, 50, 53f
  to characterize true findings, 50, 57f
Magnification specimen radiography, 178
Magnified images, on monitor, 60
Magnifier, for viewing calcifications, 32, 37,
  60–61
Male breast cancer, 279, 280, 285b,
  285f–287f
  inflammatory, ultrasound imaging of, 148f
  sentinel node biopsy in, 235
Mammography
  acquisition in. *See* Digital mammography;
    Screen-film mammography (SFM).
  after reduction mammaplasty, 271,
    274f–275f
  after wire placement, 169
    MRI-guided, 219
  age of patient and, 302
  artifacts in, 6, 9f–11f
    simulating calcifications, 70–71, 71f–72f
  benign findings on, probable, 37, 39b, 84,
    288, 290, 290b, 291f, 292
  calcifications on. *See* Calcifications.
  contrast agent in, 293–294, 295f–297f
  core biopsy and, 177, 178f–179f, 180, 180t,
    181, 182f
    correlation with pathology report, 183,
      184
    follow-up mammography, 186
  density on. *See* Density of breast.
  development over time, 28, 29f, 31f, 37
  diagnostic. *See* Diagnostic mammography.
  follow-up
    after percutaneous biopsy, 186
    after radiation therapy, 236t, 239–240,
      241f–246f, 243b
    non-compliance with, 290
    of indeterminate calcifications, 84

Mammography—*cont'd*
  of probably benign findings, 37, 39b, 84,
    288, 290
  in breast-conserving therapy, 236, 236t,
    237f, 239, 240, 240f, 241f–246f
  in men
    normal, 280
    of breast cancer, 280, 285f–287f
    of gynecomastia, 280, 281f–284f, 282t
  interpretation in
    approach to, 28, 32, 32t, 34t, 35f–36f,
      38f–39f
      BI-RADS code and, 37, 39b
      history in, 28, 32, 33f, 37
      positions in breast and, 32, 34f
    comparison with old films, 28, 29f, 31f,
      32, 34t, 37, 317
    key elements of, 50, 58
    obscured masses in, 28
    qualifications for, 12b
      for digital images, 18
    quality assurance for, 12–13, 14b
    viewing conditions for, 8, 12f, 28, 37,
      316–317
    views in. *See* Views, mammographic.
  key elements of, 21–22, 50, 58
  nipple discharge and, 292, 292t
  normal findings in, 26, 27f, 28, 28b, 29f–30f
    with palpable mass, 150, 213
  of autologous flaps, 271, 272f–273f, 276f
  of breast cancer. *See* Breast cancer,
    mammography of.
  of breast edema, 294, 296, 298f–299f
  of diabetic mastopathy, 309
  of findings undetected with ultrasound,
    150
  of implant in breast, 253f, 255, 256b,
    256f–258f, 259, 260f–261f, 262t
    after subcutaneous mastectomy, 271
    ruptured, 255, 256b, 256f–258f
    of injected silicone, 254
  of mass(es), 90–92, 91f, 91t, 92b. *See also*
    specific diagnosis.
    approach to, 32, 34, 34t, 35f–36f, 37,
      38f–39f
    correlating ultrasound with, 92, 94, 95f
    report on, 94, 95b
  of Mondor's disease, 306, 310f
  of trichinosis, 311, 311f
  one-view finding in, 151, 164, 316
    MRI evaluation of, 211, 215f
  postoperative findings on, 225, 226b,
    226f–230f, 229
  pre-biopsy work-up with, 163
  probably benign findings on, 37, 39b, 84,
    288, 290, 290b, 291f, 292
  quality assurance in, 1–2, 1b, 12–14, 12b,
    13b, 14b, 14t, 15b
  screening. *See* Screening mammography.
  suboptimal, MRI instead of, 213–214
  timing of, after menses, 2
  training in, 1, 12, 12b, 13b
  ultrasound and. *See* Ultrasound,
    mammographic findings and.
  views in. *See* Views, mammographic.
Mammography Quality Standards Act of 1992
  (MQSA), 1–2, 1b, 12–14, 12b, 13b, 14b,
  14t, 15b
  digital images and, 17, 18, 18b
  follow-up on abnormalities and, 186
  implants and, 255
  magnification and, 3
  viewing conditions and, 8

Margins
  of mass, 90, 91, 91f, 91t, 92, 94, 94t
    on ultrasound image, 134, 134t
    surgical, 231, 236
Markers, metallic, 313f–314f, 314–315. *See
  also* Clips.
  available types of, 181
  BBs as, 169, 176f
  before neoadjuvant chemotherapy, 155,
    156f–158f
  in biopsy cavity, 155, 159f
  MRI-compatible, 181, 190, 313f
  of scar, 32, 80, 100, 101f–102f, 229
  to correlate ultrasound with mammogram,
    150–151, 151f
Masking, 8, 28
Mass(es), 90–131. *See also* Breast cancer.
  associated findings with, 92, 92b
  calcifications associated with, 92, 92b, 93f.
    See also Calcifications.
  clinical presentation of, 25–26
  computer-aided detection of, 18, 19, 20, 21f
  definition of, 90, 91
  density of, 91t, 92, 94
  desmoid tumor as, 309, 311b, 311f
  diabetic mastopathy with, 308–309, 310b
  epidermal inclusion cyst as, 128, 271, 276f
  fat necrosis as, post-surgical, 271, 276f
  fat-containing, 92, 120, 120b, 121f–125f,
    122. *See also* Oil cyst(s).
  galactocele as, 288, 290f
  fluid-containing, 122, 124, 126, 126b,
    126f–130f, 128. *See also* Cyst(s).
  galactocele as, 128, 130f, 280, 288, 290f
    ultrasound imaging of, 140, 140b
  granulomatous mastitis as, 306
  hormone-associated densities vs., 303
  implant-associated, 255, 258f
    after removal, 262, 264f
    after subcutaneous mastectomy, 271
  in cyst, 171. *See also* Intracystic carcinoma;
    Intracystic papilloma.
  in male breast, 279
  indistinct margins of, 90, 116–118, 117b,
    117f–120f, 120
  inflammatory breast cancer with, 296, 300
  key elements of, 131
  mammography of, 90–92, 91f, 91t, 92b
    approach to, 32, 34, 34t, 35f–36f, 37,
      38f–39f
    correlating ultrasound with, 92, 94, 95f
    report on, 94, 95b
  margins (borders) of, 90, 91, 91f, 91t, 92,
    94, 94t
    on ultrasound image, 134, 134t
  palpable. *See* Palpable mass.
  probably benign, 37, 39b, 288, 290b, 291f
  rounded or expansile, 90, 91f
    benign, 106b, 110, 111f–116f
    differential diagnosis of, 32t, 106b, 144b
    malignant, 28, 32t, 105–106, 106b,
      107f–110f, 108b, 109–110, 109b
    multiple, differential diagnosis of, 109b
    probably benign, 37, 39b, 288, 290b, 291f
    ultrasound imaging of, 134, 134t,
      145–146, 146b, 146f, 147
  shape of, 91, 91f, 91t, 92, 94, 94t
  spiculated. *See* Spiculated mass.
  ultrasound of. *See* Ultrasound, of mass(es).
  vs. density, 34, 90
  vs. nipple, 136
  vs. sternalis muscle, 26
Mastalgia, cyclic, 303. *See also* Pain, breast.

Mastectomy, 231, 233. *See also*
  Reconstruction, breast.
  for coumarin necrosis, 302
  implants after, 247, 249, 252
    latissimus dorsi flap for, 271
    tissue expander for, 270
  in pregnancy, 287
  preoperative MRI and, 236
  prophylactic, 235
  reconstruction after, 233, 247, 249,
    270-271, 272f-273f
  recurrence in site of, 249
  salvage, 247, 248b
  subcutaneous, 247, 249
    implant in case of, 271
  with occult primary tumor, 305
Mastitis. *See also* Abscess; Infection.
  abscess subsequent to, 126, 152
  axillary adenopathy in, 303
  causes of, 297b, 301
  cellulitis in, 126, 128f, 301
  edema in, 151, 294, 297b, 301
  granulomatous, 306, 308
  lactational, 288, 289f
  MRI of, 300
  percutaneous biopsy causing, 185
  plasma cell. *See* Secretory disease.
  tuberculous, 301, 304
  vs. inflammatory cancer, 300
Mastopexy, 271
Mean glandular dose, 2
Medial-lateral (ML) view, 41t
Medially exaggerated craniocaudal (XCCM)
    view, 40t, 41t, 47, 52f, 54f
Mediastinal lymph nodes
  breast edema and, 299f
  MRI of, 193
Medical physicists
  duties of, 14, 15b
    in digital mammography, 18, 18b
  MQSA qualifications for, 1, 12, 13b, 18, 18b
Mediolateral oblique (MLO) view, 5-6, 6f-7f
  in digital mammography, 16f
  normal, 26, 27f, 29f-31f
Medroxyprogesterone, 302, 303
Medullary cancer, 106, 108f
  atypical, 106
  in men, 280
  ultrasound imaging of, 146, 146f
Men. *See* Gynecomastia; Male breast cancer.
Menarche, early, 25
Menopause
  late, breast cancer risk and, 25
  MRI and, 190
Menstrual cycle
  breast pain associated with, 303
  cyst changes and, 122, 137
  mammography and, 2
  MRI and, 190, 191b
    enhancement and, 201, 204f
    with fibroadenoma, 110
Metallic materials. *See also* Foreign body(ies);
    Markers, metallic.
  acupuncture needle tips, retained, 312, 313f
  MRI and, 181, 190, 192f, 315
Metastasis(es), 109. *See also* Lymph nodes;
    Lymphadenopathy; Occult metastases.
  distant, staging and, 232t
  micrometastases, 235
  to breast, 109-110, 110f
  to skin, in locally advanced breast cancer,
    300
Microcalcifications. *See also* Calcifications.

biopsy of
  stereotactic, 178, 179f, 182f
  ultrasound-guided, 173
BI-RADS definition of, 135
computer-aided detection of, 19, 21f
DCIS with absence of, MRI for, 213
dust artifacts and, 10f
implant capsule with, 257f
in autologous flap, 271
in biopsy site, 239, 240
in biopsy specimen, 85f, 86f
inflammatory breast cancer with, 300
magnification mammography of, 3, 240
male breast cancer with, 287f
mass associated with, 92, 92b, 93f
  in sclerosing adenosis, 103
  radial scar as, 103, 105f
  tubular carcinoma as, 99
  ultrasound-guided biopsy of, 173
needle localization and, 165f, 167f
Paget's disease of nipple with, 305
recurrent breast cancer with, 246
specimen radiography of, 178, 179f
ultrasound of, 142, 144-145, 149, 149f,
  160
Microinvasive carcinoma, calcifications in, 82
Microlobulated mass, 91, 93f
  fibroadenoma as, 112f
  invasive ductal carcinoma as, 106, 147f
  medullary cancer as, 108f
  on ultrasound image, 134, 134t
    as malignant finding, 144, 145f, 147f
    as suspicious finding, 142
  papilloma as, 114, 115f
Micrometastases, 235
Micropapillary DCIS, calcifications in, 62, 67,
  82
Milk. *See* Galactocele; Lactating breast.
Milk ducts. *See* Duct(s).
Milk fistula, 288
Milk of calcium, 73, 75, 76f-77f, 77, 77t, 85f
  missing from pathologic slides, 168
Mixed echo pattern, 134, 134t
ML (medial-lateral) view, 41t
MLO (mediolateral oblique) view, 5-6, 6f-7f
  in digital mammography, 16f
  normal, 26, 27f, 29f-31f
Moles, technologist's marks on, 32
Molluscum contagiosum, 301
Mondor's disease, 305-306, 309b, 310f
Motion artifacts
  in mammography, 6
  in MRI, 197, 197f, 197t, 198
MQSA. *See* Mammography Quality Standards
    Act of 1992 (MQSA).
MRI. *See* Magnetic resonance imaging
    (MRI).
MRI-guided procedures
  biopsy as, 217, 219, 219b, 221, 221f
  needle localization as, 217, 219, 219b, 220f,
    221
Mucinous carcinoma, 106, 108f
  MRI of, 206, 211f
  ultrasound imaging of, 146, 146f, 147
Multicentric breast cancer
  breast conservation precluded by, 236,
    237f
  MRI of, 214, 218f
  radiation therapy and, 233
  sentinel node biopsy of, 235
Multifocal breast cancer, MRI of, 214, 217f,
  238f
Mumps orchitis, 280

N
Necrosis
  coumarin-induced, 294, 301-302, 301b
  heparin-induced, 302
Necrotic cancer
  calcification of, 62, 66f
  fluid in, 124
  vs. cyst, 137, 140, 147
Needle biopsy. *See* Core needle biopsy; Fine-
    needle aspiration.
Needle localization, 155, 158f-159f, 163. *See
    also* Excisional biopsy; Specimen
    radiography; Surgical excision.
  clip placement prior to, 177, 178f-179f,
    180t, 181, 182f
  implants and, 257f, 259
  in breast-conserving therapy, 236
  local anesthesia for, 164
  MRI-guided, 217, 219, 219b, 220f, 221
  stereotactic, 168
  ultrasound-guided, 168-169, 171f-172f, 176f
  wire fragments left by, 315
  x-ray-guided, 164-166, 165f, 166b
    after galactography, 294
    specimen radiography after, 165f,
      166-168, 166b, 167b, 167f
    calcifications and, 168, 168t, 169f-170f
Neoadjuvant chemotherapy. *See*
    Chemotherapy, neoadjuvant.
Neurofibromatosis, 315, 316f
Nipple. *See also* Areola.
  calcifications in, 61
  cracked, infection entering through, 126,
    288
  inverted, 26, 34
    in secretory disease, 79
  mammographic appearance of, 34
  Paget's disease of, 305, 305b, 306f
    calcifications in, 61, 88f, 305
  post-radiation swelling of, 239
  reconstruction of, 271
  relocation of, in reduction mammmaplasty,
    271, 274f-275f
  retraction of, 92
    in Paget's disease, 305, 306f
    inflammatory cancer with, 300
  subcutaneous mastectomy and, 249
  ultrasound image of, 136, 137f
Nipple discharge, 26, 292-294, 292t,
    293f-297f. *See also* Galactography.
  bloody, 114, 211, 292
    in pregnancy, 285
  in male breast cancer, 280
  MRI in evaluation of, 211
  papillary carcinoma with, 106
  papilloma(s) with, 114, 205, 292, 292t, 293,
    293f, 294, 295f-297f
Noise, image, 6, 17, 18
Non-Hodgkin's lymphoma, 117. *See also*
    Lymphoma.
Nursing. *See* Lactating breast.
Nutrition, breast pain and, 303

O
Obesity. *See also* Weight loss.
  breast cancer and, 24
  hidradenitis suppurativa and, 315
Obscured mass, 91
Occult breast cancer. *See also* Breast cancer,
    missed by mammography.
  mammographically occult, 28, 37, 47, 315
    in core biopsy site, 183
  MRI of, 189, 190f, 210, 213

Occult breast cancer.—*cont'd*
    multicentric or bilateral, 214, 218f
    multifocal, 214, 217f, 238f
    with axillary node metastases, 213, 216f
    manifested as axillary metastases, 304–305, 304f–305f
    sonographically occult, MRI of, 213
Occult metastases, to lymph nodes
    not detected on ultrasound, 149
    sentinel node biopsy and, 234
OD (optical density), 5, 6, 17
Oil cyst(s), 73, 74f, 122, 124f
    intradermal, in steatocystoma multiplex, 122
    post-biopsy, 225, 229f
    post-surgical, 271
Optical density (OD), 5, 6, 17
Oral contraceptives
    granulomatous mastitis and, 306
    MRI enhancement and, 201, 204f
Orchitis, mumps, 280
Osteogenic sarcoma, 82, 305, 309f
Outcome data
    for percutaneous biopsy, 186
    mandated review of, 1, 2, 12–13, 14b
Ovarian cancer, family history of, 25

P

Paget's disease of nipple, 305, 305b, 306f
    calcifications in, 61, 88f, 305
Pain, breast
    causes of, 26
        abscess as, 301
        coumarin necrosis as, 302
        cyst(s) as, 137, 303
        galactography as, 293
        hormone therapy as, 302
        implant as, 255
        mammography as, 2
        mastitis as, 288, 301
        Mondor's disease as, 306
    cyclic, 303
    focal, 303
    in male, 279
    therapies for, 303
Pain control
    after core biopsy, 180
    before core biopsy, bleeding and, 185
    for cyclic mastalgia, 303
Palpable mass
    asymmetric, 32, 34
    biopsy of
        by fine-needle aspiration, freehand, 171, 173
        with normal mammogram and ultrasound, 150
    diagnostic mammography with, 37, 40
    exclusion from "probably benign" category, 290
    foreign-body granuloma as, 81, 82f
    implants and, 255
    on history sheet, 32, 33f
    recurrent breast cancer as, 246–247, 247f–248f
    spot compression of, 47, 56f
    ultrasound evaluation of, 92, 134
        in young patients, 150
        with no findings, 150, 150f
    undetected by mammography, 150
    undetected by ultrasound, 150, 150f
Papillary carcinoma, 106, 109f
    calcifications in, 82

Papillary carcinoma—*cont'd*
    core biopsy suggestive of, 183, 184
    in men, 280
    papilloma progressing to, 292
    papillomas with, 116
    vs. fibroadenoma, 143, 146
Papilloma, 113–114, 115f, 292
    carcinoma developing from, 292
    core biopsy with, 184
    ductoscopy of, 294
    galactography of, 115f, 116, 205, 294, 295f–297f
    intracystic, 124, 126, 294, 297f
        ultrasound imaging of, 140, 141f
        vs. cyst, 140
        vs. intracystic carcinoma, 109, 109f, 140
    MRI of, 198, 199, 205, 208, 208f, 210, 294
    nipple discharge associated with, 114, 205, 292, 292t, 293, 293f, 294, 295f–297f
    vs. papillary carcinoma, 106, 109f
Papillomatosis
    core biopsy with, 184
    juvenile, 113, 114
Paraffin injections, 254, 259, 262, 263f, 264
Parasitic diseases, calcifications in, 311, 311b, 311f
Parity
    breast cancer risk and, 25
    breast density and, 136
PASH (pseudoangiomatous stromal hyperplasia), 118, 120, 120f, 184
Pathology report
    on core biopsy, mammography and, 183, 184
    on excisional biopsy, calcifications and, 168, 168t, 169f–170f
Peak kilovoltage (kVp), 2–3, 3b
Peau d'orange, 26, 151, 232t, 294
    infection with, 301
    inflammatory cancer with, 300
    post-radiation, 239
Pectoralis muscle. See also Chest wall.
    implant and, 253, 253f, 254, 254f, 255
    in male, 280
    on mammogram, 6, 6f–8f, 26, 27f, 29f
        spiculated mass behind, 37
    on MRI, with invasion, 217f, 236, 239f
    on ultrasound image, 134, 136, 137f
    trichinosis in, 311, 311b, 311f
Pellets, ultrasound-visible, 313f, 314
Phantom image
    in digital mammography, 18
    in screen-film mammography, 6, 8f, 13b, 14, 14b, 14t
    in ultrasound imaging, 133
Phototimer. See Automatic exposure control (AEC).
Phyllodes tumor, 110, 113, 113f–114f
    excision of, 183
    MRI of, 205
Physical examination. See Breast examination, clinical.
Physicians. See Radiologists.
Physicists, medical
    duties of, 14, 15b
    in digital mammography, 18, 18b
    MQSA qualifications for, 1, 12, 13b, 18, 18b
Phytoestrogens, 303
Pixels, 15, 17
Plasma cell mastitis. See Secretory disease.

Pleomorphic calcifications, 60, 62, 65f, 67
    at biopsy or trauma site, 80, 81, 240, 240f
    biopsy of, 84, 87f
    differential diagnosis of, 32t
    exclusion from "probably benign" category, 290
    in axillary lymphadenopathy, 304
    in breast cancer, 28, 32t, 93f
    in computer-aided diagnosis, 18
    in DCIS, 83f, 92, 93f, 95
        adjacent to implant, 257f
    in invasive ductal cancer, 95, 96f
        as round mass, 107f
    in pregnancy-associated breast cancer, 285
    in recurrent breast cancer, 246, 246b
    radiologist's search for, 37
    segmental distribution of, 69f
    stability of, 82, 84
    ultrasound imaging of, 88f, 143
Pneumocystography
    of aspirated cyst, 169, 171, 174f
    of intracystic mass, 140, 171
        carcinoma as, 109
        papilloma as, 141f
Pneumothorax, risk of
    with ultrasound-guided biopsy, 164, 171, 173, 175f, 185
    with ultrasound-guided needle localization, 168
PNL (posterior nipple line), 6, 6f–7f
Popcorn-like calcifying fibroadenoma, 79–80, 79f, 110, 143f
    MRI of, 205
Positioning of patient
    for MRI, 193, 193f
    for screen-film mammography, 5–6, 6f–7f
    for ultrasound imaging, 133–134
    of cyst, 138
Positions in breast
    describing, 32, 34f
    on label of ultrasound, 92, 94b
Posterior acoustic enhancement. See Acoustic enhancement.
Posterior nipple line (PNL), 6, 6f–7f
Postoperative appearance. See also Scar, post-biopsy; Trauma, surgical.
    key elements of, 249
    normal changes in. See also Scar.
        mammographic, 225, 226b, 226f–230f, 229
        MRI, 229, 231, 231b
        ultrasound, 229, 230f–231f
    of abscess, 289f
    of residual tumor, 236, 239, 240, 240f
    radiation changes superimposed on, 239
Power Doppler ultrasound, 155, 160. See also Doppler ultrasound.
    of cyst, 138, 139f, 140
    of lymphatics, in breast edema, 152f
    of round cancer, 138, 139f
    retroareolar vascularity on, 136
Pregnancy
    benign breast conditions in, 280, 287–288, 287b, 289f–290f
        fibroadenoma as, 280, 287
        lactating adenoma as, 116, 116f, 280, 287, 288
    bloody nipple discharge in, 292
    density of breasts in, 28, 302
    enlargement of breasts in, 280
    probably benign breast conditions in, 290
    radiation therapy and, 233

Pregnancy-associated breast cancer, 285, 287, 287b

Preoperative needle localization. *See* Needle localization.

"Probably benign" findings, mammographic, 37, 39b, 84, 288, 290, 290b, 291f, 292

Progestins
    breast cancer risk and, 25
    for breast pain, 303
    medroxyprogesterone as, 302, 303

Projections. *See* Views.

Prolactin-producing tumors, nipple discharge and, 292

Pseudoaneurysm, after core biopsy, 186

Pseudoangiomatous stromal hyperplasia (PASH), 118, 120, 120f, 184

Pseudogynecomastia, 279-280, 282t

Pseudolesions, fatty, on ultrasound image, 143

Pulse sequences, MRI, 189, 193, 194, 198
    for imaging silicone implants, 264

Punctate calcifications, 71
    indeterminate for malignancy, 84, 85f
    new, 87f

Q

QC technologist, 13-14, 14t

Quality assurance, 1-2, 1b, 12-14, 12b, 13b, 14b, 14t, 15b
    for digital mammography, 18, 18b

Quality control tests, 13-14, 14t, 15b
    for digital mammography, 18, 18b

R

Radial scar, 36f, 103, 104f-105f, 105b
    as precursor to tubular carcinoma, 99, 103, 184
    calcifications in, 103, 105f
    on core biopsy, 183-184

Radiation, as breast cancer risk factor, 2, 25, 247

Radiation dose
    in digital mammography, 17, 18
    in screen-film mammography, 2

Radiation therapy, 229, 231, 233. *See also* Breast-conserving therapy.
    after excision of DCIS, 82
    as risk factor for breast cancer, 25, 247
    calcifications subsequent to, 80-81, 80f
        in sutures, 315
    contraindications to, 231, 233, 233b
        pregnancy as, 287
    edema of breast caused by, 151, 294
    electron beam boost following, 239-240, 243f, 315
    follow-up imaging after, 236t, 239-240, 241f-246f, 243b, 246
    for desmoid tumor, 309
    for inflammatory breast cancer, 300
    for intramammary lymph node metastases, 234, 235
    key elements of, 249
    local recurrence after, 233, 233b
    MRI enhancement following, 231b
    scarring after, 154f, 227f
    treatment failure following, 246-247, 246b, 247f-248f

Radiographic guidance. *See* X-ray–guided procedures.

Radioisotope tracers
    for lymphoscintigraphy, 235f
    for sentinel node biopsy, 233, 234

Radiologic technologists
    MQSA qualifications for, 1, 12, 13b, 18, 18b
    QC technologist, 13-14, 14t

Radiologists
    MQSA qualifications for, 12, 12b
        for digital mammography, 18, 18b
        review of outcomes with, 13, 14b

Radiopaque materials, on skin, 70, 71f
    to mark ultrasound finding, 150-151

Raloxifene, 302

Rapid acquisition with relaxation inhibition (RARE), 193, 194b

Recalls, screening
    BI-RADS category for, 37
    double reading and, 18-19, 20
    with digital vs. screen-film technique, 17

Receiver operating characteristic (ROC) curve, 17

Reconstruction, breast, 233, 247, 249, 270-271, 272f-273f. *See also* Implants.
    after desmoid tumor excision, 309
    contralateral reduction following, 233, 271

Recurrent breast cancer, local
    after breast-conserving therapy, 233, 233b, 246-247, 246b, 247f-248f, 248b
    at biopsy site, 240, 245f-246f
    calcifications in, 80f, 81, 236, 240, 244f
    after subcutaneous mastectomy, 271
    extensive intraductal component and, 92
    in TRAM flap, 271, 276f
    MRI of, 214

Reduction mammaplasty, 271, 274f-275f
    contralateral, after reconstruction, 233, 271

Refractive shadows, ultrasound of cyst and, 138

Regional calcifications, 70

Renal cell carcinoma, metastatic to breast, 109, 110f

Reserpine, duct ectasia and, 294f

Residual tumor, after surgery, 236, 239, 240, 240f, 246, 246b, 247, 248b

Resolution. *See* Spatial resolution.

Retroareolar lesions. *See also* Subareolar lesions.
    galactography of, 296f
    inflammatory cancer with, 148f
    neurofibroma as, 316f
    nipple inversion caused by, 34
    views of, 47, 55f

Retroareolar vascularity, 136

Retromammary fascia, 136

Reverberation artifacts
    implants with, 253f, 262, 265f
    internal cyst echoes produced by, 140

Reverse oblique view, 47, 55f

Rheumatoid arthritis, axillary adenopathy in, 303, 303f, 304

Rib(s)
    chondrosarcoma of, 308f
    on ultrasound image, 136, 137f

Ring-down shadow, of metallic marker, 150, 151f

ROC (receiver operating characteristic) curve, 17

Rolled view laterally (RL), 41t

Rolled view medially (RM), 41t

Rolled views, 40-41, 40b, 40t, 42f-43f, 50f-51f
    abbreviations for, 41t

Round calcifications, 71, 73f
    indeterminate for malignancy, 84, 85f
    new, 87f

Round mass. *See* Mass(es), rounded or expansile.

S

Saline expander, 271

Saline implants, 252
    mammography of, 255, 257f
        with residual silicone, 261f
        with rupture, 255, 256f

Saline outer/silicone inner implants, 253b, 255

Sarcoma, 117, 305, 307f-309f
    angiosarcoma as
        MRI of, 305
        vs. pseudoangiomatous stromal hyperplasia, 120, 184
    osteogenic, 82, 305, 309f

Scar. *See also* Architectural distortion; Radial scar.
    implant removal causing, 262, 264f
    marker of, 32, 80, 100, 101f-102f, 229
    post-biopsy, 100, 100b, 101f-102f, 225, 226b, 227f-229f, 240, 244f
        epidermal inclusion cyst in, 271
        MRI of, 206, 208, 214, 229, 240
        ultrasound imaging of, 153, 154f, 229, 230f-231f
    with radiation effects, 239, 241f

Scattered calcifications, 61, 70
    simulating a group, 82, 82b
    with radiolucent centers, 73

Scattered fibroglandular density, 28, 28b

Scattered radiation
    grid and, 2, 4, 5
    in magnification mammography, 5
    in slot scanning, 17

Scirrhous breast cancer, vs. diabetic mastopathy, 309

Sclerosing adenosis, 103
    calcifications in, 62, 85f, 103

Sclerosing lesions, on core biopsy, 183-184

Sclerotic fibroadenoma, 110

Screen-film cassettes, 2, 4-5, 4f. *See also* Film.
    artifacts associated with, 6, 10f
    label of mammogram referring to, 8

Screen-film mammography (SFM)
    breast pain from, 2
    digitization of images from, 19, 19f-20f, 20
    equipment for, 2-5, 2f, 3b, 4b, 4f
        quality assurance for, 12, 13b
    film labeling in, 8, 12b
    film processing in, 5, 5t
        artifacts caused by, 6, 10f-11f
        quality assurance for, 13-14, 14t
    film viewing in, 8, 12f, 28, 37, 316-317
    focal spot in, 3-4, 3t, 4f
    image quality in
        breast cancer detection and, 1
        quality assurance for, 14, 14b, 14t, 15b
        variables affecting, 5-6, 5t, 6f-11f
    image receptor in, 2, 4-5, 4b, 4f
    magnification mode of. *See* Magnification mammography.
    positioning in, 5-6, 6f-7f
    quality assurance in, 1-2, 1b, 12-14, 12b, 13b, 14b, 14t, 15b
    magnification and, 3
    radiation dose from, 2
    spatial resolution in, 3-4, 4f, 5
    views in. *See* Views.

Screening mammography
    breast cancer identified on, 28
    computer-aided, 18-20
    digital vs. screen-film, 17
    double reading in, 18-19, 20
    guidelines for, 1, 1b, 24

Screening mammography—*cont'd*
  mortality reduction and, 1, 2
  "probably benign" findings in, 37, 39b, 84, 288, 290, 290b, 291f, 292
  recalls in
    BI-RADS category for, 37
    double reading and, 18–19, 20
    with digital vs. screen-film technique, 17
  to monitor cyst, 137
  views in, 5–6, 6f–7f, 37
    distance from nipple on, 34, 35f, 40
    vs. diagnostic mammography, 37, 40, 40t
Screening MRI, 210–211, 213b, 214f
Screening ultrasound, 149, 160–161
Sebaceous cyst, 128, 129f
Second reader, 18–19, 32
Secretory disease, calcifications in, 70, 77, 78f, 79
  vs. DCIS, 62, 65f, 68f, 77, 79, 79t
Sedentary lifestyle, breast cancer and, 24
Segmental calcifications, 67, 69f, 70
Sentinel lymph node (SLN) biopsy, 82, 233–235, 233t, 234b, 235f
Seroma, 124, 127f
  after excisional biopsy, 225, 228f, 230f–231f
  MRI of, 206, 231f
SFM. *See* Screen-film mammography (SFM).
Shadow. *See* Acoustic shadowing; Edge shadowing; Summation shadow.
Short tau inversion recovery (STIR) MRI, 264
SID (source-to-image distance), 3, 3t, 4
Signal-to-noise ratio
  in digital mammography, 17
  in screen-film mammography, 3–4
  in slot scanning, 17
Silicone implants. *See* Implants.
Silicone injections, 254, 259, 262, 263f, 264, 313f
  granulomas associated with, 81, 82f, 254, 259
  MRI of breast with, 213
  screening and, 211
SIO (superior-inferior oblique) view, 47, 55f
Skin
  calcifications in, 61, 73, 74f–75f, 75b, 82, 164
    in autologous flap, 271
  dimpling of, 26
  heparin-induced necrosis of, 302
  lesion of, vs. calcified breast lesion, 70, 71f
  locally advanced breast cancer and, 300
  neurofibromatosis-related lesions of, 315, 316f
  radiopaque materials on, 70, 71f
    to mark ultrasound finding, 150–151
  retraction of, 26, 92
    on ultrasound report, 135
  thickening of. *See also* Peau d'orange.
    abscess with, 126, 153f
    after reduction mammaplasty, 271
    asymmetric, 34
    breast cancer with, 148f, 149
    breast edema with, 151, 152f–153f, 294, 296, 300
      as peau d'orange, 294
    in Paget's disease of nipple, 305
    male breast cancer with, 280
    post-biopsy, 225, 226b
    post-radiation, 239, 241f–242f
    pregnancy-associated breast cancer with, 285
  ultrasound imaging of, 135, 148f
  ultrasound image of, 136, 136b, 136f

Skin folds, on film, 6, 8f
SLN (sentinel lymph node) biopsy, 82, 233–235, 233t, 234b, 235f
Slot-scanning techniques, 17
"Snowstorm," on ultrasound image, of silicone, 255, 261f, 262, 262t, 264, 265f–267f
Sonography. *See* Ultrasound.
Source-to-image distance (SID), 3, 3t, 4
Soy foods, 303
Spatial resolution
  of digital mammography, 17
  of magnification mammography, 60
  of MRI, 193, 194, 194b, 198, 199
  of screen-film mammography, 3–4, 4f, 5
  of ultrasound, 133
Specimen radiography. *See also* Needle localization.
  in breast-conserving therapy, 236
  of core, 177–178, 179f
  of implant-associated calcifications, 257f
  with needle localization
    key elements of, 186
    MRI-guided, 220f
    removal of wire fragments and, 315
    ultrasound-guided, 169, 176f
    x-ray–guided, 165f, 166–168, 166b, 167b, 167f
      calcifications and, 168, 168t, 169f–170f
Specimen ultrasound, 169, 236
Speckle artifact
  calcifications lost in, 149, 149f
  cyst image and, 138, 139f–140f
  vs. metallic marker, 155, 159f
Spiculated mass, 90, 91, 91f, 94–105, 95b
  computer-aided detection of, 18
  desmoid tumor as, 309, 311b
  differential diagnosis of, 32t, 95b. *See also* *specific diagnosis.*
  exclusion from "probably benign" category, 290
  in axilla, 37
  in breast cancer, 28, 32t
  mammographic appearance of, 32, 34, 36f, 37
    on magnification view, 50, 57f
    on spot compression view, 45f–46f, 51f
  MRI of, 199, 200f, 206, 208, 217f, 238f–239f
    intraductal papilloma as, 294
  Paget's disease of nipple with, 305
  post-biopsy, 225, 226f, 229, 229f, 240
  ultrasound image of, 134, 134t, 144, 145f
    acoustic spiculation in, 92
    as biopsy scar, 153, 154f
    as inflammatory cancer, 148f
    as medullary cancer, 146f
    with implant, 259f
Spoiled gradient echo MRI, 193–194, 194b
Spot compression, 40b, 40t, 41, 43f–46f, 51f–52f
  close to chest wall, 47
  for assessing mass, 91
  of axillary breast tissue, 37, 39f
  of palpable mass, 47, 56f
  retroareolar, 47, 55f
  with implants, 255, 257f, 259
  with magnification, 50, 61, 91
  of implant capsule, 255, 257f
Squamous cell carcinoma, 120
Staging of breast cancer
  MRI in, 213–214, 213b, 216f–218f, 229

Staging of breast cancer—*cont'd*
  sentinel node biopsy in, 82, 233–235, 233t, 234b, 235f
  TNM classification for, 229, 232t
Staphylococcus aureus infection, 297b, 301
Static discharge, image quality and, 6, 11f
Steatocystoma multiplex, 122
Step oblique views, 41
Stepladder sign, 262t, 264, 267f
Stereotactic core needle biopsy, 177–178, 178f–179f, 180t. *See also* Core needle biopsy.
  calcifications displaced by, 181, 183
  cancellation of, 164
  carbon marking after, 180
  clip placement with, 177, 178f–179f, 180t, 181, 182f, 183
  complete lesion removal by, 180–181, 183
  complications of, 177, 185
  epithelium displaced by, 183
  excision based on, 183, 184
  follow-up to benign findings in, 185
  implants and, 259
  Mondor's disease following, 306
  pathologic-mammographic correlation with, 183
  patient comfort after, 180
  removal of markers and, 314
  tumor size underestimated by, 183
  vs. ultrasound-guided biopsy, 177
Stereotactic needle localization, preoperative, 168
Sternalis muscle, 26, 27f, 37
STIR (short tau inversion recovery) MRI, 264
Subareolar ducts, 136
Subareolar lesions. *See also* Retroareolar lesions; Secretory disease.
  abscess as, 126, 128, 128f, 152, 153f, 288, 301
    recurrent, 301
  in male breast
    breast cancer as, 280, 285f–286f
    gynecomastia as, 279, 280, 281f–284f
  Paget's disease of nipple with, 305, 306f
  papilloma as, 114, 116
  sebaceous cyst as, 129f
Sulfur colloid, technetium Tc 99m, 233
Summation shadow, 34, 35f, 40, 40t
  rolled view and, 41, 42f–43f
  spot compression and, 41, 44f
  step oblique views and, 41
Superior vena cava (SVC) syndrome, breast edema in, 294, 299f
Superior-inferior oblique (SIO) view, 47, 55f
Supervising physician, 12, 14
Supraclavicular lymph nodes
  as sentinel nodes, 234
  MRI of, 193
  TNM staging and, 232t
Surgical excision, 229, 231, 233. *See also* Breast-conserving therapy; Excisional biopsy; Lumpectomy; Needle localization.
  after core biopsy, 180–181, 182f, 183
  controversial, 183–184, 184b
  noncompliance with, 186
  specific indications for, 183, 183b
  of desmoid tumor, 309
  of granulomatous mastitis, 308
  of inflammatory breast cancer, 300
  residual tumor left by, 236, 239, 240, 240f, 246, 246b, 247, 248b
Surgical trauma. *See* Trauma, surgical.

Sutures, retained in breast, 314f, 315
SVC (superior vena cava) syndrome, breast edema in, 294, 299f
Sweat glands, hidradenitis of, 315
Symmetry, of glandular tissue, 28, 29f-30f, 32.
    See also Density of breast, asymmetric.
Syphilis, 301

T

T1. *See* T1-weighted imaging.
T2. *See* T2-weighted imaging.
Tamoxifen
    breast density and, 303
    for breast pain, 303
TCG (time-compensated gain) curve, 134, 137, 138f
TDLU (terminal ductal lobular unit), 62f
    fibroadenoma arising from, 110
Teardrop sign, 262t, 268f-269f, 269
Technetium Tc 99m sulfur colloid, 233
Technologists, radiologic
    MQSA qualifications for, 1, 12, 13b, 18
    QC technologist, 13-14, 14t
Technologist's marks, 32
Tent sign, 32, 34, 57f
    in invasive lobular carcinoma, 98
    missed, 316
Terminal ductal lobular unit (TDLU), 62f
    fibroadenoma arising from, 110
Terminal ducts, 26, 27f
Terminology. *See* BI-RADS lexicon.
Tethering, by tumor, 92
Thrombophlebitis, 305-306, 309b, 310f
Thyroid disease, diabetic mastopathy in, 308
Time-compensated gain (TCG) curve, 134, 137, 138f
Tissue expander, 233, 247, 270, 271
Tissue flap, autologous, 233, 247, 270-271, 272f-273f
TNM staging classification, 229, 232t
Training, in mammography, 1, 12, 12b, 13b
Transverse rectus abdominis myocutaneous (TRAM) flap, 247, 270-271, 272f-273f, 276f
Trauma
    breast edema caused by, 294, 299f
        post-biopsy, 151
    calcifications caused by, 80-81, 80f, 80t
    desmoid tumor associated with, 309, 311b
    fat necrosis caused by, 100, 103, 225
    hematoma or seroma caused by, 124, 127f
        with edema, 299f
    oil cyst caused by, 73, 74f, 122
    surgical. *See also* Postoperative appearance.
        calcifications and, 80-81, 80f, 80t
        desmoid tumor and, 309, 311b
        fat necrosis and, 100, 103
        oil cyst and, 73, 74f, 122
        thrombophlebitis in breast and, 306
        thrombophlebitis in breast caused by, 306
Treatment failure, 246-247, 246b, 247f-248f, 248b
Tree static, 6, 11f
Triangulation of lesion, 40, 40t, 41, 47f-51f
    for planning biopsy, 91, 163-164
Trichinosis, 309, 311, 311b, 311f
Trilucent implants, 252-253
Tuberculosis, 301, 304
Tubular adenoma, 288
Tubular carcinoma, 98-99, 99f-100f
    radial scar as precursor to, 99, 103, 184
Turbo spin echo (TSE) MRI, 193, 194b

Turner's syndrome, 280, 281f
T1-weighted imaging, 189, 193-194, 194-195, 194b, 195f
    of silicone implants, 264, 269
T2-weighted imaging
    of benign vs. malignant lesions, 198, 199, 201, 201t, 202f
    of lactating breast, 285
    of normal breast, 195f, 196
    of silicone implants, 264, 269
    protocols for, 193, 194b

U

Ulceration
    in granulomatous mastitis, 306
    in Paget's disease of nipple, 305
Ultrasound, 133-161. *See also* Acoustic enhancement;Acoustic shadowing; Acoustic spiculation.
    artifacts in, 133-134
        cyst imaging and, 137, 138, 138f-139f, 140
        edge shadowing as, 144, 145f
            with implant, 253f, 264
        reverberation as
            internal cyst echoes and, 140
            with implant, 253f, 262, 265f
        speckle as
            calcifications lost in, 149, 149f
            cyst image and, 138, 139f-140f
    benign features in, 92, 140-143, 141b, 142f-143f
        probably benign, 288
    BI-RADS descriptors for, 134-135, 134t
    breast cancer screening with, 149, 160-161
    breast pain evaluation in, 303
    confirming presence of lesion with, 40, 40t, 41, 44f, 48f, 51f
    Doppler. *See* Doppler ultrasound.
    intraoperative, 169, 181
    key elements of, 161
    labeling of image, 92, 94b, 134, 134b
    malignant features in, 92, 94b, 144-147, 144b, 144f-148f, 146b, 149
    mammographic findings and, 136-149
        correlation with, 92, 94, 95f, 143, 150-151, 151f
        cystic, 136-138, 137b, 138f-141f, 140b
        of benign solid masses, 140-143, 141b, 142f-143f
        of calcifications, 149, 149f
        of malignant solid masses, 144-147, 144b, 144f-148f, 146b, 149, 149b
        probably benign, 288
    marking biopsy cavity with, for electron beam boost, 240, 315
    neoadjuvant chemotherapy and, 155, 156f
    nipple discharge and, 292-293, 292t, 293f-294f
    normal breast anatomy on, 135-136, 135f-137f, 136b
    of biopsy cavity, 153, 154f, 181
    of biopsy scar, 153, 154f
    of breast cancer. *See* Breast cancer, ultrasound of.
    of breast edema, 135, 136, 151, 152f, 296
        with abscess, 152, 153f
        with post-biopsy scar, 154f
    of calcifications, 84, 88f, 92, 142, 144-145, 147, 147f
    of diabetic mastopathy, 309
    of duct ectasia, 293f-294f
    of fat necrosis, post-surgical, 271, 276f

Ultrasound—*cont'd*
    of gynecomastia, 280, 282f-284f
    of implants, 253f, 255, 256f
        ruptured, 256f, 259, 262, 262t, 264, 265f-267f
    of lymph nodes, 26
    of mass(es), 90, 92, 93f, 94, 94b, 94t, 95f.
        See also specific diagnosis.
        artifactual, 134, 137
        benign findings, 140-143, 141b, 142f-143f
        BI-RADS terminology for, 134-135, 134t
        correlating mammography with, 92, 94, 95f, 160
        cystic vs. solid, 134, 136-138, 138f-139f, 140
        invisible on mammography, 160
        malignant findings, 144-147, 144f-148f, 146b, 149
        palpable, 92
            in dense breast, 150
            in recurrent cancer, 246-247, 247f-248f
        report on, 94, 95b
        suspicious findings, 142, 144b
    of Mondor's disease, 306
    of MRI-detected lesions, 217
    of nonpalpable findings, 92, 94
    of silicone injections, 259, 262
    of specimen, 169, 236
    of young patients, 150
    pellets visible on, 313f, 314
    positioning of patient for, 133-134
    postoperative findings on, 229, 230f-231f
    pre-biopsy work-up with, 163
    "probably benign" category in, 292
    scanners for, 133
    taller than wide, 106, 144, 144f, 145
    technique of, 133-134
    undetected findings with
        calcifications, 145f, 147
        lymph node metastases, 149
        mammographically detected, 150
        palpable, 150, 150f
Ultrasound-guided procedures
    clip placement as, 94, 95f, 313f
        with core biopsy, 175f-176f
    core needle biopsy as, 173, 175f-176f, 177
        Mondor's disease following, 306
        of MRI-detected lesion, 217
        pneumothorax caused by, 164, 171, 173, 175f, 185-186
        with implant, 259, 259f
    fine-needle aspiration as
        of abscess, 288, 289f
        of cyst, 169, 173f-174f
        of solid mass, 173, 175f-176f, 177
    marker placement as
        before excisional biopsy, 155, 159f
        before neoadjuvant chemotherapy, 155, 156f
        for correlation with mammogram, 150-151
    Mondor's disease following, 306
    needle localization as, 168-169, 171f-172f, 176f
        after stereotactic biopsy, 181
    percutaneous biopsy as, neoadjuvant chemotherapy and, 155, 156f
    pseudoaneurysm treatment as, 186

V

Vacuum-assisted biopsy, 155, 159f. *See also* Core needle biopsy.
  atypical hyperplasia in, 177, 183
  complications of, 177
  epithelium displaced by, 183
  MRI-guided, 221, 221f
  removal of markers and, 181, 314
  stereotactic. *See* Stereotactic core needle biopsy.
  ultrasound-guided, 173, 177
Vascular calcifications, 81, 81f, 316
Vascular invasion, recurrence and, 233
Vasovagal reaction, biopsy-induced, 177, 185
Viewing conditions, 8, 12f, 28, 37, 316-317
Views, mammographic
  abbreviations for, 41t
  implants and, 255, 256b, 256f, 258f
  in diagnostic mammography, 37, 40, 40b, 40t
    to characterize true lesion, 40, 50, 56b, 57f

Views, mammographic—*cont'd*
    to confirm or exclude lesion, 40-41, 40b, 40t, 42f-46f
    to localize lesion, 40, 40t, 41, 47f-51f
      in specific locations, 40t, 41, 47, 52f-56f
  in screening mammography, 5-6, 6f-7f, 37
    distance from nipple on, 34, 35f, 40
  labeling of mammogram with, 8
Views, MRI, 194
Vitamin B$_6$, 303
Vitamin E, 303

W

Warfarin. *See* Coumarin necrosis.
Weight loss, vs. breast edema, 296, 301f
Wire. *See* Needle localization.

X

XCCL (laterally exaggerated craniocaudal) view, 40t, 41t, 47, 52f-53f
XCCM (medially exaggerated craniocaudal) view, 40t, 41t, 47, 52f, 54f

X-ray mammography units, 2-5, 2f, 3b, 3t, 4b, 4f
  for digital imaging, 15
  slot scanning with, 17
X-ray-guided procedures
  clip insertion as, for electron beam boost, 240, 315
  fine-needle aspiration as, 173
  needle localization as, 164-166, 165f, 166b
    after galactography, 294
    specimen radiography after, 165f, 166-168, 166b, 167b, 167f
      calcifications and, 168, 168t, 169f-170f
  stereotactic biopsy as, 177, 178f-179f

Y

Young patient
  density of breasts in, 302
  palpable mass in, ultrasound evaluation of, 150
  recurrence of breast cancer in, 233, 246